HANDBOOK OF PSYCHIATRIC DIFFERENTIAL DIAGNOSIS

Stephen M. Soreff, MD
Chief of Psychiatry, Mercy Hospital
Attending Psychiatrist, Maine Medical Center
Portland, Maine

George N. McNeil, MD
Training Director
Department of Psychiatry, Maine Medical Center
Portland, Maine

with contributions by

Walter R. Christie, MD
Assistant Chief of Psychiatry
Director of Inpatient Services
Maine Medical Center
Portland, Maine

Charles V. Ford, MD
Professor of Psychiatry
Vice Chairman for Psychiatric
 Education
University of Arkansas for
 Medical Sciences
Little Rock, Arkansas

and a foreword by

Thomas P. Hackett, MD
Chief of Psychiatry
Massachusetts General Hospital
Boston, Massachusetts

PSG PUBLISHING COMPANY, INC.
LITTLETON, MASSACHUSETTS

Library of Congress Cataloging in Publication Data

Main entry under title:
Handbook of psychiatric differential diagnosis.

Includes index.
1. Mental illness--Diagnosis. 2. Diagnosis, Differential.
I. McNeil, George N. II. Title. [DNLM: 1. Diagnosis, Differential. 2. Mental
Disorders--diagnosis. WM 141 S713h]
RC473.D54S67 1986 616.89'075 86-27535
ISBN 0-88416-541-8

Published by:
PSG PUBLISHING COMPANY, INC
545 Great Road
Littleton, Massachusetts 01460

Printed in the United States of America

International Standard Book Number: 0-88416-541-8

Library of Congress Catalog Card Number: 86-27535

Last digit is print number: 9 8 7 6 5 4 3 2 1

Dedicated to the Physician in every Psychiatrist and the Psychiatrist in every Physician.

CONTENTS

FOREWORD

The phases and faces of psychiatry have been many during the course of the last half century. Throughout there has remained a firmament in which psychiatry has remained rooted. Whether psychoanalyst, community psychiatrist, psychosomaticist, or geropsychiatrist, most of us have held fast to our early training in medical school as the taproot of our professional life. We are fortunate in this decade to have seen medicine rather than social science, behaviorism, or political action become the framework of psychiatric practice.

An integral part of the medical framework is the making of enlightened diagnoses by the careful application of clinical skills including observation, examination, and the use of laboratory science. Differential diagnosis is the hallmark of medical practice. I am glad to see that it has been honored by having this worthy volume given over to its mastery. Drs Soreff and McNeil have written a book that elucidates the principles of differential diagnosis in an understandable and reasonable way. It is clear that these authors and their contributors have been on the line. They demonstrate that participation in clinical psychiatry requires accurate diagnosis, which, of course, depends for its authority on a thorough, relevant consideration of differential diagnostic possibilities.

One of the virtues of the method employed in this text is that it stimulates the reader to thoughtful formulation of diagnostic possibilities and does not force him into hard and fast diagnostic categories. Some textbooks shoehorn that reader into a rigid schema of differential diagnostic possibilities, precluding speculation or easement. The Kraepelinian tendency is to set down a classification that is all-inclusive, taking every variation, exception, and clinical oddity into account. It is my belief that the good clinician should be able to tolerate a fair amount of uncertainty in selecting diagnostic possibilities. Room should always be left for the unusual case that may represent a truly new condition or a unique variation on a traditional model. I would hope that the philosophy of the differential diagnostician would be to identify the obvious and to separate it from the less obvious in order to allow the unknown to be recognized.

Jean Martin Charcot, the great French neurologist said, "to learn to treat disease, one must learn how to recognize it. The diagnosis is the best trump in the scheme of treatment." I cannot think of a better benediction with which to launch the reader on his voyage through this text.

Thomas P. Hackett, MD
Psychiatrist in Chief
Massachusetts General Hospital
Eben S. Draper Professor of Psychiatry
Harvard Medical School
Boston, Massachusetts

PREFACE

This book takes the most common psychiatric symptoms and provides a comprehensive approach to their diagnosis. It is rooted in three concepts. First, symptoms represent the point of departure for diagnosis. Second, proper diagnosis is a key to treatment. Third, psychiatric symptoms emerge from a variety of struggles, conditions, and illnesses. To appreciate these one must apply a truly biopsychosocial model of illness.

We approach symptoms from three directions: clinical features, pathogenesis, and differential diagnosis. After the symptom has been defined and highlighted by a case example, the feature section examines it along five parameters: the patient's mood, thoughts, and behavior, the physical examination and laboratory studies, and the interviewer's reaction. These five dimensions serve to better define the clinical problem.

The pathogenesis section is a bridge between symptom and differential diagnosis. It emphasizes the interplay of four powerful determinants: psychodynamics, biologic factors, genetics, and environment.

The differential diagnosis section includes the following critical areas: nonpsychotropic drugs, psychotropic drugs, alcohol, other abused substances, medical illnesses, surgical complications, physical trauma, and psychiatric illness. While we find the distinction between "medical" and "psychiatric" illness to be artificial, our current state of knowledge seems to warrant its use.

In essence, the book offers a method to determine a diagnosis starting with the presenting symptom. It furnishes an approach which views the symptom within the context of the patient in all his biopsychosocial complexity and leads to a specific diagnosis from the host of pharmocologic, medical, surgical, and psychiatric causes.

S.M.S.
G.N.Mc

ACKNOWLEDGMENTS

We are indebted to our colleagues who have provided us with support, information, ideas, and encouragement. The secretarial assistance, as well as the word-processing wizardry of Joan Aldrich and Gloria Moline, made this whole endeavor possible. The Health Science Library at the Maine Medical Center through Robin Rand and Diane Winand, as well as the library at Mercy Hospital under Mary Anne Toner, have kept us current, up-to-date, and in good reference. The supporting work by Susan Hodges and Nancy Ludwig has proved also to be of great value.

INTRODUCTION

Differential diagnosis lies close to the heart of the practice of medicine. Indeed, much of medical thinking is based upon the process of ruling out various disorders, and lengthy differentials have evolved for problems such as fever of unknown origin or acute monoarticular arthritis.

Psychiatry has been somewhat different. Until recently its practitioners have typically eschewed the "medical model." Psychiatric diagnosis was a vague descriptive art. The various symptoms were explained largely in psychological terms, and biologic causality was given short shrift. To the extent that such causality was established (eg, the role of *Treponema pallidum* in general paresis of the insane), the disease and the patient became the domain of the internist.

While biologic psychiatry remains in its infancy there has been striking change. Investigation into the nature and actions of neurotransmitters, for example, has added to this objective-descriptive art the leaven of modern science. It may be argued that psychiatry is at a developmental stage akin to that of medicine at the time of the discovery of insulin. Nonetheless, psychiatry is irrevocably headed in a direction that will bring it closer to the medical mainstream and that will stress the question of differential diagnosis. It is with this in mind that we developed the idea for this book.

Increasingly, psychiatrists are called upon to assist in the management of the medically ill. The growth and success of the consultation-liaison subspecialty attests to this, and numerous texts have been published that address this growth. Almost invariably such texts approach differential diagnosis from the standpoint of the diseased organ system (eg, "Psychiatric Symptoms in the Patient with Renal Disease"). While this may be enormously helpful to the hospital-based psychiatrist fortunate enough to have an established medical diagnosis, it is less helpful to others. What of the office-based psychiatrist seeing a patient who has never consulted an internist? Indeed, what of the internist seeing a patient who has been previously well but who complains of depression? In this setting one begins the process of differential diagnosis, not with a diseased organ, but with a *symptom*.

We have identified a group of psychiatric symptoms commonly seen in the practice of medicine. It has been estimated that anxiety and depression, for example, are the fifth most common cause of outpatient visits and that the majority of these patients are seen by nonpsychiatrists.* Each has been assigned a chapter heading, and each is discussed (1) from an objective-descriptive standpoint (the description of syndromes remains important both in psychiatry and the rest of medicine), (2) from the standpoint of symptom pathogenesis, and (3) from the standpoint of differential diagnosis.

The sections on differential diagnosis contain brief clinical overviews of the various disease states. Here the discussions of psychiatric disease will invariably fall short of satisfying the psychiatrist, and the discussions of other organic disease will fall short of the rigor required by the internist. This seems unavoidable in a work that should not be seen as a comprehensive text of either psychiatry or general medicine, but rather one which points the way to such works. On the other hand, it is our hope that the psychiatrist will profit, for example, from a brief clinical review of hyperthyroidism and that the primary care physician will likewise benefit from an overview of schizophrenia. We also hope that medical students and junior house officers will find our integrative approach useful. We certainly have found it so and have learned much in our writing.

Stephen M. Soreff, MD
George N. McNeil, MD

* Rosenblatt RA, Cherkin DC, Schneeweiss R, et al: The content of ambulatory medical care in the United States. *N Engl J Med* 1983;309:892-897.

1 Anxiety

George N. McNeil

ANXIETY A condition frequently characterized by somatic symptoms of sympathetic autonomic arousal and marked by subjective feelings ranging from foreboding to stark terror.

Anxiety in some degree is a universal part of the human experience. In its milder forms it rarely comes to the attention of the clinician and warrants little intervention. In its more severe forms it can cause major disruption in patients' lives and may serve as an indicator of serious underlying disease.

Case report A 32-year-old married mother of three was seen by her family doctor at the urging of her husband. She complained of episodes during which she experienced tremor, rapid, pounding heart beat, air hunger, and, frequently, an urgent need to defecate. Associated with these symptoms was fear of imminent death and an intense desire to flee.

Between "attacks" the patient became increasingly worried about recurrent episodes (indeed, the problem seemed to occur with growing frequency). She developed growing concern over potential embarrassment from suffering such an episode in public. Such worries gradually dominated her life, and she gradually restricted her activities until she rarely left the "safe" confines of her home.

FEATURES

Mood

The mood of the anxious patient might be described as fearful, although such fear may at times assume the proportions of panic or terror.

The patient described above admitted to feeling "like I would die." Other patients are terrified that their experience is a harbinger of psychosis (while this might on occasion come to pass, most anxious patients may be reassured that they are not "going crazy.")

The nonpsychotic anxious patient recognizes the illogic of his fears, agrees with the logic of family and other helpers who would reassure him, yet is unable to control the perverse and senseless symptoms. Tiring of her idiosyncrasy, the husband of the patient described above became critical, dismissing the problem as "all in your head," and charging her to "pull yourself together." It is hardly surprising that this patient, like many with anxiety disorders, became secondarily depressed.

The *psychotically* anxious patient (see "Psychiatric Diagnosis" below) is apt to manifest mood that is bizarre or inappropriate. A 21-year-old manic-depressive woman, for instance, was seen in the emergency room, showing intense agitation, irritability and giddy, expansive mood consistent with her delusion that she was the Virgin Mary.

On the other hand, psychotic anxiety may be masked by sphinxlike flatness that belies all feeling. A 28-year-old schizophrenic man, beset with the ill-defined delusion that people were mocking him and were in league against him, appeared devoid of emotion. A 32-year-old schizophrenic man reported blandly to his therapist a fear that the therapist wished to kill him

Anxiety, secondary to *organic brain syndromes*, is apt to be marked by *lability* of mood. Giddiness may give way to tears or to belligerence without apparent provocation.

Seen in the context of agitated depression, anxiety is heavily colored by depressed mood. Preeminent here are feelings of worthlessness, of despair, and ennui. Somewhat less prominent may be the evidence of anger (see Chapter 2).

Thought

Anxious patients commonly complain of "confused" thinking. Such complaints require scrutiny. On the face of it, "confusion" leads one to consider psychotic disorders. The *schizophrenias* have as perhaps their cardinal symptom a disturbance in thought. The schizophrenic patient complaining of confusion may be experiencing thought blocking (wherein thoughts are repeatedly blocked or "chopped off" in midstream) or intrusive thinking (thoughts that seem to the patient to be forced upon him from an outside source). His thought may be colored by delusions and hallucinations. In short, he may feel overwhelmed by the disparity between logical thought and the web of illogical, psychotic, primary process thought in which he finds himself.

The confused thought of the *manic patient* may also have a distinct character. Such patients are notable by the profusion of their thoughts. Thinking is rapid, expansive, and lacking in focus. It may be confusing to the patient and to the interviewer as well. Here again, thought content may be marked by delusions and hallucinations. In practice, the confusion of the manic patient and the schizophrenic patient may be difficult to distinguish.

Anxiety, as manifested in *agitated depression*, may also be accompanied by "confusion." Although such confusion may be born out of psychotic disturbance (eg, mood-congruent delusions such as "my insides are rotting"), it may equally well reflect the all-pervasive nature of the depression. A 49-year-old woman, for instance, was seen for major depression with agitated features. As she paced and wrung her hands she described an overwhelming sense of hopelessness that led to virtual paralysis of decision making in her life. Domestic and financial matters that normally would have been routine became clouded ("confused") by the depressed state. Here the confusion, and the agitation, responded to specific treatment of the depression.

The confusion of the anxious patient without affective or psychotic illness is qualitatively different. Conspicuously absent are the psychotic thought experiences of the manic or schizopohrenic patient. Absent also are the disturbances in orientation, memory, and intellect typically seen in the patient with organic brain syndromes (see below). Upon close inquiry, one learns that the confused state here is a state of *distraction*. So preoccupied is the patient with his anxiety and the various protective measures that have evolved around it that careful reasoning is impaired. The woman presented briefly at the beginning of the chapter complained of just such confusion, and the insidious restriction in her activity took growth from this.

Finally, as noted above, the patient with anxiety as a product of *organic brain syndrome* may also have thought processes best described as confused. Here careful mental status examination shows the confusion to be a product of frank, cognitive deficit. The patient may, indeed, not recall the events that brought him to treatment. In the extreme case, he may not recall the three conventional data of orientation testing (date, place, name). The thought content of these patients may also be colored by delusions or hallucinations. While these introduce a possible source of a diagnostic error, the derangement of cognition should serve as a key differential point.

Behavior

The behavior of the anxious patient generally reflects a state of readiness for "fight or flight" (see "Psychodynamic Explanation", below). The patient is in a state of arousal manifested not only by an increase in mental activity (see above), but often by a parallel increase in motor activity. He may pace the floor, unable to sit still; or if sitting he may fidget restlessly with hands and feet. Frequent sighing is common and may indicate subtle hyperventilation (at other times, frank hyperventilation may be seen, with complaints of air hunger or "a weight on my chest"). Not surprisingly, appeal for relief is quite apt to be part of the behavioral picture seen by the physician.

Attention to the patient's behavior is crucial to the diagnosis of a number of disorders associated with anxiety. The patient with *panic disorder* manifests (or describes to the physician) arousal and agitation commensurate with the state of mortal fear in which he finds himself. Frank flight from the situation in which panic occurs is common. Between panic episodes, such patients commonly exhibit lower grade, sustained behavioral symptoms of generalized anxiety, as described above. Frequently, agoraphobic behavior (*agoraphobia*: literally, "fear of the marketplace") evolves as the patient, in anxious anticipation of panic episodes, gradually constricts his activities to the safety of his home.

The *phobic disorders* are virtually defined by the unusual, avoidant behavior of patients so afflicted. The patient with agoraphobia associates the intense discomfort of anxiety with being in crowds or public places. Defensively, he evolves behavior that allows him to avoid such places. (The maladaptive nature of this behavior is obvious. The woman presented at the beginning of the chapter had become virtually housebound, unable to shop, attend church, and do other things previously important to her.)

In like manner, the patient with social phobia assiduously avoids situations in which he might be subject to scrutiny by others, which in turn might lead to embarrassment. The patient with simple phobia similarly shows avoidance of a phobic object or situation (the spectrum of such objects and situations is apparently limitless and has provided lexicographers fertile ground; witness mysophobia [fear of dirt], peccatiphobia [fear of sinning], etc).

Obsessive-compulsive disorder also is manifest in striking behavior. Indeed, the disorder is defined, in part, by the ritualized behavior that afflicted patients seem condemned to repeat, despite all conscious desire and reason, in order to mitigate their anxiety. Clearly, not all compulsive behavior warrants psychiatric diagnosis. The play of children is often colored by compulsive ritual (eg, "step on a crack, break your mother's back"). And we see compulsion elevated to an adult art form by the professional athlete who postures ritualistically at the foul line or in the batter's box. On the other hand, the patient who feels compelled to wash his hands myriad times daily and who finds this a source of trouble and embarrassment may well warrant this diagnosis.

The *somatoform disorders* have as a common behavioral correlate the frequent, often relentless pursuit of medical care. This may persist despite all manner of careful evaluation and reassurance. In the face of dissappointment and hostility, patients with these disorders frequently end up "doctor shopping." In the extreme, this leads to a class of medical mendicants, ʾwandering from tertiary care setting to tertiary care setting at considerable personal expense.

Of the *dissociative disorders*, psychogenic fugue has perhaps the most striking behavioral correlates. Patients with this disorder manifest sudden, unexplainable wandering from their usual setting with inability to recall their past.

One particular behavioral aspect of *posttraumatic stress disorder* bears mention. With growing attention to this disorder following the Vietnam conflict, it has been noted that a significant number of patients so afflicted present with legal difficulties. Assaults, armed robberies, and other felony offenses may be associated with the disorder. Walker recently described two such cases and pointed out the importance of distinguishing posttraumatic stress disorder from antisocial personality disorder in this setting.[1] He notes, as key points of differential diagnosis, the absence of antisocial behavior prior to age 15 in the patient with posttraumatic stress, as well as the clear presence of guilt and anxiety in this disorder.

Agitated depression may present behavior quite akin to that of patients with primary anxiety. Patients with this disorder may show extreme restlessness, pacing, sighing, and wringing of the hands. Attention to other aspects of the mental status examination and to the history of present illness is vital to proper diagnosis.

Similarly, the agitated behavior seen in *mania* might on casual inspection be mistaken for primary anxiety. The mildly manic (hypomanic) patient might easily be so mistaken. As mania becomes more florid, however, distinctive behaviors emerge. The manic patient may involve himself in ill-advised and often calamitous financial schemes or social liaisons. He may become irritable; angry, violent behavior may ensue. He often eschews sleep to pursue relentless (and often unproductive) activity. Again, careful attention to history and complete mental status examination are essential to accurate diagnosis and treatment of this eminently treatable affective disorder.

The behavior of patients with anxiety secondary to *schizophrenia* is apt to be bizarre. Acts may be carried out in response to delusions (eg, the patient who proselytizes in the subway in the belief that he is the Messiah) or to hallucinations (eg, the patient who mutilates himself in deference to voices commanding such an act). Patients responding to paranoid delusions are likely to show great suspiciousness and a marked sense of vigilance. They may respond dramatically to the most subtle threat. A medical student, for example, sat too close to a paranoid schizophrenic patient, who proceeded to attempt to throttle him with his necktie, crying, "You're the devil!" This vignette bears clear witness to the caveat that the paranoid patient literally be given plenty of room.

Behavior in patients with an *organic brain syndrome* is less likely to be a product of hallucinations or delusions than it is to be born out of impaired judgment. A cardinal area of deficit in organicity, judgment is that intangible commodity that governs the myriad decisions we make daily and which, if functioning well, gets us through each day with minimal dislocation. With judgment intact, one's behavioral response to thirst is to drink something potable. The patient with organic brain syndrome may drink from his urinal.

Some organic disorders have fairly specific behavioral correlates. *Complex partial seizures* (temporal lobe epilepsy) are manifest in a change in the level of consciousness (cessation of preictal activity, staring) and in semipurposeful behavior, such as picking at buttons. More complex, purposeful behavior, ranging from the playing of a musical recital to the commission of a crime, has been reported in association with temporal lobe seizures. While it cannot be said with certainty that these behaviors are not the product of seizure activity, it is generally agreed that such phenomena are, at best, quite rare.[2]

There is, on the other hand, a well-recognized *inter*ictal behavior pattern associated with temporal lobe seizures. Affected patients commonly experience a deepening and increased lability of emotions. They become quick to anger and may exhibit frank aggressive behavior. Increased preoccupation with religion is also commonly seen, and multiple religious conversions are not unusual. "Hypergraphia" is also commonly reported, with patients keeping voluminous diaries attentive to boring detail. Altered sexual appetite and practice is also reported in this disorder, with either decrease or increase in sexual drive as well as transvestism, fetishism, and other perverse practices as variants.

Disease of the frontal lobes, of whatever etiology, may result in fairly specific behavior. Bear and Arana divide the frontal lobe disorders into those associated with disease of the convexity and those associated with disease of the orbital surface of the frontal lobe.[3] Convexity lesions are commonly associated with retardation of motor activity, apathy, and shallow, depressed affect. More likely to be confused with primary anxiety is the syndrome associated with disease of the orbital surface of the frontal lobes. Afflicted patients tend to show a general loss of social control; and sexual, aggressive, and other unattractive impulses may be expressed without appropriate censorship. Emotional outbursts, lewd, sexually explicit speech and behavior, such as open masturbation, may make such patients a major management problem. At the same time, the extremes of behavior lead readily to the discrimination of the disorder from primary anxiety.

Huntington's disease may also be associated with loss of impulse control, leading to sexual promiscuity or to aggressive behavior. Alcoholism may also ensue. Although the disease is more commonly associated with depression (and frequent suicide), anxiety may be seen, particularly in concert with paranoid delusions.

Physical Examination and Laboratory Findings

Certain physical findings may be made in virtually all anxiety syndromes and are thus of little differential diagnostic value. These are signs that are generally associated with stimulation of the sympathetic autonomic nervous system. Such signs include rapid pulse, increase in systolic and diastolic blood pressure, mydriasis, piloerection, diaphoresis, and fine tremor.

Hyperventilation[4] may accompany anxiety disorders and is noted to be a common occurrence in *panic disorder* and in *generalized anxiety disorders*.[4] In the throes of acute anxiety, frequently the patient can be noted to have an increased rate of respiration. At other times, hyperventilation is more subtle and may be marked only by deep, sighing respiration. Study of arterial blood gases reveals that in patients with hyperventilation not due to underlying medical disorder, blood pH is elevated and both Pco_2 and bicarbonate are low (the latter being low to a greater or lesser extent depending on the duration of hyperventilation). In the extreme one may observe the tetanic contractions of carpopedal spasm and elicit a positive Chvostek's sign.

Caution must be used in interpreting the significance of hyperventilation, and thorough history and physical examination are essential. The patient with rapid respiratory rate may be responding to acute hypoxia or to metabolic acidosis. Either state may be associated with a number of medical disorders which will be discussed below. If the clinician is rushed into a premature diagnostic closure by factors such as the patient's youth, general good health, or history of psychiatric disorder, even obvious medical illness may be missed with disastrous consequence. (A more detailed discussion of physical findings and pertinent laboratory tests will be found below under "Differential Diagnosis.")

Interviewer's Reaction

Patients with nonpsychotic anxiety generally succeed in making emotional contact with the interviewer and commonly convey to the physician a sense of their discomfort. Since such patients commonly present in the role of the supplicant, it is understandable that they evoke in us the need to do something helpful. The pervasive use of minor tranquilizers in Western culture bears witness both to the overwhelming prevalence of anxiety and to the nearly reflex response of physicians.

Anxiety associated with virtually all but the most transient disorders (eg, *adjustment disorder, acute bereavement*) is apt to run a somewhat chronic course. Confronted with this and with the all too common failure of treatment with minor tranquilizers, the physician is apt to feel confounded by the patient—betrayed by the patient's inability (which sometimes seems more like unwillingness) to get better. Office visits may become associated with dread and some degree of loathing. Common is an intense desire to be rid of the patient.

Interviewing the patient with anxiety secondary to major affective disease tends to evoke other distinctive responses. The despair and hopelessness of the patient with *agitated depression* tend to be infectious; it is rare not to feel some degree of the depression. The patient with *mania* may amuse the interviewer with his banter and jocularity. However, amusement usually gives way quite rapidly to irritation at the cloying, manipulative, often hostile behavior of the manic patient.

The anxiety of the *psychotic patient* is frequently not felt by the interviewer. Walled off behind a flattened facade or disguised by bizarre thought and behavior, the anxiety is frequently not present in easily understandable form.

The *paranoid patient* represents a notable exception to this. Angry, suspicious, sometimes openly hostile, he is apt to elicit considerable anxiety in the interviewer. The severely paranoid patient is very difficult to interview with equanimity, and some degree of circumspection in the interviewer is quite appropriate.

PATHOGENESIS

Psychodynamic Explanation

The physiologic changes attendant upon anxiety led Freud to classify it as one of the *actual* neuroses. No doubt influenced by his training in neurology, he saw in anxiety not the product of a psychological process but the product of biologic forces gone awry. According to his early postulates, anxiety arose when sexual energies were not given adequate outlet, whether by conscious abstinence or by repression of such energy.

It is ironic that this early theory, formally recanted by Freud in 1926, seems to have been elevated by some contemporary movements to a position of dogma. Doing whatever feels good or "doing your own thing" have thus, with their attendant excesses, been unfortunately associated with psychiatry.

The publication of *Inhibitions, Symptoms, and Anxiety* (1926) represents a major turn in psychodynamic thinking about anxiety.[5] Freud now reasoned that anxiety arose not from repression of sexual instincts but from a failure of that repression. He reasoned that sexual and other forbidden impulses, threatening to burst from the confines of the unconscious, constitute a threat to the organism. Anxiety, he reasoned, is a signal of such impending threat.

We noted earlier that anxiety may be symptomatically identical to the "fight-or-flight" response evoked by fear of physical danger. The difference, then, between anxiety and fear is that the latter is a response to palpable, external threat, while the former is a response to threat from within. One *fears* attack from a man brandishing a weapon. One is rendered *anxious* by forces that become identified only by psychoanalysis or its equivalent as impulses arising from the unconscious.

Psychodynamic rationale may be helpful in understanding several variants of anxiety disorder. The ritualistic behavior and thought seen in *obsessive-compulsive disorder* may be seen as attempts to contain anxiety arising (as noted above) from prohibited unconscious impulses. (One is reminded, for example, of the feverish prayers of Victor Hugo's archdeacon Claude Frollo, tormented by lust for the gypsy Esmeralda in *The Hunchback of Notre Dame* .)

Phobic anxiety may be understood by invoking the mechanisms of symbolization and displacement. Here anxiety is tempered by displacing it from its source to a more neutral, symbolic object or situation. The patient described in the case at the beginning of the chapter suffered from agoraphobia. Ostensibly, public places were the source of her anxiety. What emerged in psychotherapy was that she was extremely threatened by what for her were unspeakable sexual impulses. The threat was then unconsciously displaced from the impulse to the setting in which she feared her passion would be disclosed. Her gradual restriction of activity to the home provided further insurance against emerging sexual impulse.

Neurochemical Factors

It has been suggested that anxiety may be mediated by excessive central nervous system noradrenergic activity.[6] Redmond has implicated noradrenergic neurons in the locus ceruleus, noting that stimulation of this area produces fearful behavior.[7] This biochemical model draws support from common observation that a state very much akin to anxiety may be produced by exogenous sympathomimetic agents (see below).

A source of intriguing speculation are recent findings suggesting the presence of benzodiazepine binding sites in the brain.[8,9] In research that has followed, and in many ways parallels, the search for endogenous opiates (which resulted in the discovery of endorphins and enkephalins), several groups have shown these receptors to be widely distributed in the brain.[10,11] What remains to be discovered is the "brain's own diazepam," a naturally occurring molecule that would make teleologic sense of the benzodiazepine receptor.

Assuming the existence of an "endogenous diazepam," one might speculate that anxiety is related to a deficiency of the substance or to some dysfunction of its membrane receptors. The future for research in this area seems to be bright.

The inhibitory neurotransmitter γ-aminobutyric acid (GABA) also seems to have a role in the mitigation of anxiety.[12,13] Again, it seems feasible that the picture of anxiety might emerge from any disturbance in the homeostatic action of GABA. (An analogous situation is known to exist in Parkinson's disease. The pathogenesis of this disorder seems to involve insult to nigrostriatal inhibitory neurons (dopaminergic neurons), which normally exert a tonic influence over the extrapyramidal motor system. Released from this influence, the extrapyramidal system becomes overactive; and the well-known neurologic stigmata emerge.) Similarly, adenosine and the adenosine receptor seem to exert a tonic inhibitory effect on neuron firing.[14] Disruption of this may be associated with symptoms of anxiety.

The precipitation of panic attacks by intravenous (IV) sodium lactate infusion is a finding of uncertain significance. Pitts and McClure first pointed out that patients prone to panic attacks quite regularly had such attacks precipitated by lactate while normal controls did not.[15] Others have found that successful pharamacotherapy of panic disorder is associated with disappearance of the lactate response.[16,17] The pathophysiology of the lactate response is unknown. It has been speculated that chelation of calcium by the lactate anion might be responsible for symptom production. However, Pitts was unable to induce panic in susceptible patients by infusion of the potent calcium chelator EDTA.[18]

Genetic and Environmental Factors

While there is considerable evidence pointing to familial clustering of anxiety, data do not exist to support anything approaching mendelian inheritance of anxiety.[19,20] One is left, instead, to wonder about the subtle interplay between genetic and environmental factors ("nature versus nurture").

A study by Dealy et al of 93 patients with either panic disorder or generalized anxiety disorder showed that 45% reported anxiety disorder in other family members.[21] In a similar survey by Clancy et al, 54% of probands reported family members with similar disorder.[22] Both studies show females to be at higher risk. More recently, Surman et al reported two sets of HLA-identical twins who were concordant for panic disorder.[23]

Dealy's group reported a 9.3% risk of alcoholism in first-degree relatives of their patient sample. They wondered whether alcoholism might not represent a variant of anxiety disorder, the substance abuse growing out of an attempt at self-medication.

How does environment lend to the development of anxiety? The somewhat benighted view of existential philosophy is that anxiety is a normal, in fact universal, response to the absurdity of human existence and the ever-present threat of annihilation. Although this view does not particularly lend itself to the treatment of anxiety, it has gained currency in an era when global destruction has become a distinct possibility.

Retreating from such cosmic views to the level of personal development, we find that anxiety has been attributed to numerous factors. Otto Rank felt that the prototype for all subsequent anxiety was the trauma of birth.[24] Certain innovations in obstetrical practice (muted noise and lighting, warm baths for the newborn) draw support from this theory.

Later developmental events or accidents may equally well militate for adult anxiety. *Separation anxiety* , for instance, may be seen as a normal occurrence in early childhood. In a milieu that enhances this response, however, it may assume pathologic proportions.

> **Case report** A 30-year-old housewife was referred for treatment of agoraphobia with panic attacks. Her activity had gradually become constricted, such that she was loathe to leave her home. Developmental history revealed that she had a lifelong solicitous concern for her mother's health. Her mother, it was learned, had repeatedly warned her during childhood of her (the mother's) imminent death. The patient dared not upset her mother for fear of hastening her demise. Such fears were reinforced by the mother's being taken away for what were later found to be psychiatric hospitalizations. By the time the patient reached school age, she was frightened to leave home, fearing her mother's death during her time at school. After a fairly long quiescent period, anxiety symptoms had re-emerged as the last of her own children became ready to start school.

This case illustrates the fact that childhood separation anxiety may well serve as a prologue to adult *panic disorder* or *agoraphobia* .[25,26] It also raises the question of interplay between genetic and environmental influences. The patient's mother, described as "always nervous," may well have suffered from psychopathology very similar to her daughter's. The patient's son, noted to be "nervous, always worried," had developed serious concern about losing his father to ill health.

Harsh, punitive child rearing may result in anxiety in later life. The agoraphobic woman described at the outset of the chapter retained from her parochial school education an unforgiving moral view. Not only were sexual and aggressive actions anathema to her, but the merest conscious impulse of this sort generated significant anxiety. As her sexuality and her anger became conscious issues in psychotherapy she became visibly anxious, chastising herself for "bad thoughts."

Castration anxiety is common, if not universal, in the oedipal child.[27] Most agree that this anxiety is associated not necessarily with fear of castration but with fear of any bodily injury or incapacity. Developmental accidents that lead to poor resolution of oedipal conflict may be associated with significant persistent castration anxiety. An 18-year-old student, for example, presented with generalized anxiety and poor school performance. It was learned that his father, a very successful attorney, had divorced his mother a year previously, leaving the patient to live with his mother. What emerged in psychotherapy was that this situation rekindled the oedipal struggle. The father had essentially been vanquished, and mother was his. Only slowly did competitive strivings with the father emerge from the unconscious. These strivings were so fraught with anxiety, with fear of retribution from the powerful father, that the patient's conscious approach had been to abjure competition and to court failure. This he had done with unfortunate success.

Myriad other developmental and environmental accidents may generate later anxiety.[28] This cause and effect is dramatically illustrated in *post-traumatic stress disorder* . This disorder has won recent attention largely because of its prevalence in Vietnam war veterans. Nowhere is disaster "outside the range of usual human experience" more likely to occur than in war.[29] However, a wide range of traumatic events, including natural disasters and man made disasters, may result in this disorder.

The subtle interplay between environment, psyche, and soma has been the focus of recent intriguing work by Lown et al.[30,31] They describe, for example, a 39-year-old man who was resuscitated from two episodes of ventricular fibrillation. The first of these occurred when he was wrestling playfully with his sexually mature daughter. At the ringing of a doorbell he uttered, "I'm sorry," and had a cardiac arrest. Thorough evaluation, including coronary angiography, revealed no underlying heart disease. Psychiatric evaluation showed him to have rigid emotional control and to be unconscious of and intolerant of sexual or aggressive feelings. Anxiety provoked by the psychiatric interview, while not outwardly apparent, took the form of increased ventricular ectopic activity.

Lown's work, while lending physiologic support to Freud's theory of signal anxiety, also speaks to long-standing questions about sudden death under overwhelming stress (*voodoo death* and similar phenomena). There have long been anecdotal accounts of deaths occurring in victims of voodoo magic. Cannon published a collection of these and postulated that death ensued from massive adrenergic discharge.[32] More recently, Jones and Robinson reported a case of extreme anxiety (without fatality) in an Australian aborigine who believed himself doomed by magic.[33] Lown's findings suggest that death from overwhelming stress or anxiety is probably secondary to cardiac dysrhythmia. The role of the sympathetic nervous system in generating this is supported by studies showing that such tachyarrhythmias are blocked by cardiac sympathectomy or β-adrenergic blockers.

DIFFERENTIAL DIAGNOSIS

Nonpsychotropic Drugs

Table 1-1 lists nonpsychotropic medicines commonly associated with symptoms of anxiety. Clearly the key to making the diagnosis of this form of secondary anxiety is the taking of a scrupulous drug history. In addition, the presence of certain medical disorders should alert the physician to the possibility of drug-induced anxiety. Asthmatic patients may well be taking preparations containing combinations of sympathomimetics and xanthine derivatives. Patients with chronic allergy might be prescribed preparations containing ephedrine. Insulin dependent diabetics might experience symptoms of hypoglycemia. Thyroid preparations may be precribed not only in the face of thyroid disease but for the highly questionable indication of weight loss.

Specific attention should be paid to self-medication with over-the-counter medicines, agents often unwittingly left out of the patient's review of drugs. "Occult" sympathomimetic use may be uncovered in the patient taking patent medicines for upper respiratory infection or for dieting.

Caffeine consumption should also be determined in the complete drug review.[14,37] While coffee consumption probably accounts for the most common etiology of caffeine toxicity, occult sources such as colas and combination pain remedies should be considered. *Caffeine withdrawal* may also be culpable. We recently saw a 42-year-old woman with well-compensated schizophrenia who drank twenty or more cups of coffee per day. After her daughter switched her to decaffeinated coffee she experienced a gradual escalation of anxiety which culminated in psychotic decompensation.

A review by Dietch of organic anxiety disorders mentions *ginseng* ingestion as part of the differential diagnosis.[38] The Far Eastern practice of using preparations of this root for their purported aphrodisiac properties is apparently finding favor in some Western subcultures.

Another disorder attributable to Far Eastern influence has been prosaically called the "Chinese restaurant syndrome."[39,40] This syndrome of

Table 1-1
Drugs Commonly Associated with Production of Anxiety

I. Nonpsychotropic preparations
  A. Sympathomimetics[34]: epinephrine, norepinephrine, isoproteronol, levodopa, dopamine hydrochloride, dobutamine, terbutaline sulfate, ephedrine, pseudo-ephedrine, over-the-counter cold and diet remedies[14,35]
  B. Xanthine derivatives: aminophylline, theophylline, caffeine (coffee, colas, over-the-counter pain remedies)
  C. Anti-inflammatory agents: indomethacin[36]
  D. Thyroid preparations: T_3, T_4, dessicated thyroid
  E. Insulin (via: hypoglycemic reaction)
  F. Corticosteroids[36]
  G. Others: nicotine[38,41], ginseng root[38], monosodium glutamate[39,40]
  H. Drug withdrawal: caffeine[37], nicotine

II. Psychotropic preparations
  A. Drugs for treatment of mood, attention deficit disorders: d-amphetamine, methylphenidate hydrochloride, tricyclic antidepressants[36,] monoamine oxidase (MAO)-inhibitors
  B. Tranquilizing drugs: benzodiazepines (paradoxical response)[36], antipsychotics (akathisia)
  C. Anticholinergic toxicity[36]: antipsychotics, antiparkinsonian agents, tricyclic antidepressants, scopolamine (over-the-counter sleep preparations)
  D. Drug withdrawal : sedative-hypnotics (including benzodiazepines), major tranquilizers[44,45], tricyclic antidepressants, antiparkinsonian agents[46,47]

III. Alcohol-related syndromes
  A. Acute intoxication
  B. Alcoholic paranoia
  C. Alcohol withdrawal
  D. Disulfiram-alcohol interaction

IV. Other drugs of abuse
  A. Sympathomimetics[34]: cocaine, d-amphetamine
  B. Anticholinergics[36]: antiparkinsonian drugs[51]
  C. Euphoriant/hallucinogens[49]: marijuana, phencyclidine hydro-chloride, LSD, psilocybin, mescaline
  D. Withdrawal states: opiates, barbiturates, other sedative-hypnotics

flushing, tachycardia, and diarrhea has been ascribed to *monosodium glutamate* commonly used in the preparation of Chinese food.

While nicotine is noted to be associated with production of anxiety, it is unlikely that doses commonly inhaled by cigarette smokers (0.05-0.2mg/cigarette) would be so associated.[38,41] On the other hand, doses of nicotine approaching the lethal dose of 50 mg may result from ingestion and inhalation of certain insecticides and may produce symptoms of anxiety (dizziness, tachycardia) or of frank nicotine poisoning (tachyarrhythmias, seizures, gastrointestinal irritability).[42] Conversely, *withdrawal* from chronic nicotine use is commonly known to produce a picture of anxiety and irritable mood.

Psychotropic Drugs

Psychotropic drugs, too, are summarized in Table 1-1. The drugs used in treating mood and attention deficit disorders presumably have in common the enhancement of adrenergic nervous activity both in the brain and peripherally. The tremendous frequency with which the *tricyclic antidepressants* are prescribed make this a particularly important diagnostic consideration. Since anxiety and depressive symptoms commonly occur in concert, the question of drug-induced anxiety takes on added meaning here. The tricyclics may produce anxiety of frankly psychotic proportions.

While the *benzodiazepine minor tranquilizers* (diazepam, etc) mitigate anxiety in the vast majority of cases, a paradoxical excitatory response has been described. This seems to be a particular vulnerability of the elderly; and it clearly warrants recognition, lest treatment involve even higher doses of the noxious agent.

The diagnosis of *akathisia* (Greek, literally: "not sitting down") due to use of antipsychotics is similarly vital. This syndrome, usually occurring days to weeks after initiation of drug therapy, is characterized by pacing, agitation, and difficulty sitting still. Patients typically feel like "jumping out of my skin." The clinical picture may readily be confused with worsening psychosis, and the resultant increase in drug dose is likely to worsen the disorder.

Anticholinergic toxicity may mimic anxiety and, in the extreme may produce frank psychosis. It is then important to recognize that many psychotropic drugs share anticholinergic properties. It is not unusual to find patients taking combinations of antipsychotics and tricyclic antidepressants. It is only slightly less common to find these patients taking antiparkinsonian agents, such as trihexyphenidyl hydrochloride, for drug-induced dyskinesias. Needless to say, such regimens constitute a fairly significant anticholinergic assault. Add to this the prescription of another atropinelike agent in the form of an antispasmodic or "gastrointestinal sedative," and the stage is set for drug toxicity. In addition to questioning the patient about the more common prescription anticholinergics, the clinician would do well to ask about use of over-the-counter sedative hypnotics which may contain scopolamine.

Withdrawal from virtually any sedative hypnotic may produce symptoms of anxiety. Even the relatively safe benzodiazepines, while undeserving of the scorn that the media have heaped upon them, may quite clearly produce tolerance and a syndrome of drug withdrawal.[43] Less commonly considered in the differential diagnosis of drug withdrawal anxiety; the antipsychotics have been so associated.[44] Some case reports have suggested that chronic antipsychotic use may produce a condition of limbic lobe "denervation hypersensitivity" to dopamine.[45] Affected patients require ever higher doses of antipsychotics to suppress psychotic anxiety and related symptoms and may show emergence of psychotic anxiety upon the slightest reduction in drug dose.

Other case reports have focused upon the perils of withdrawing antiparkinsonian drugs prescribed for the management of dyskinesias induced by antipsychotics. While earlier studies suggested this could be done with relative impunity, more recent work cites the risk not only of recurrent dyskinesia but of anxiety and, on occasion, frank psychosis.[46,47]

Finally, withdrawal of tricyclic antidepressants has also been noted to produce clinical anxiety. This is a common problem when the dose is reduced precipitously. As with the other drug withdrawal states, obtaining a complete history is the most critical step in differential diagnosis.

Physical examination is apt to give little specific help with the question of psychotropic drug-induced anxiety. Most likely are nonspecific signs of anxiety (tachycardia, elevated blood pressure). Evidence of anticholinergic activity (mydriasis, dry mucous membranes, decreased bowel sounds) may help the diagnosis, but even these signs are relatively nonspecific. Many centers have laboratories equipped to confirm (or refute) the presence of psychotropic drugs in the blood.

Alcohol

The faces of acute alcohol intoxication are many and are so common that they hardly need description. Typically, acute drunkenness is unlikely to be confused with disorders producing anxiety. In atypical patients, ingestion of even small amounts of alcohol may lead to agitated, often combative behavior ("pathological intoxication") with a distinct flavor of anxiety. *Alcoholic paranoia* is another relatively rare state associated with ongoing alcohol consumption. Affected patients harbor paranoid delusions (and attendant anxiety), often involving the belief that a spouse is unfaithful. These diagnoses are, of course, supported by a history of ongoing alcohol consumption, by typical physical findings (slurred speech, ataxia, alcohol on the breath, etc) and, if need be, by laboratory measurement of blood alcohol.

Alcohol withdrawal may in its own right be associated with anxiety. Early in the period of abstinence, anxiety may be associated with tremulousness, nausea, irritability, and occasionally with visual or auditory hallucinations or with seizures ("rum fits"). This entire spectrum occurs in the setting of a clear sensorium. Conversely, the patient who develops frank *delirium tremens* invariably has derangement of sensorium as well as marked agitation. In addition to tachycardia and elevation of blood pressure, fever is a distinctive physical sign of this potentially fatal disorder.

An additional alcohol-related syndrome that bears mention here is the interaction of alcohol with disulfiram. Prescribed precisely because of its noxious interaction with alcohol, disulfiram (Antabuse) is a common adjunct in the treatment of alcoholism. Interacting with alcohol by blocking acetaldehyde dehydrogenase, the drug produces flushing, tachycardia, sweating, nausea, hyperventilation, decreased blood pressure and, rarely, circulatory collapse. Again, the history of drug use (often denoted by medical identification bracelets) is crucial to this diagnosis.

Similar to the alcohol-disulfiram interaction is the interaction between alcohol and metronidazole. This agent, commonly used to treat *trichomonas* infections and amebic infestation, is often not considered as a potential synergist with alcohol.

While the mechanisms of alcohol-related anxiety are no doubt complex, Coffman and Petty have reported findings that may, in part, explain these phenomena.[48] Comparing chronic alcoholics with controls, they found that alcoholism was associated with a significant depression of plasma γ- aminobutyric acid (GABA); and they deduced that brain levels of this inhibitory neurotransmitter were similarly depressed.

Other Drugs of Abuse

Abuse of various drugs (Table 1-1) may produce a state of anxiety, and the careful medical history includes inquiry into such practices. Amphetamines and cocaine, by virtue of their sympathomimetic action, produce a spectrum of anxiety that includes frank psychosis.

Anxiety associated with use of euphorohallucinogens (mescaline, tetrahydrocannabinol [THC], psilocybin, LSD) is also represented in a spectrum.[49] The hallucinatory, often paranoid, response to these agents is commonly associated with toxic doses (low doses being associated simply with euphoria). By the same token, the "bad trip" may be a product of the psychological make-up of the drug abuser and/or the milieu in which the drug is taken (a supportive, nonthreatening setting lessening the likelihood of the idiosyncratic anxious response). Although proof of this assertion is difficult, it is often suspected that these agents provoke the flowering of latent functional psychoses.

Phencyclidine hydrochloride abuse may evoke a wide range of symptoms, from a schizophrenialike withdrawal to a state of moderate anxiety, to a state of agitated (and oft dangerous) rage.[49] Its association with disordered thinking and blunting or dissociation of affect place this agent in the differential considerations for severe, psychotic anxiety.[50]

Similarly, the anticholinergic agents have won increasing favor as drugs of abuse. Bereft of significant euphoriant activity, these agents are associated at high doses with the anxiety of a toxic psychosis.[51] Among the anticholinergics that have been adapted to this perverse use are the antiparkinsonian agents trihexiphenidyl (Artane) and benztropine mesylate (Cogentin), mainstays of the psychiatrist's pharmacopeia.

Withdrawal from numerous illicit or abused drugs may also produce anxiety. The autonomic state of arousal in the abstinent opiate addict is well known. Anxiety, muscle twitching, dizziness, nausea, sweating, and hyperactive deep tendon reflexes all characterize barbiturate withdrawal. Before giving way to generalized seizures these symptoms might be mistaken for those of a less urgent disorder. While not associated with the mortality of barbiturate withdrawal, abstinence syndromes have been described with a wide range of sedative hypnotics. Even the benzodiazepines have been held culpable, although the media have perhaps overdramatized the perils of diazepam (Valium) withdrawal.

While the history is perhaps most crucial to the diagnosis of anxiety secondary to drug abuse, physical examination may be of help. Needle tracks or thrombosed superficial veins may suggest parenteral use of opiates, amphetamines, cocaine, or nearly any soluble agent (some, alas, may be injected in less-than-soluble states). Skin abscesses may indicate subcutaneous injection ("skin popping"). Since parenteral drug use is often associated with hepatitis, sepsis, or endocarditis, physical stigmata of these disorders should be carefully considered. Finally, the popularity of nasal insufflation ("snorting") of cocaine should lead the suspicious clinician to look for ulceration or perforation of the nasal septum.

Medical Disorders

Myriad illnesses may be associated with some or all of the classic symptoms of anxiety.[38,52-54] Most are unlikely to be missed by the clinician practicing careful history taking and physical examination. The more arcane may require special diligence and a high suspicion of organic illness. Table 1-2 outlines medical disorders to be considered in the differential diagnosis of anxiety.

Cardiopulmonary disorders Chest pain, shortness of breath, and rapid pulse are common symptoms of primary anxiety. They are also common symptoms of cardiac or pulmonary disease, and as such they warrant careful consideration.

Atherosclerotic coronary artery disease is likely to present with chest pain (location and radiation are variable), shortness of breath, and diaphoresis. Patients typically appear anxious and may note a feeling of foreboding. The history may be helpful in distinguishing this potentially life-threatening disorder from primary anxiety. Association of symptoms with physical activity, while by no means an absolute indicator, leads one toward the diagnosis of structural heart disease. Similarly, the presence of "coronary risk factors" (hypertension, smoking, diabetes, hyperlipidemia) logically leads one away from a primary psychiatric diagnosis. The patient's age and gender also enter into the logical consideration of coronary artery disease. However, the assumption that the young female does not suffer from this disease is fraught with risk and should be tempered by other data from history, physical examination, and laboratory examination.

In a series of 588 patients presenting to an emergency room with chest pain, Levene found that the description of pain, as well as its site and radiation, were useful discriminators.[55] Pain that was described as "squeezing" or as "pressure" was usually associated with coronary artery disease (CAD). "Stabbing" or "throbbing" pain was more likely to be associated with anxiety, although it did not preclude structural heart disease. Central (substernal) chest pain was more likely to be associated with CAD or esophageal disease than with anxiety. And patients with CAD were more likely to report multiple areas of radiation than were patients with anxiety.

Physical examination of the patient with CAD may not be very helpful. Barring the presence of rhythm disturbances, congestive failure, or a new murmur (as found with papillary muscle dysfunction or ruptured ven-

Table 1-2
Medical Disorders Presenting with Symptoms of Anxiety

I. Cardiopulmonary disorders
  A. Atherosclerotic heart disease with angina, myocardial infarction[55]
  B. Congestive heart failure (of any etiology)
  C. Mitral valve prolapse syndrome[56,58]
  D. Other disorders with tachyarrhythmias
  E. Hyperdynamic β–adrenergic state[59,60]
  F. Atrial myxoma[61]
  G. Pulmonary embolus
  H. Pneumothorax
  I. Acute asthma
  J. Chronic obstructive lung disease or other lung disease in exacerbation

II. Endocrine disorders
  A. Hyperthyroidism[54]
  B. Cushing's syndrome[54]
  C. Hypoglycemia[54]
  D. Hypoparathyroidism[62]
  E. Pheochromocytoma[54]
  F. Carcinoid syndrome
  G. Postmenopausal syndrome
  H. Diabetic ketoacidosis or other metabolic acidosis

III. Gastrointestinal disorders
  A. Peptic ulcer disease
  B. Reflux esophagitis
  C. Gallbladder disease
  D. Ulcerative, granulomatous colitis
  E. Parasitic infestation
  F. "Pancreatic cholera," other episodic diarrhea[66]

IV. Infectious disease
  A. Septicemia
  B. Meningitis
  C. Encephalitis

    D. Neurosyphilis

    E. Sydenham's chorea[67]

V. Metabolic disorders
- A. Uremia
- B. Liver failure[68]
- C. Hypokalemia[69,70]
- D. Hypocalcemia
- E. Low serum magnesium
- F. Acute hypoxia
- G. Other metabolic acidosis
- H. Acute intermittent porphyria[72]

VI. Diseases of the central nervous system
- A. Complex partial seizures (temporal lobe epilepsy)[70,73]
- B. Transient ischemic attacks
- C. Stroke with dysphasia[69]
- D. Subarachnoid hemorrhage
- E. CNS vasculitides
- F. CNS tumor
- G. Myasthenia gravis[82]
- H. Wilson's disease[84]
- I. Vitamin B_{12}, thiamine, nicotinic acid deficiencies
- J. Degenerative diseases (Alzheimer's disease, Huntington's chorea, multiple sclerosis, etc)
- K. Benign essential tremor, other tremor
- L. Ménière's disease

VII. Toxins, heavy metals
- A. Lead
- B. Mercury[85]
- C. Manganese[85]
- D. Organophosphate insecticides, "nerve gases" (anticholine-sterases)[85]

VIII. Anemias (iron, vitamin B_{12}, folate, and other deficienceis; other anemias)

IX. Nonspecific response to illness, surgery

tricular septum), examination may yield no more than nonspecific signs (rapid pulse, elevated blood pressure, diaphoresis).

Electrocardiography should be done if coronary artery disease is being considered. The presence of ST segment lowering (ischemic pattern) or elevation (infarction pattern), or of significant Q waves all help to confirm the diagnosis. A normal ECG does not rule out CAD, however. Hospitalization, with serial ECGs and myocardial enzyme determinations, myocardial scanning, or other studies may be necessary to clarify the diagnosis and should be undertaken if myocardial infarction is being considered. If CAD with angina is to be ruled out, a stress ECG may be diagnostic. Coronary angiography remains for now the "gold standard" for diagnosing CAD. Even a normal angiogram might be regarded with some caution, however, since coronary spasm has been found to produce angina in the absence of coronary stenosis.

Congestive heart failure in its florid form is unlikely to be mistaken for primary anxiety. Tachypnea and agitation are but part of a clinical picture that should not be missed by the careful clinician. History taking may reveal underlying heart disease or other systemic disease (eg, anemia, hyperthyroidism) associated with congestive failure. The differential diagnosis of congestive heart failure in itself is extremely broad. The interested reader should consult one of the comprehensive texts on internal medicine or cardiology. The patient may also complain of increasing dyspnea on exertion or of orthopnea or paroxysmal nocturnal dyspnea. Physical examination may reveal tachycardia, an S3 gallop rhythm, rales, dependent edema, hepatomegaly, and abnormal jugular venous distention. The chest film classically shows cardiac enlargement and may show pulmonary venous congestion.

Mitral valve prolapse (MVP) has received growing attention from both psychiatrists and nonpsychiatric physicians. The syndrome, associated with physical findings of midsystolic click and late systolic murmur, is often found incidental to routine physical examination. However, not all cases are clinically silent, and patients may experience tachyarrhythmias, shortness of breath, and chest pain secondary to MVP.[56-58]

Panic disorder and mitral valve prolapse have been found to coexist in a significant number of patients, leading to speculation about which represents the primary disorder.[56] Clearly, physical examination is a useful means of diagnosing MVP. In some patients the murmur is elicited only in certain positions (eg, sitting). In others, the systolic click may be the sole manifestation of the disorder. Echocardiography of affected patients shows redundancy of the posterior mitral valve leaflet with ballooning of the leaflet back into the left atrium during systole.

Tachyarrhythmias due to any underlying cardiac disorder may be mistaken for the "palpitations" of primary anxiety. While this diagnosis is readily made in the older patient with known heart disease, it may be a source of consternation in the younger patient. Paroxysmal atrial tachycardia, for instance, is often seen in young people without known heart disease. Its association with stress and fatigue make it likely to be confused with simple anxiety. The diagnosis may be confirmed by ECG (24-hour portable monitoring may be needed to document the arrhythmia). The ECG finding of anomalous atrioventricular excitation (Wolff-Parkinson-White syndrome and others) should make the clinician increasingly suspicious of the occurrence of paroxysmal tachyarrhythmias. The classic ECG findings here include a shortened PR interval (0.1 second) and a slurred upstroke on the QRS complex (delta wave).

Cardiologists have long been perplexed by a syndrome variously called "soldier's heart," "cardiac neurosis," "neurocirculatory asthenia," and "Da Costa's syndrome." Currently called *hyperdynamic β-adrenergic state*, this syndrome includes tachycardia, complaints of anxiety, and cardiac awareness.[59,60] It may be provoked by isoproterenol infusion and blocked by β-adrenergic blockers. Diagnosis may hinge upon the patient's response to these agents.

Wharton has reported a case of left *atrial myxoma* presenting with mixed anxiety and depression and with transient neurologic deficits that were felt for some time to be pscychogenic.[61] After more than 2 years of joint follow-up by an internist and various consultants (including a psychiatrist), atrial myxoma was considered and was confirmed by echocardiogram.

Anxiety might be mimicked by any of a number of pulmonary disorders which result in acute embarrassment of ventilation and/or perfusion. The air hunger and agitation associated with these disorders might readily be ascribed to psychogenic hyperventilation unless the problem is given careful scrutiny.

Pneumothorax may occur in healthy, young people in the absence of trauma and illustrates the importance of physical examination. Auscultation of the chest should reveal the rather striking absence of breath sounds on the affected side.

The *acute asthmatic attack* is not likely to be missed. One usually obtains a past history of such attacks, and expiratory wheezing is often evident even without resort to the stethoscope.

The patient with *chronic obstructive lung disease* or other chronic lung disease in exacerbation is likely to present with air hunger and agitation. If hypoxia or carbon dioxide retention are severe, such patients may show frank delirium. Here again, the past history of lung disease is usually available. Physical examination often shows stigmata of chronic lung disease (eg, "barrel chest," variable auscultatory findings). The chest film should reveal evidence of chronic lung disease and may show evidence of acute infection or other causes of decompensation. Arterial blood gases should reveal hypoxia and may show hypercarbia.

The discussion of anxiety in the setting of chronic lung disease would not be complete without attention to the anxiety commonly felt by these patients secondary to their disease. The patient with severe chronic lung disease has often experienced the terrifying subjective experience of smothering or of drowning in his own secretions. Such terror is an excellent substrate for the sort of existential anxiety commonly felt by these patients. In this setting the doctor is apt to be viewed as a talisman against these mortal fears, and it is not surprising that such patients commonly form intense dependent ties to their physicians.

Pulmonary embolism in its classic presentation is not likely to be missed. The history of sudden pleuritic chest pain with hemoptysis, the finding of a pleural friction rub and of an accentuated pulmonic component of the second heart sound, the wedge-shaped density on chest film and the pattern of right ventricular strain on ECG taken together, these findings make the diagnosis quite easy. Unfortunately, we are often not beneficiaries of the classic presentation. For the patient presenting with vague chest pain and air hunger alone, this very serious problem may readily be missed. Not always is there an apparent source of embolism (eg, a deep vein thrombosis of the leg). Frequently the physical examination is not conclusive. If embolism is suspected, arterial blood gases (showing hypoxia) should be done as should radionuclide lung scanning and, if need be, pulmonary arteriography.

Endocrine disorders Of the endocrinopathies, *hyperthyroidism* is one of the most easily mistaken for anxiety. Affected patients are likely to complain of jitteriness. Weight loss and heat intolerance may be noted. Physical findings typically include tachycardia, tremor, diaphoresis, and brisk deep tendon reflexes. Skin and hair may be of fine texture, and there may be either diffuse or nodular enlargement of the thyroid gland. Patients with hyperthyroidism secondary to Graves' disease may exhibit exophthalmos. Laboratory determination of high levels of circulating thyroid hormones confirms the suspicion of hyperthyroidism.

Cushing's syndrome may be seen in a number of settings. Originally described by Cushing in patients with pituitary basophilic adenomas (producing high levels of adrenal corticotropin), the disorder is also seen with primary tumors or hyperplasia of the adrenal cortex. Today, given the popular use of adrenal steroids in treating many medical disorders, the syndrome is frequently iatrogenic. Anxiety secondary to Cushing's syndrome is variable but may be of frankly psychotic proportions ("steriod psychosis").

Correct diagnosis of Cushing's syndrome is often yielded to the careful historian. The medication history is of particular import. Physical examination may show any or all of the following: hypertension, hirsutism, truncal obesity, purple striae, and pronounced dorsal fat pad ("buffalo hump"). The relatively rare patient with a pituitary adenoma may show a bitemporal visual field deficit. Laboratory findings include increased plasma cortisol and urinary 17-hydroxycorticosteriods and, frequently, an elevated blood sugar.

The anxiety seen with hypoglycemia is in part mediated by the sympathetic autonomic discharge provoked by low blood sugar. There may also be a direct CNS response, neuronal tissue being highly dependent upon adequate nurturant supplies of glucose. Again, anxiety may vary from mild to frankly psychotic levels.

Hypoglycemia is most apt to be seen in the setting of insulin-dependent diabetes, where it results from carbohydrate intake inadequate for a given dose of insulin. The history of diabetes is usually readily available to the clinician but may not be in the case of the psychotic patient seen without benefit of family members and other historians. Here a high index of suspicion, coupled with a determination of blood sugar (a crude but rapid assessment can be made with readily available dip sticks), will yield the proper diagnosis.

Although perhaps overdiagnosed, hypoglycemia may be seen as a response to dietary carbohydrate challenge and might be suspected in the patient with postprandial anxiety. In affected patients a prolonged glucose tolerance test usually shows late, significant hypoglycemia.

Rarely, hypoglycemia is due to an insulin-secreting islet cell tumor of the pancreas. Again, diagnosis depends first upon documentation of low blood sugar. More refined testing (eg, insulin levels, tolbutamide stimulation) is then indicated.

While hyperventilation may reflect uncomplicated anxiety, it may represent, among other things, a physiologic response to metabolic acidosis. *Diabetic ketoacidosis* typically is manifest not only in rapid Kussmaul respiration, but in a distinctive fruity smell to the patient's breath.

Additional physical findings are likely to include poor skin turgor and dry mucous membranes. Other stigmata of diabetes (eg, retinopathy) may be found. Blood sugar, serum acetone, and arterial pH determinations are diagnostic here.

Hypoparathyroidism may be discovered by serendipity from multiple channel analysis (eg, SMA 12) of blood samples. If present, physical findings reflect the state of neuromuscular excitability in the hypocalcemic patient and may include carpopedal spasm and a positive Chvostek's sign. Since primary parathyroid insufficiency is rare, the clinician should look for a history of thyroid surgery and search for the scar suggestive of this. While surgical technique usually involves assiduous avoidance of the parathyroid glands, this remains the major cause of hypoparathyroidism.[62] Emotional symptoms are a varied but frequent concomitant to hypoparathyroidism. Such changes include depression, irritability, and anxiety that may vary from mild to psychotic proportions.[62]

Anxiety associated with *pheochromocytoma* can be explained on the basis of abnormally high levels of circulating catecholamines. The rare patient afflicted with this problem usually presents with hypertension and typically complains of headache, excessive sweating, and palpitations.[63] While physical examination often yields no more than the finding of increased blood pressure, the occasional patient will have provocation of the syndrome upon palpation of the abdomen and resultant pressure upon the tumor. More commonly, the diagnosis yields only to a high index of suspicion and the finding of increased urinary levels of the catecholamine metabolite vanillylmandelic acid (VMA).

Also exceedingly rare, *carcinoid syndrome* typically presents with cutaneous flushing which can be provoked by exercise, stress, eating, or tumor manipulation.[64] Tachycardia, hypotension, and wheezing commonly accompany the flushing. Elevated urinary levels of the serotonin metabolite 5-hydroxyindoleacetic acid (5-HIAA) suggest the presence of the serotonin-secreting tumor (or tumors) associated with this syndrome.

Considerably more common, yet imperfectly understood, *menopause* may produce a range of emotional symptoms which include anxiety and irritability. Commonly associated with a change in menstrual cycle and with symptoms of vasomotor instability ("hot flashes"), the syndrome is presumed secondary to ovarian failure and lowered levels of circulating estrogens. While clinical diagnosis often obviates the need for laboratory confirmation, histopathologic study of vaginal epithelium (as by Pap smear) often shows loss of estrogen effect. High serum or urinary levels of follicle-stimulating hormone (FSH) reflect the lack of ovarian feedback inhibition of the pituitary.

Gastrointestinal (GI) disorders The anxious patient with GI symptoms presents a common dilemma. Aerophagia with bloating and belching is a common, if unconscious concomitant of anxiety. Similarly, crampy abdominal pain, flatulence, and loose stools ("irritable bowel syndrome") are common in the anxious, stressed patient. Yet the diagnosis of "functional" GI disorder is properly a diagnosis of exclusion. Alas, even the patient with well-documented psychological conflict is not immune (indeed, may have impaired immunity) to structural disease.[65]

Peptic ulcer disease has long been linked with anxiety. The activation of ulcer disease by stress has been widely described, and observations of gastric secretion as a function of stress lend some insight into the pathogenesis of the disorder.

Typically, the afflicted patient will describe burning epigastric pain, relieved by food or antacids. (More ominous symptoms, such as melena or hematemesis, if present, lead the clinician quite rapidly away from the consideration of functional illness.) Physical examination may be inconclusive, often yielding little more than epigastric tenderness. Diagnosis usually hinges on radiologic examination of the upper GI tract with barium contrast. Endoscopy may be equally revealing.

Reflux esophagitis typically presents with intermittent substernal "burning," often brought on by large meals and/or a recumbent position. Diagnosis is largely dependent upon fluoroscopic studies of the patient swallowing barium.

Gallstones are an extremely common affliction of middle and late age. In the patient presenting with fever and right upper quadrant abdominal pain the distinction from functional anxiety is easy. It is somewhat less easy in the patient who presents merely with episodic belching and bloating (particularly the younger patient who tends not to be seen as a candidate for gallstones). Clearly, the more closely the history approximates the typical story of fatty food intolerance the more straightforward the diagnosis becomes. Physical examination is immensely helpful if the patient is icteric or exhibits tenderness over the gallbladder (rarely, a hydroptic gallbladder may be palpated). Diagnosis is usually confirmed by radiologic contrast studies or ultrasound examination.

Inflammatory bowel disease , having established its chronic relapsing course, is unlikely to be mistaken for primary anxiety. At first appearance, however, the cramping, diarrhea, and tenesmus associated with ulcerative colitis and related disorders might be so interpreted. The occurrence of bloody diarrhea should dissuade one from diagnosing functional illness, as should the presence of fever, arthritis, or other systemic symptoms associated with inflammatory bowel disease. Proper diagnosis is usually achieved with sigmoidoscopy and barium enema.

Diarrhea of infectious origin is usually of an acute nature unlikely to be ascribed to anxiety. Careful stool examination for parasites, such as amebae, may be very important, as may careful culturing of stool. Of the fairly common pathogens that often defy laboratory detection, and often present as a rather chronic, intermittent disorder, *Giardia lamblia*, bears mention. This protozoan may cause quite nonspecific intestinal complaints, and its elusive nature lends to the mistaken diagnosis of functional disorder. The organism has an affinity for residence in the duodenum, and while cysts may be found in stool samples, duodenal aspiration may be necessary for proper diagnosis.

Among other disorders associated with episodic diarrhea, *pancreatic cholera* is a fascinating, albeit extremely rare condition.[66] Associated with high levels of vasoactive intestinal peptide (VIP) produced by non-β-islet cell tumors of the pancreas, the syndrome is marked by voluminous watery diarrhea. Of interest to the psychiatrist is the use of lithium carbonate to treat this disorder.[66] Lithium presumably acts by inhibiting VIP-sensitive adenylate cyclase in the gut, a mechanism probably analogous to the drug's effect upon antidiuretic hormone (ADH) and thyroid-stimulating hormone (TSH).

Infectious disease While they should not lead to serious diagnostic difficulties, infectious diseases may at first blush be mistaken for primary anxiety. *Septicemia* of any sort may be heralded by restlessness and a sense of foreboding. This usually gives way to fever and various other constitutional symptoms unlikely to be ascribed to a functional cause.

Infections of the central nervous system obviously are quite likely to produce mental symptoms, among them anxiety. In considering the possibility of *meningoencephalitis* the clinician should look for fever, stiff neck, or other signs of meningeal irritation. He should also test mental status, with careful attention to the patient's sensorium. Perturbation of judgment, orientation, memory, affect, or other cognitive functions suggest some sort of organic brain dysfunction. Many argue that if meningoencephalitis is so much as considered, then lumbar puncture should be done (barring evidence of increased intracranial pressure). Careful examination of cerebrospinal fluid (CSF) for cells, protein, glucose, and infectious organisms is then called for. Special examination for unusual pathogens such as amebae *(Naegleria)* or *Cryptococci* may be warranted.

While neurosyphilis has all but completed the transformation from societal scourge to medical curiosity, the "great masquerader" bears mention here. In its fullest expression this disorder is extremely unlikely to pass for functional anxiety and is marked by intellectual deterioration, memory loss, and other signs of dementia. Early in its development, however, the disorder may present with increasing irritability or insidious personality change. These developments usually give way to a frankly psychotic picture wherein mania or paranoid disorders may be mimicked. Neurologic examination may be of considerable diagnostic help if focal deficits are present. The classic unreactive pupil of Argyll-Robertson may be seen as may signs of *tabes dorsalis* (loss of vibratory and position sense, dysesthesias). Though less telling than these classic signs, virtually any focal deficit might be caused by gumma formation in the brain or spinal cord. Positive blood serology (eg, rapid plasma reagin [RPR] or the more specific fluorescent treponemal antibody assay) strongly supports this diagnosis, and screening serology should perhaps still be considered in the routine psychiatric evaluation given the simplicity of the test and the seriousness of missed diagnosis. Spinal fluid examination of affected patients also shows positive serology as well as increased protein and cell counts.

Sydenham's chorea (Saint Vitus' dance) is a relatively common concomitant of acute rheumatic fever in children, whereas it is rare in adults.[67] It may appear in the absence of carditis, arthritis, etc, and be the only manifestation of this poststreptococcal illness. Symptoms are apt to develop insidiously; anxiety and emotional lability may precede choreiform movement. Correct diagnosis is unlikely without the presence of the movement disorder. Other physical evidence of rheumatic fever (polyarthritis, fever, rash, signs of pancarditis) clearly support the diagnosis, as does serologic evidence of recent streptococcal infection (high antistreptolysin titer).

Metabolic disorders Numerous metabolic disturbances are associated with symptoms akin to anxiety. While most of these disorders have associated signs and symptoms readily distinguishable from anxiety, brief mention will be made of each.

Hyperventilation secondary to metabolic acidosis has been mentioned in the discussion of diabetic ketoacidosis. A similar response may be seen in other metabolic acidoses. *Lactic acidosis* is usually seen in the context of major medical illness and is a fairly common sequela to circulatory collapse. It may present in less dramatic fashion in patients taking the oral hypoglycemic agent phenformin hydrochloride. Presumptive diagnosis is made clinically and supported by the finding of a large serum anion gap. It is confirmed by arterial pH determination and the finding of high serum lactate levels.

Renal failure is another common cause of metabolic acidosis. If hyperventilation is seen as a response to this, it is likely to be in the context of clear historical, physical, and laboratory evidence of kidney disease. Affected patients usually appear unequivocally ill. They are likely to be hypertensive. In chronic renal failure the skin may show "uremic frost." Serum urea nitrogen, creatinine, and electrolyte determinations are confirmatory.

Salicylate poisoning is a fairly common cause of metabolic acidosis and is not unusual in a psychiatric setting. While hyperventilation may be the only physical evidence of the disorder, the history of overdose can usually be obtained. Blood salicylate levels confirm the diagnosis. Oil of wintergreen (methyl salicylate), because of its distinctive odor, sometimes is an agent of childhood poisoning. The odor of wintergreen on or about the intoxicated youngster may be a critical diagnostic clue.

Hepatic failure is associated with a broad spectrum of mental abnormalities, ranging from anxiety and irritability to delirium or frank coma.[68] Usually there is a history of liver disease as well as a rapid fluctuation of the mental state, suggesting an organic pathogenesis. Mental status examination usually shows clouding of the sensorium. Neurologic findings of ataxia, hyperreflexia, and inability to maintain wrist extension (asterixis or "liver flap") may be present. The patient's breath may smell of the musty *fetor hepaticus* . In the laboratory, serum liver function tests are markedly deranged. Serum ammonia levels are elevated and the EEG is felt by some to be diagnostic of this type of encephalopathy.

Hypokalemia has also been noted to mimic anxiety.[69,70] At serum potassium levels of 2.5 mEq/L or less, muscle weakness may be expected to occur.[71]

As levels become yet lower, embarrassment of respiratory muscles may supervene as may serious cardiac rhythm disturbance. Hypokalemia of this degree is most often seen in patients taking diuretics without adequate potassium replacement. It may also be seen after prolonged vomiting or diarrhea (and may thus complicate the course of anorexia nervosa), in cases of adrenal overactivity, and in other less common settings. Diagnosis is suggested by the appearance on ECG of diffuse T wave lowering and of U waves. It is confirmed by serum potassium determination.

Magnesium deficiency is an uncommon occurrence usually associated with rather severe malnutrition (as seen in some alcoholics, in malabsorption syndromes, and in frank starvation). Symptoms of the disorder resemble those of hypocalcemic tetany, and laboratory confirmation is made by determining the serum magnesium level.

Acute intermittent porphyria is a disorder of heme synthesis, inherited as an autosomal dominant trait and manifested most strikingly by recurrent crises of abdominal pain and by highly variable emotional symptoms. The genetic taint is commonly thought by some to have been present in the Hanoverian rulers of England and may have accounted for the episodic madness of George III. Affected patients often have a long history of anxiety or emotional lability. More striking emotional symptoms may include personality change, psychosis, and clouding of consciousness that may progress to frank coma. Lending to diagnostic confusion is the fact that emotional symptoms may be seen in the absence of abdominal crisis. Similarly, neurologic deficits, including muscle weakness, peripheral neuropathy, or cranial nerve palsies, may be unassociated with abdominal symptoms.

The diagnosis of acute porphyria is made by detection of abnormally high levels of specific heme precursors in the urine. Urine samples obtained during crisis may change upon exposure to light from normal color to a dark red-brown, due to photoconversion of these precursors to pigmented products.

Disease of the central nervous system It comes as little surprise that diseases of the CNS, particularly in the early stages of their development, often simulate the syndrome of anxiety. Often, only the passage of time makes clear the organic underpinnings of these disorders.

Perhaps the prototype of disorders existing at the interface of psychiatry and neurology, *complex partial seizures* have been noted to resemble primary anxiety.[70,73] The behavioral correlates of this disorder were described earlier in this chapter. While the interictal pattern of emotional lability and excitement may dominate the clinical picture, the temporal lobe epileptic usually presents with brief lapses in consciousness, during which semipurposeful or automatic behavior is carried out. Thus the seizure pattern per se is unlikely to be mistaken for anxiety.

It is not unusual for complex partial seizures to coexist with a generalized seizure disorder. Thus the history of major motor seizures is often obtained. On the other hand, there is debate about the relationship between temporal lobe seizure disorder and a schizophrenialike psychosis seen at times late in the course of the seizure diathesis.[74] A causal relationship has been put forth to support aggressive treatment of the cerebral dysrhythmia, including consideration of surgical excision of the seizure focus.[75] While causality remains unclear, it is generally agreed that a low percentage of patients with temporal lobe epilepsy (TLE) develop a syndrome akin to schizophrenia. Appearance of psychotic anxiety in patients with a history of seizure disorder should lead to consideration of this phenomenon.

Clinical suspicion of TLE can be confirmed by finding focal, anterior temporal spike or slow wave discharge on the EEG. Recording from these relatively deep cortical areas may be enhanced by the use of nasopharyngeal leads.

Vascular disorders of various types may be confused with functional anxiety. Perhaps most perplexing of these disorders, *transient ischemic attacks* are associated with brief loss of neurologic function, which is frequently resolved by the time the patient sees his physician. Such attacks are due to cerebral ischemia too brief to cause infarction.[76] Needless to say, the associated neurologic deficit is, in itself, a source of considerable anxiety to the afflicted patient. This, coupled with the frequently normal neurologic examination, may lead to improper diagnosis of "anxiety state" or "conversion disorder," and to improper clinical management. Correct diagnosis depends upon avoidance of premature diagnostic closure. While physical findings may be nil, one's index of suspicion is raised by the presence of a carotid bruit or other evidence of atherosclerosis.

Frank occlusion of a cerebral vessel usually leads to readily recognizable neurologic deficit. An exception to this rule is a stroke resulting in *dysphasia* .

The patient with vascular compromise to the posterior, superior temporal lobe (Wernicke's area) is likely to suffer a *fluent aphasia* . While he may be able to comprehend others, he cannot repeat the words of an examiner. His production of speech is smooth and at times frankly rapid; yet its content is apt to be confusing or nonsensical. Strokes in this area of the cortex are often unassociated with involvement of the motor cortex, and the isolated abnormality of speech may be mistaken for functional thought disorder.

Lesions involving Broca's area (lower portions of the motor strip and adjacent temporal cortex) produce *nonfluent or expressive aphasia* in patients whose comprehension is apt to be unimpaired. Such patients may become extremely anxious as a result of their impairment.[69] The usual coexistence of hemiparesis, due to involvement of adjacent motor cortex, is a major help in correct diagnosis.

Systemic lupus erythematosus (SLE) may be associated with a cerebral vasculitis which, in turn, may produce an array of emotional symptoms. Irritability, obsessional states, and paranoid anxiety have been described, as has a delirious state difficult to distinguish from steroid psychosis (SLE is commonly treated with corticosteroids).[77] At least 15% of affected patients will also experience seizures with this disorder, and focal neurologic deficits may be seen. There are quite likely to be stigmata that reflect disease involvement of other organ systems, this being a virtually protean systemic illness. Photosensitive skin eruption, arthritis, and Raynaud's phenomenon are commonly seen. Laboratory support for the diagnosis is found in an elevated sedimentation rate and in positive assays for antinuclear antibodies. More specific is the finding of LE cells in peripheral blood.

While *subarachnoid hemorrhage* tends quite rapidly to produce clouding of consciousness, its early evolution may be marked by anxiety, foreboding, and agitation. The history of sudden, severe headache should alert one to the possibility of this problem, as should the fairly rapid evolution of confusion. Stiff neck and other meningeal signs may initially be absent but virtually always develop within hours.[78] In the absence of contraindications, lumbar puncture should be carried out. The presence of bloody spinal fluid strongly supports the diagnosis.

Degenerative disease of the CNS may be heralded by prominent symptoms of anxiety. Common examples of such degenerative disorders include Alzheimer's disease, multiple sclerosis, and Huntington's chorea.

Alzheimer's disease (senile dementia) is an extremely common dementing disorder that may occur at any age (hence presenile dementia), but is usually seen in senescence. While it has typical neuropathologic features, antemortem diagnosis is principally a matter of ruling out other forms of dementia. The disorder begins insidiously, and early deficits in cognitive function may not be readily apparent. The patient, on the other hand, may well perceive subtle deficits and may react by manifest anxiety, depression, or simply by exaggeration of pre-existent psychopathology.

As the disease progresses, memory loss, impaired judgment, and other deficits associated with dementia color the mental status. Laboratory examination should be carried out to rule out treatable causes of dementia (eg, hypothyroidism, vitamin B_{12} deficiency, syphilis, frontal lobe tumor). Careful consideration should be given to the possible presence of depression ("pseudodementia"). In the final analysis, positive laboratory findings in the patient with Alzheimer's disease will be limited to cortical atrophy, noted best by computed tomography (CT).

Multiple sclerosis is a chameleonlike illness with a highly variable course. Mental disturbance has been noted with 50% or more of patients afflicted with the disease. The often vague and evanescent nature of the neurologic deficits associated with the illness often results in early conjecture about somatization or other functional disturbance.[79]

Correct diagnosis often awaits the appearance of incontrovertible neurologic deficits, and it is the clinical waxing and waning of such deficits which tends to establish the diagnosis.

Huntington's chorea is a rare degenerative disorder inherited as an autosomal dominant.[79] In its full flower, it presents inexorable dementia and chorea. However, the movement disorder may be quite absent early in the illness (which usually becomes evident in midlife), and emotional symptoms ranging from irritability and anxiety to psychosis may be harbingers of the disorder.

Affected patients are usually aware of a family history of this devastating illness, and the early expression of the disorder may rapidly give way to profound depression. Suicide is a common outcome.

Diagnosis of Huntington's chorea depends upon the positive family history and the observation of clinical signs of disease. It has been suggested that challenging suspected patients with levodopa (the disease seems to be mediated by dopamine hypersensitivity of the basal ganglia) and causing latent symptoms to emerge can help to establish early diagnosis and aid genetic counseling, etc. Opponents of this procedure see it as an unnecessarily premature confirmation of doom for affected patients and point to the tremendous psychological burden imposed upon the patient by such knowledge.

Nutritional deficiencies affecting the CNS may present with prominent symptoms of anxiety. As a rule, however, adjunctive findings are sufficient to avoid the improper diagnosis of functional illness.

Vitamin B_{12} deficiency is manifested by peripheral neuropathy as well as embarrassment of the corticospinal tracts and posterior columns. Early in its course, the disease may not produce signs of long tract involvement, and complaints of paresthesias alone may lead to the erroneous diagnosis of functional illness.

Emotional symptoms are common and are highly varied in this disorder. They range from irritability, anxiety, and emotional lability to frank psychosis ("megaloblastic madness").

The patient who has had gastric resection or who for any other reason might have decreased secretion of stomach acid and of intrinsic factor (necessary for small intestinal absorption of vitamin B_{12}) should raise one's suspicion for this disorder. Similarly, patients with disease or resection of the ileum may suffer malabsorption of this essential vitamin. Patients with surgically created "blind loops" of bowel may have abnormal overgrowth of certain gut bacteria that compete for available vitamin B_{12}.

Similarly, the patient with fish tapeworm (*diphylobothrium latum*) infestation from ingestion of raw fish may suffer vitamin B_{12} deficiency due to the high vitamin B_{12} demands of the parasite.

In the absence of these historic clues, the finding of corticospinal tract impairment (weakness, spasticity, positive Babinski reflexes) or of posterior column deficits (loss of vibratory, position sense) points to the consideration of this disorder. While neurologic and mental abnormality may precede hematologic disturbance, the hemogram may be of great use. The finding of a macrocytic anemia with hypersegmentation of neutrophils is strongly supportive of the diagnosis, which can be confirmed by serum vitamin B_{12} determination.

Thiamine deficiency due to malnutrition (beriberi) is uncommon in the Western world. Instead, it is usually encountered in the setting of chronic alcoholism, wherein it may lead to Wernicke's encephalopathy and its sequela, Korsakoff's psychosis.

The mental changes encountered in Wernicke's encephalopathy are varied and may include nervousness, irritability, apathy, or depression.[80] Memory and intellectual function are commonly impaired. Associated neurologic findings are critical to the diagnosis and include impaired conjugate gaze, nystagmus, ataxia, and evidence of peripheral neuropathy. Signs of myocardial disease (beriberi heart disease) may be present. Clinical suspicion of Wernicke's encephalopathy represents a medical emergency, immediate treatment with thiamine being indicated.

Pellagra results from dietary deficiency of nicotinic acid or its precursor tryptophan and is likely to be seen only in cases of dietary protein deficiency.[81] In its full form, the disease is marked by the "four D's" of dermatitis, diarrhea, dementia, and death. This florid syndrome may be preceded by nonspecific emotional symptoms including nervousness, fatigue, or depression.

In the face of the typical erythematous, sunburnlike rash and of a painful, beefy-red tongue, the diagnosis of pellagra is made easier. Complaints of nausea, vomiting, and diarrhea are usual. Neurologic deficits are variable and most commonly include impairment of memory, cognition, and level of consciousness.

The early stages of *myasthenia gravis* may readily be mistaken for anxiety or other functional disorders. Emery and Szymanski report a patient followed for 2 years in psychotherapy before myasthenia gravis was diagnosed.[82] The patient's vague complaints of fatigue and weakness had been variously ascribed to anxiety, depression, and conversion disorder before she was admitted to the hospital in myasthenic crisis with acute respiratory failure.

While correct diagnosis of this disorder may be confounded by ambiguous physical findings, one should look for easy tiring upon sustained or repeated muscular action (eg, sustained looking at the ceiling may produce the telling ptosis of the eyelids). Clinical suspicion may be supported by IV administration of edrophonium chloride (Tensilon). Myasthenic weakness is immediately relieved by this maneuver. Electromyography may offer further substantiation of the diagnosis.

Early *Wilson's disease* has a highly variable presentation. While signs of liver dysfunction may dominate the picture, more often neurologic disturbance heralds the disorder.[83] Early findings may include intention tremor, dysarthria, and incoordination. At times, no such "hard signs" are to be found; and personality change or other emotional alteration may be solitary findings.

Rao et al report the case of a 9-year-old boy with recurrent abdominal colic, which led to the impression of anxiety and school phobia.[84] He had no signs of basal ganglion disease and no stigmata of liver disease. He did not have a Kayser-Fleischer ring (a ring of brownish pigment at the periphery of the cornea pathognomonic for Wilson's disease), and a family history of illness suggesting autosomal recessive inheritance was not obtained. Correct diagnosis was attendant upon laboratory evaluation. Abnormal liver function tests led to liver biopsy, which finally led to a determination of serum and urinary copper and of serum ceruloplasmin. Wilson's disease was confirmed by low levels of serum ceruloplasmin and copper, and high urinary copper.

Fine *tremor* may be seen as part of the anxiety syndrome and must be distinguished from tremor of other etiology. The tremor at rest seen with disease of the basal ganglia (eg, Parkinson's disease) should be ruled out, as should the intention tremor associated with cerebellar disease. Familial or hereditary tremor should be considered. Finally, certain mimics of primary anxiety (hyperthyroidism, sympathomimetic drugs, alcohol withdrawal, etc) may exhibit prominent tremor.

One of us was recently alerted by a patient to an increasing preoccupation by the lay press with Meniere's disease. This disorder of inner ear function, classically manifested by tinnitus, neural hearing loss, and vertigo, has apparently been mistaken for generalized anxiety or even panic disorder. The patient in question suffered from the latter and needed assurance that her doctor had considered the full range of differential diagnosis.

Toxic disorders Poisoning with various toxins and heavy metals may produce symptoms of anxiety.

Lead poisoning, while usually considered a disorder of children, may be seen in adults with occupational exposure to lead. A local junkyard worker, exposed to fumes from burning automobile batteries, has been followed in our clinics with chronic lead poisoning. In other parts of the country cottage industry alcohol distilling may be done in discarded automobile radiators, another source of lead.

Early lead intoxication may be marked by loss of appetite, constipation, and colicky abdominal pain (lead colic). At higher blood levels, irritability and restlessness might be confused with anxiety. These symptoms may be concomitant, however, with ataxia, dizziness, and peripheral neuropathy. They may give way, moreover, to frank delirium and/or seizures. The diagnosis is supported by the presence of a black "lead line" at the gingival margins. It may be confirmed by serum or urinary lead levels.

Chronic *mercury poisoning* is usually seen in the setting of industrial exposure (Lewis Carroll's Mad Hatter was so afflicted). It has been seen in Japan as a result of chronic ingestion of fish exposed to industrial pollutants. The disorder may be heralded by tremor and nonspecific personality change. Progressive symptoms are said to range from irritability and ease of embarrassment to withdrawal and psychosis.[85]

Manganese intoxication is also likely to be associated with exposure, either in mining or manufacture of the metal. "Manganese madness" tends to be ushered in by headache, irritability, and arthralgias.[85] These symptoms may then give way to frank psychosis, with hallucinations and disordered sensorium. This syndrome may be accompanied by signs of basal ganglion dysfunction (resting tremor, cogwheel rigidity, masklike facies, etc) identical to those seen in Parkinson's disease.

Organophosphate insecticides and certain *nerve gases* have in common the inhibition of cholinesterase enzymes. Poisoning with these agents results then in a surfeit of cholinergic activity, the effect of which is striking both at the level of the neuromuscular junction and of the brain.

Patients exposed to these agents may first complain of symptoms not readily distinguished from anxiety: numbness of extremities, dizziness, chest tightness, excessive sweating (the typical excess salivation is less consonant with functional anxiety).[85] Gastrointestinal upset is common. With more advanced poisoning, muscle fasciculation may be seen in a setting of weakness. Paralysis may ensue. Restlessness may give way to delirium, convulsions, and coma. Suspicion of anticholinesterase poisoning may be supported by clinical response to the administration of atropine sulfate.

Anemias The tired patient complaining of dizziness and rapid pulse may be describing symptoms of anemia. Unless carefully considered, his symptoms might be ascribed to anxiety. Careful history taking might reveal a source of blood loss. Acute loss is more likely to produce symptoms. With insidious decline in packed cell volume, physiologic adaptation may occur until anemia is quite marked. The history may also highlight the presence of chronic disease, autoimmune disorder, or other disease associated with anemia.

A complete exposition of the anemias is beyond the scope of this chapter. While etiologies vary quite widely, the anemias have in common a decrease in packed red cell volume (hematocrit). The resulting decrease in oxygen-carrying capacity of the blood results in the symptoms described above. Physical examination may reveal pallor and tachycardia. Orthostatic hypotension may be present, particularly in cases of acute blood loss with decreased intravascular volume. Myriad other physical findings are associated with the various types of anemia. Thorough examination should include a search for stigmata of various nutritional deficiencies (eg, vitamin B_{12}), of chronic disease or endocrine dysfunction, and of lymphoid dysfunction (spleen and lymph nodes should be carefully palpated). Occult sources of blood loss should be considered (rectal examination with stool guaiac is essential).

Laboratory confirmation of anemia is readily obtained with hemoglobin and/or Hct determination. Further refinement of the diagnosis is attendant upon examination of red cell morphology, determination of red cell indices, serum iron, iron-binding capacity, and a number of more specific tests.

Nonspecific response to illness, surgery

There are individuals, doctors—and nurses—for example, whose very existence is a constant reminder of our frailties. We cannot picture a time when birth and life and death shall be separated from that "grizzly troop" which we dread so much and which is ever associated in our minds with "physician and nurse."[86]

No man with any self-respect cares to be taken off guard, in mufti so to speak. Sickness dims the eye, pales the cheek, roughens the chin, and makes a man a scarecrow, not fit to be seen by his wife, to say nothing of a strange woman all in white or blue or gray. Moreover, she will take such unwarrantable liberties with a fellow, particularly if she catches him with fever.[87]

Long before the heyday of consultation psychiatry, Sir William Osler had an intuitive grasp of the anxiety that is generated by medical illness. He noted the patient's association between illness and its ultimate expression: death. And he noted the compromise of normal psychological defenses by illness.

Helene Deutsch observed the frequent occurrence of anxiety in surgical patients and offered a psychoanalytic explanation.[88] General anesthesia, she reasoned, is equated by the unconscious with death; while surgery per se is associated with primitive fears of mutilation (castration anxiety).

Anxiety of some degree is extremely common in the face of major medical illness. Several groups have studied anxiety in the setting of the coronary care unit (CCU).[89-91] Rating anxiety by use of a brief questionnaire, Vetter et al assessed 338 patients upon admission to such a unit.[91] They found that women in general were more anxious than men and that myocardial ischemia had a higher correlation with anxiety than myocardial infarction. They also found that admission to a CCU was no more likely to be associated with anxiety than emergency admission to another part of the hospital.

The high correlation of medical emergency with anxiety may well be related less to the severity of illness than to its acuity. Confronted with a sudden, perhaps calamitous, change in homeostasis, the ego may be unable to summon adequate defenses, with resultant emergence of anxiety. A report by Lansky and Gendel on patients with childhood malignancy (a calamitous disorder, even if not very acute) highlights such failure of normal defenses.[92] These authors describe a phenomenon of marked regression to a state of early infantile symbiosis. Affected children exhibited marked separation anxiety.

While virtually any medical emergency is likely to generate anxiety, perhaps none does so to the extent seen with acute respiratory compromise. The patient with pneumothorax or acute bronchospasm experiences acute air hunger and may describe a sense of suffocation or even drowning. These metaphors help to explain the severity of the anxiety seen with these disorders. Ironically, the symptoms of anxiety may be exacerbated in the acutely asthmatic patient by routine treatment, which usually includes epinephrine.

Anxiety in the preoperative setting is not only common but is perhaps adaptive. Janis studied the relationship between postoperative outcome and preoperative anxiety, and found that patients with moderate preoperative anxiety had fewer postoperative psychiatric complications than patients with either low or high preoperative anxiety.[93] Goble et al studied patients admitted for cardiac pacemaker implantation, finding that high preoperative anxiety was associated with dissatisfaction with operative outcome.[94]

Postoperative anxiety may represent an exacerbation of long-standing psychiatric disturbance (see section on psychiatric diagnosis below) or may, in the extreme, take the form of psychosis. Studies by Titchener and others have concluded that the stresses of surgery may precipitate any of the functional psychoses (see below) or a delirious state.[95]

Postoperative delirium has been found to occur more often in the elderly (in whom there may be an underlying subtle organic deficit) and has been found to be highly dependent upon sensory stimulation.[96] Underscoring the importance of sensory input, Weisman and Hackett described psychosis occurring after eye surgery ("black patch delirium").[97] Prior to recent advances in preoperative preparation and postoperative management, psychosis in patients after open heart surgery had an incidence of 50% or more.[98] Such dire statistics have been improved considerably by attention to the milieu of the recovery room and intensive care unit. Attempts now are made to maximize orienting stimuli, not the least of which is the presence of a familiar doctor, nurse, or family member.

Before leaving the topic of anxiety seen in the setting of a medical—surgical unit, added mention should be made of the problem of alcohol withdrawal. It is not at all unusual for routine medical or surgical admissions to be complicated by an abstinence syndrome (the early signs of which might be mistaken for anxiety). Often there is no suspicion of alcoholism, the history indicating only "social drinking." At times the occurrence of a generalized seizure is the first clue of the use of euphemism in the drinking history.

Trauma Anxiety secondary to trauma may be divided into disorders with brain damage and disorders without such damage. Specific brain lesions associated with anxiety have been discussed under neurologic disorders.

Posttraumatic personality disorder is characterized by striking personality change in a patient without focal neurologic deficit but with evidence that cerebral damage has occurred.[99] Affected patients have been described by Goldstein as showing irritability, impulsiveness, and catastrophic anxiety in the face of stress.[100]

In contrast, the *postconcussion syndrome* (or posttraumatic syndrome) is seen in the absence of demonstrable brain damage. Associated mental changes are less pervasive than those of posttraumatic personality disorder. Commonly seen with this disorder are headaches, generalized anxiety, lassitude, insomnia, decreased tolerance to alcohol, and difficulty with concentration.[101] The psychological underpinnings of this disorder remain a point of debate, and some observers have suggested that the severity of symptoms seems inversely related to the degree of trauma.

Anxiety is a cardinal symptom of *posttraumatic stress disorder* (traumatic neurosis). This disorder is seen as a sequela to trauma that is "outside the range of usual human experience."[29] Such trauma may be physical (eg, injury from auto accidents, fire, or natural disaster), or emotional (eg, sudden, catastrophic loss of loved ones). Physical and emotional assaults are clearly combined in cases of torture, concentration camp experience, etc.

Posttraumatic stress is characterized by episodic re-experience of the traumatic event ("flashbacks" or recurrent dreams). Such episodes may be associated with marked anxiety, equalling, for example, the anxiety experienced in wartime combat. The disorder is further characterized by withdrawal from usual activities and from significant persons. Sleep disturbance, difficulty in concentrating, hypervigilance, and guilt over surviving the traumatic event may all be associated.

Psychiatric Disorders

"Functional" anxiety can be conveniently, if somewhat arbitrarily, divided into nonpsychotic, psychotic, and affective syndromes (see Table 1-3). Accurate diagnosis is important, since these disparate forms of anxiety carry widely different prognoses and still different mandates for treatment.

Nonpsychotic anxiety (neurotic anxiety). While this diagnosis no longer enjoys a place of its own in the psychiatric nomenclature, it subsumes a number of current diagnoses. These share common symptoms of apprehension, foreboding, and sympathetic autonomic arousal (as outlined earlier in the chapter). They also imply an exclusion of any disorder associated with psychotic symptoms (see below).

Table 1-3
Differential Diagnosis of the Anxious Patient:
Psychiatric Diagnosis

I. Anxiety without associated psychotic symptoms (primary anxiety)
   A. Panic disorder (acute anxiety)[102,103]
   B. Generalized anxiety disorder (chronic anxiety)[104]
   C. Phobic disorders
      1. Agoraphobia[107]
      2. Social phobia[108]
      3. Simple phobia[109]
   D. Obsessive-compulsive disorder[108]
   E. Posttraumatic stress disorder[29]
   F. Somatoform disorders[113—115]
   G. Dissociative disorders[117]
   H. Adjustment disorder, acute grief[105]

II. Anxiety secondary to major affective disorder (psychotic features may or may not be present)
   A. Major depression (agitated)[118]
   B. Mania[119]

III. Anxiety secondary to other psychotic disorders
   A. Schizophrenia and related disorders[120]
   B. Paranoid disorders[122]

Panic disorder [102].Patients suffering from this disorder experience episodic attacks of sheer panic. These are associated with intense apprehension. Affected patients often admit to fears of dying or of "going crazy" during an attack. The attacks, which are usually self-limited to a matter of minutes, are commonly marked by visceral symptoms of anxiety: dyspnea and hyperventilation, chest tightness, palpitations, dizziness, sweats, etc. While the episodes are often unrelated to the patient's activity, they may become associated with a given setting or situation, in which case phobic symptoms may develop (see below).

In the face of episodic panic, the patient may develop significant anticipatory anxiety. Thus, the coexistence of acute anxiety (panic attacks) and *chronic or generalized anxiety* is not unusual. This is clinically important since treatment of panic attacks and of generalized anxiety differs. Panic disorder often responds dramatically to imipramine hydrochloride while responding more poorly to diazepam and other antianxiety agents commonly used to treat generalized anxiety.[103] While psychotherapy is an important factor in the treatment of both acute and generalized anxiety, the presence of panic disorder argues for the addition of drug therapy with imipramine or other selected antidepressants.

The coexistence of panic disorder with mitral valve prolapse has been discussed. Clearly the diagnosis of panic disorder involves the exclusion of this and other organic problems as the basis for anxiety symptoms. Complaints of panic may also be seen with schizophrenia and major depression.

Generalized anxiety is diagnosed in the face of persistent anxiety lasting longer than 1 month in a patient over 18 years of age.[104] Symptoms common to the disorder include motor tension (muscle tension, fatigue, shakiness, etc), autonomic hyperactivity (palpitations, vasomotor instability, sweating, diarrhea, etc), apprehensiveness, and vigilance (often assuming the form of distractibility, insomnia).

Generalized anxiety must be distinguished from panic disorder, with which it may coexist (see above). The diagnosis of generalized anxiety should not be made if persistent anxiety is secondary to schizophrenia, affective disorder, or another anxiety disorder, such as obsessive-compulsive disorder (see below).

Adjustment disorder with anxious mood may present with many of the findings seen in generalized anxiety (motor tension, autonomic overactivity, etc)[105]. Usually, however, the symptom complex is not as fully developed; the presence of recent psychosocial stress is clear; and the duration of the disorder is less than 1 month.

The *phobic disorders* are characterized by a persistent and irrational fear of an object, situation, or activity.[106] In the face of the phobic stimulus, affected patients develop anxiety, and elaborate measures of avoiding this stimulus are often set up.

Depending upon the nature of the feared stimulus, several types of phobia may be diagnosed. It is important to note that in all types of phobic disorder the patient is aware of (and usually troubled by) the irrational nature of his fear. The patient suffering from agoraphobia experiences anxiety in the face of being alone, in a crowd, or in public places.[107] Avoidance of these situations often leads to insidious loss of function, and affected patients may become homebound. Activity in public may be tolerated only in the presence of another supportive individual (sometimes called a "phobic partner").

Agoraphobia may be preceded by panic disorder, and it seems at times that the phobic anxiety represents a learned response to repeated panic episodes that have occurred in public. In such cases *agoraphobia with panic attacks* may be diagnosed, and pharmacologic treatment of the panic attacks may be a mainstay of therapy.

Symptoms of avoidance or withdrawal, suggestive of agoraphobia, may be seen in schizophrenia, in paranoid disorders, affective disorders, and obsessive-compulsive disorder. Agoraphobia should not be diagnosed if avoidance symptoms are secondary to one of these disorders.

Diagnosis of *social phobia* is based on a persistent irrational fear of social situations in which the patient might be subject to scrutiny by others.[108] Such situations might include dining in public, and speaking or performing in public. Some degree of anxiety is normally generated by these activities. Diagnosis of phobic disorder then depends on the degree of distress generated by the feared activity. Affected patients commonly describe a fear of embarrassment in such settings and again, avoidance of the feared situation evolves.

Social phobia should be distinguished from appropriate, nonphobic anxiety. In addition, anxiety and avoidant behavior may be seen in schizophrenia, major depression, obsessive-compulsive disorder, paranoid disorder, and avoidant personality disorder. Social phobia should not be diagnosed if phobic avoidance is due to any of these disorders.

A phobic response to situation or objects other than those subsumed under agoraphobia and social phobia may merit the diagnosis of *simple phobia*.[109] Simple phobia may be associated with virtually any stimulus, but common stimuli include animals, heights (acrophobia), and closed spaces (claustrophobia). Simple phobias are not unusual in children and often remit spontaneously before adulthood. They are rarely disabling and often are not brought to the clinician's attention.

Schizophrenic patients may exhibit avoidance anxiety on the basis of delusional thinking about an object or situation. Simple phobia should not be diagnosed in this case. Similarly, simple phobia should not be diagnosed where anxious avoidance of dirt or contamination is a product of obsessive-compulsive disorder.[108]

Anxiety may be a prominent feature of *obsessive- compulsive* disorder, a disturbance marked by obsessions (persistent, recurrent thoughts or ideas that intrude themselves upon consciousness and are troubling or repugnant) and/or compulsions (actions performed to forestall some future mishap or to insure some future event; while the patient may recognize his rituals as senseless, he cannot curtail them without considerable anxiety).[110,111] Patients suffering from this disorder are likely to be distressed by it and may suffer significant impairment of social function. In the extreme, obsessions and compulsions may dominate the patient's intellectual and motor activity.

Obsessive-compulsive symptoms may be seen as part of a schizophrenic disorder or a major depression, in which case the diagnosis should rest with the underlying disorder.[112] The stereotyped behavior and utterances seen in Gilles de la Tourette's syndrome should also be distinguished from obsessive-compulsive disorder.

Posttraumatic stress disorder has been discussed (see "Trauma"). Anxiety associated with this disorder is distinguished by the history of an overwhelming stress and of flashback phenomena in which the traumatic event is relived.

The *somatoform disorders* are commonly associated with anxious mood (and with depression). These disorders are distinguished by complaints of physical dysfunction which are found to be without organic basis. Common to these disorders is the insidious development of hostility between patient and physician as symptoms defy both physical diagnosis and treatment.

There are several subcategories of somatoform disorders. In *somatization disorder* one finds a markedly positive review of systems (14 symptoms for women, 12 for men).[113] These multiple symptoms are noted to have their onset prior to age 30 and must have been present for several years prior to diagnosis. The disorder usually has its onset in adolescence.

Somatization disorder may be confused with physical disorders having vague, multiform presentation (eg, multiple sclerosis, systemic lupus). It should also be distinguished from schizophrenia, wherein there may be multiple somatic delusions (the complaints in somatization disorder are not delusional).

When complaints of pain dominate the clinical picture, and when no organic basis for this is found, the diagnosis of *psychogenic pain* may be entertained.[114] To support this diagnosis one should be able to demonstrate psychological factors in the genesis of the pain (eg, pain following on the heels of a conflict-laden life event or pain resulting in evasion of unpleasant activity or in other secondary gain).

Hypochondriasis may be associated with considerable anxiety.[115] Central to this diagnosis is abnormal preoccupation with bodily sensations, such that there develops an unrealistic fear of bodily illness. As with other somatoform disorders, thorough physical evaluation reveals no basis for this fear; and affected patients often become involved in angry relationships with multiple physicians.

Conversion disorder is diagnosed when a loss or alteration of function cannot be attributed to physical disease.[116] Classic examples of such loss include sensory or motor dysfunction that can usually be shown to have no neuroanatomic basis. A note of caution is in order here. For example, the patient presenting with stocking/glove dysesthesia may be presumed to have conversion symptoms, but one should recall that diabetic neuropathy and other polyneuropathy may present similarly. Long-term follow-up of patients with diagnosed conversion disorder reveals a sobering incidence of organic illness. Psychogenic vomiting and false pregnancy may also represent conversion symptoms. While the classic conversion disorder is accompanied by bland acceptance of symptoms (*la belle indifference*), this is not invariably present, and some degree of associated anxiety is common. As with psychogenic pain disorder, the conversion symptoms can be demonstrated to arise out of psychological conflict. Crucial to differential diagnosis is the exclusion of mental illness. Schizophrenia may have associated conversion symptoms but should be distinguished by its psychotic features (see below).

Given the storm and stress that the somatoform disorders create for patients and their physicians, an extra word of caution seems in order: *The somatizing patient is not feigning symptoms* . To the patient the symptoms are as "real" as if they were a product of physical illness, and any attendant anxiety or depression is *bona fide* . The somatizing patient stands in contrast to the *malingerer* , who consciously fabricates symptoms and who would be expected to experience anxiety only in the face of discovery. Symptoms may be assumed to spring from unconscious conflict and are thus truly beyond the scope of conscious control. While somatization is likely to be perceived by the clinician as offensive, it is born out of unconscious *defensive* activity on the part of the patient.

The *dissociative disorders* include a number of relatively rare syndromes (*psychogenic fugue, psychogenic amnesia, multiple personalities*) that involve lacunae of memory loss. Anxiety may not be particularly salient in these disorders. On the other hand, *depersonalization disorder* may be associated with significant anxiety. [117] Central to this disorder are one or more episodes of depersonalization. These are experiences wherein the patient has an altered sense of himself. He may describe feeling "strange" or "mechanical" or "spaced out." He may feel that his extremities are changing in size or that he is observing himself from a distance ("out-of-body experience").Symptoms of *derealization* often go hand in hand with these symptoms. Here the patient describes a troublesome alteration in perception, not of himself, but of his surroundings. He will note, for example, that objects appear particularly small, distorted, or otherwise unreal. Such experiences are a source of discomfort and, frequently, of anxiety. While mild depersonalization is quite common (occurring in up to 70% of young adults), diagnosis of depersonalization disorder presumes that symptoms have interfered with the patient's social or job functioning.

Symptoms of depersonalization are not unusual in schizophrenia, and the more pervasive symptoms of this disorder should be sought (see below). Underlying affective disorder should also be ruled out (see below). Organic brain disease may also be associated with depersonalization. Seizure disorders should be considered with particular care. Preictal events (aura) may closely mimic this disorder. Ictal phenomena in psychomotor (temporal lobe) epilepsy may have a marked flavor of depersonalization.

Anxiety may be a prominent feature of the *affective disorders* (see chapter 2), but as such it usually has a role clearly secondary to the mood disturbance. Depression or its polar opposite, mania, usually dominate the clinical picture.

The patient with *agitated depression* [118] may pose a bit of a diagnostic dilemma. Such patients may complain chiefly of restlessness, pacing, and a vague sense of foreboding. Sighing and handwringing are commonly seen in such cases. It is extremely important to question such patients about depressed mood, feelings of hopelessness, worthlessness, and ideas of suicide. The patient with depression is likely to give positive answers to these queries, unlike the patient with uncomplicated anxiety. Furthermore, the depressed patient is apt to be distinguished by a history of appetite loss, weight loss, sleep disturbance, and loss of sex drive.

Failure to elicit the history of major depressive symptoms may lead to inappropriate treatment of agitated depression by prescription, for example, of minor tranquilizers. Such treatment, at best, does not address the depressive disorder. At worst it may exacerbate the depression.

The *manic patient* is likely to present in an excited, anxious state; yet ancillary symptoms are usually so pronounced as to preclude the diagnosis of uncomplicated anxiety.[119] The manic patient's mood is notably elevated, at times frankly euphoric, and is apt to lapse into periods of irritability. Physical activity is increased and may become frantic; simultaneously there is a diminished need for sleep. The rate of speech is increased, and the patient's train of thought may fly off on tangents. Hallucinations and delusions may be present. Most commonly these fit the grandiose, expansive feelings enjoyed by the manic patient. Given this pervasive range of symptoms it is not surprising that the manic patient often exercises poor judgment, and a history of ill-conceived business or interpersonal decisions is common.

Anxiety is a marked component of the *schizophrenic disorders* . Indeed, it is here that the pain of anxiety may be felt at the most profound levels possible. A commonly held psychodynamic view is that the schizophrenic's sense of self is so nebulous that he feels at risk of losing that self, of literally being swallowed up by anyone allowed to come close. Such fears of incorporation or annihilation are, of course, accompanied by intense anxiety.

Schizophrenic anxiety is qualitatively as well as quantitatively different from the nonpsychotic anxiety discussed above. Its most distinctive feature is its inextricable relationship to psychotic thinking. The schizophrenic patient commonly suffers from frightening delusions. These are unshakable beliefs involving mind control, persecutory plots, or other frightening notions. While usually patently illogical to the clinician, these beliefs are rigidly held by the patient.

Hallucinations are also commonly experienced by the schizophrenic patient and are an understandable source of anxiety. Also central to this diagnosis is a disturbance of thinking marked by bizarreness, illogic, and by a train of thought that cannot be followed by the nonpsychotic observer (looseness of associations). At times the patient may experience abrupt cessation of a train of thought (thought blocking).

The schizophrenic patient suffers deterioration in his level of function.[120] Also central to the diagnosis is a certain degree of chronicity. The newer nosology requires at least 6 months of continuously active illness for the diagnosis of schizophrenia to be made.

It is beyond the scope of this chapter to discuss in detail a putative spectrum of schizophrenic illness (see chapter 3). Brief mention is made, however, because anxiety may figure prominently in all these disorders. *Schizophreniform disorder* is distinguished entirely by the duration of psychotic disturbance (less than 6 months).[121] *Paranoid disorders* are marked by the presence of delusions of jealousy or persecution in an otherwise unremarkable mental state.[122] Conspicuously absent is the bizzareness of behavior and thought of the schizophrenic. *Brief reactive psychosis* is a disorder, lasting no more than 2 weeks, occurring in response to overwhelming stress.[123] Associated psychotic symptoms may include delusions, hallucinations, and disordered thought that is indistinguishable from that of the schizophrenic. Central to this diagnosis is the patient's full return to the premorbid level of function.

SUMMARY

Anxiety is so common as to be virtually a daily part of life. On the other hand, it may be symptomatic of a broad range of physical and psychological disturbances. Careful attention to the patient's history as well as to physical and laboratory findings may be necessary for proper diagnosis of this protean symptom. As with other nonspecific symptoms, sheer passage of time may be required for the emergence of a correct diagnosis.

REFERENCES

1. Walker JI: Viet Nam combat veterans with legal difficulties: a psychiatric problem? *Am J Psychiatry* 1981;138:1384-1385.
2. Delgado-Escueta AV,Mattson RH, King L, et al: The nature of aggression during epileptic seizures. *N Engl J Med* 1981;305:711-716.
3. Bear D, Arana G: Nonfunctional disorders of emotion. *Neurol Neurosurg Weekly Update* 1978;1:2-7.
4. Waites TF: Hyperventilation: chronic and acute. *Arch Intern Med* 1978;138:1700-1701.
5. Freud S, in Strachey (ed): *Inhibitions, Symptoms, and Anxiety.* New York, WW Norton, 1959.
6. Hoehn-Saric R: Neurotransmitters in anxiety. *Arch Gen Psychiatry* 1982;39:735-742.
7. Redmond DE: New and old evidence for the involvement of a brain norepinephrine system in anxiety, in Fann WE, Karacan AD, Pokorny AD, et al (eds): *Phenomenology and Treatment of Anxiety* . New York, Spectrum, 1979, pp 153-203.
8. Mohler H, Okada T: Benzodiazepine receptor: demonstration in the central nervous system. *Science* 1977;198:849-851.
9. Braestrup C, Nielsen M: Neurotransmitters and CNS disease. *Lancet* 1982; 2:1030-1034.
10. Braestrup C, Squires R: Specific benzodiazepine receptors in rat brain characterized by high-affinity H-diazepam binding. *Proc Natl Acad Sci USA* 1977;74:3805-3809.
11. Gavish M, Snyder SH: Gamma aminobutyric acid and benzodiazepine receptors. *Proc Natl Acad Sci USA* 1981;78:1939-1942.
12. Snyder SH, Enna SJ, Young AB: Brain mechanisms associated with therapeutic actions of benzodiazepines: focus on neurotransmitters. *Am J Psychiatry* 1977;134:662-664.

13. Enna SJ: GABA pharmacology and neuropsychiatric illness, in Hales RE, Frances AJ (eds): *American Psychiatric Association, Annual Review* , Washington, American Psychiatric Press, 1985, vol 4.
14. Snyder SH, Sklar P: Behavioral and molecular actions of caffeine: focus on adenosine. *J Psychiatr Res* 1984;18(2):41-106.
15. Pitts FN, McClure JN: Lactate metabolism in anxiety neuroses. *N Engl J Med* 1967;277:1328-1336.
16. Kelly D, Mitchell-Heggs N, Sherman D: Anxiety and the effects of sodium lactate assessed clinically and physiologically. *Br J Psychiatry* 1971;119:129-141.
17. Liebowitz MR, Klein DF: Assessment and treatment of phobic anxiety. *J Clin Psychiatry* 1979;40:486-492.
18. Pitts FN: Personal communication, reported in Liebowitz MR, Klein DF: Assessment and treatment of phobic anxiety. *J Clin Psychiatry* 1979;40:486-492.
19. Crowe RR, Pauls DL, Slymen DJ, et al: A family study of anxiety neurosis. *Arch Gen Psychiatry* 1980;37:77-79.
20. Pauls DL, Bucher KD, Crowe RR, et al: A genetic study of panic disorder pedigrees. *Am J Hum Genet* 1980;32:639-644.
21. Dealy RS, Ishiki DM, Avery DH, et al: Secondary depression in anxiety disorders. *Compr Psychiatry* 1981;22:612-618.
22. Clancy J, Noyes R, Hoenk PR, et al: Secondary depression in anxiety neurosis. *J Nerv Ment Dis* 1978;166:846-850.
23. Surman OS, Sheehan DV, Fuller TC, et al: Panic disorder in genotypic HLA identical sibling pairs. *Am J Psychiatry* 1983;140:237-238.
24. Weiner MF: Other psychodynamic schools, in Kaplan HI, Sadock BJ (eds): *Comprehensive Textbook of Psychiatry*, ed 4. Baltimore, Williams & Wilkins Co, 1985, pp 452-453.
25. American Psychiatric Association: *Diagnostic and Statistical Manual of Mental Disorders,* ed 3. [DSM-III] Washington, American Psychiatric Association, 1980, p 231.
26. Liebowitz M, Klein DF: Differential diagnosis and treatment of panic attacks and phobic states. *Annu Rev Med* 1981;32:583-599.
27. Meissner WN: Theories of personality and psychopathology: psychoanalysis, in Kaplan HI, Sadock BJ (eds): *Comprehensive Textbook of Psychiatry,* ed 4. Baltimore, Williams & Wilkins Co. 1985, p 361.
28. Coakley D, Woodford-Williams E: Effects of burglary and vandalism on the health of old people. *Lancet* 1979;2:1066-1067.
29. American Psychiatric Association: *Diagnostic and Statistical Manual of Mental Disorders*, ed 3. Washington, American Psychiatric Association, 1980, p 236.
30. Lown B, Femte JV, Reich P, et al: Basis for recurring ventricular fibrillation in the absence of coronary artery disease and its management. *N Engl J Med* 1976;294:623-629.
31. Lown B, DeSilva RA, Reich P, et al: Psychological factors in sudden cardiac death. *Am J Psychiatry* 1980;137:1325-1335.

32. Cannon WB: Voodoo death. *Psychosom Med* 1957;19:182.
33. Jones IH, Robinson I: Severe illness with anxiety following a reputed magical act on an Australian aboriginal. *Med J Aust* 1977;2:93-96.
34. Weiner N, in Gilman AG, Goodman LS, Rall TW, et al: *The Pharmacological Basis of Therapeutics*, ed 7. New York, MacMillan, 1985, pp 145-180.
35. Rall TW, in Gilman AG, Goodman LS, Rall TW, Murad F: *The Pharmacological Basis of Therapeutics*, ed 7. New York, Macmillan Publishing Co, Inc, 1985, p 590.
36. Drugs that cause psychiatric symptoms. *Med Lett Drugs Ther* 1981;23:9-12.
37. White B, Lincoln CA, Pearce NW, et al: Anxiety and muscle tension as consequences of caffeine withdrawal. *Science* 1980;209:1547-1548.
38. Dietch JT: Diagnosis of organic anxiety disorders. *Psychosomatics* 1981;22:661-669.
39. Kwok RHM: Chinese restaurant syndrome. *N Engl J Med* 1968;278:796.
40. Allen D, Baker G: Chinese restaurant asthma. *N Engl J Med* 1981;305:1154.
41. Jaffe JH: Drug addiction and drug abuse, in Gilman AG, Goodman LS, Rall TW, et al: *The Pharmacological Basis of Therapeutics*, ed 7. New York, Macmillan Publishing Co, Inc, 1985, p 555.
42. Friedman PA: Poisoning and its management, in Petersdorf RG, Adams RD, Braunwald E, et al (eds): *Harrison's Principles of Internal Medicine*, ed 10. New York, McGraw-Hill Book Co, 1983, p 1270.
43. Benzodiazepine withdrawal. *Lancet* 1979;1:196.
44. Gallant DM, Edwards GC, Bishop MP: Withdrawal symptoms of antipsychotic compounds: clinical confirmation in chronic schizophrenics. *Am J Psychiatry* 1964;121:491-493.
45. Chouinard G, Jones BD, Annable L: Neuroleptic induced supersensitivity psychosis. *Am J Psychiatry* 1978;135:1409-1410.
46. Klett JC, Caffey EM: Evaluating the long-term need for anti-parkinsonian drugs by chronic schizophrenics. *Arch Gen Psychiatry* 1972;26:374-379.
47. Manos N, Gklouzepas J, Logothetis J: The need for continuous use of antiparkinsonian indication with chronic schizophrenic patients receiving long-term neuroleptic therapy. *Am J Psychiatry* 1981;138(2):184-188.
48. Coffman JA, Petty F: Plasma GABA levels in chronic alcoholics. *Am J Psychiatry* 1985;142:1204-1205.
49. Grinspoon L, Bakalar JB: Drug dependence: nonnarcotic agents, in Kaplan HI, Sadock BJ (eds): *Comprehensive Textbook of Psychiatry*, ed 4. Baltimore, Williams & Wilkins Co, 1985, pp 1003-1015.
50. Rosen A: Case report: symptomatic mania and phencyclidine abuse. *Am J Psychiatry* 1979;136:118-119.

51. Linn L: Other psychiatric emergencies, in Kaplan HI, Sadock BJ (eds): *Comprehensive Textbook of Psychiatry*, ed 4. Baltimore, Williams & Wilkins Co, 1985, p 1325.
52. Walker JI: The anxious patient. *J Fam Pract* 1981;12:733-738.
53. Davis J, Nasr S, Spina N, et al: Anxiety: differential diagnosis and treatment from a biologic perspective. *J Clin Psychiatry* 1981;42:4-14.
54. MacKenzie TB, Popkin MK: Organic anxiety syndrome. *Am J Psychiatry* 1983;140:342-344.
55. Levene OL: Chest pain: prophet of doom or nagging neurosis? *Acta Med Scand (Suppl)* 1981;644:11-13.
56. Pariser S, Pinta ER, Jones BA: Mitral valve prolapse syndrome and anxiety neurosis/panic disorder. *Am J Psychiatry* 1978;135:246-247.
57. Crowe RR, Pauls DL, Venkatesh A, et al: Exercise and anxiety neurosis: comparison of patients, with and without mitral valve prolapse. *Arch Gen Psychiatry* 1979;36:652-653.
58. Mehta D, Mehta S: Psychiatric symptoms and mitral valve prolapse syndrome, letter. *Am J Psychiatry* 1978;135:1001-1002.
59. Catron DO, Hodgetts PG: The hyperdynamic beta adrenergic state: a case report. *J Fam Pract* 1977;5:660-661.
60. Gorlin R: The hyperkinetic heart syndrome. *JAMA* 1962;182:823-829.
61. Wharton RN: Atrial myxoma masquerade. *Am J Psychiatry* 1977;134:1441-1442.
62. Arnaud CD: The parathyroid glands, hypercalcemia, and hypocalcemia, in Wyngaarden JB, Smith LH (eds): *Cecil Textbook of Medicine*, ed 17. Philadelphia, WB Saunders Co, 1985, pp 1443-1444.
63. Cryer PE: The adrenal medulla and the sympathetic nervous system, in Wyngaarden JB, Smith LH (eds): *Cecil Textbook of Medicine*, ed 17. Philadelphia, WB Saunders Co, 1985, p 1410.
64. Cryer PE: The carcinoid syndrome, in Wyngaarden JB, Smith LH (eds): *Cecil Textbook of Medicine*, ed 17. Philadelphia, WB Saunders Co, 1985, p 1413-1414.
65. Stein M, Schiavi RC, Camerino M: Influence of brain and behavior on the immune system. *Science* 1976;191:435-440.
66. Pandol SJ, Korman LY, McCarthy DM, et al: Beneficial effect of oral lithium carbonate in the treatment of pancreatic cholera syndrome. *N Engl J Med* 1980;302:1403-1404.
67. Bisno AL: Rheumatic fever, in Wyngaarden JB, Smith LH (eds): *Cecil Textbook of Medicine*, ed 17. Philadelphia, WB Saunders Co, 1985, pp 1529-1530.
68. Scharschmidt BF: Acute and chronic hepatic failure with encephalopathy, in Wyngaarden JB, Smith LH (eds): *Cecil Textbook of Medicine*, ed 17. Philadelphia, WB Saunders Co, 1985, p 846.
69. Storey P: The excited patient. *Practitioner* 1978;230:217-220.
70. Walker JT: The anxious patient. *J Fam Pract* 1981;12:733-738.

71. Andreoli TE: Disorders of fluid volume, electrolyte and acid-base balance, in Wyngaarden JB, Smith LH (eds): *Cecil Textbook of Medicine*, ed 17. Philadelphia, WB Saunders Co, 1985, p 533.

72. Bissell DM: Porphyria, in Wyngaarden JB, Smith LH (eds): *Cecil Textbook of Medicine*, ed 17. Philadelphia, WB Saunders Co, 1985, p 1156.

73. Herman BP: Interictal psychopathology in patients with ictal fear: a quantitative investigation. *Neurology* 1982;32:7-11.

74. Bear D, Arana G: Nonfunctional disorders of emotion. *Neurol Neurosurg Weekly Update* 1978;1:2-7.

75. Slater E, Beard AW, Glithero E: The schizophrenia-like psychosis of epilepsy. *Br J Psychiatry* 1963;109:95.

76. Mohr JP: Transient ischemic attacks, in Rowland LP (ed): *Merritt's Textbook of Neurology*, ed 7. Philadelphia, Lea & Febiger, 1984, p 160.

77. Steinberg AD: Systemic lupus erythematosus, in Wyngaarden JB, Smith LH (eds): *Cecil Textbook of Medicine*, ed 17. Philadelphia, WB Saunders Co, 1985, p 1929.

78. Brust JCM: Subarachnoid hemorrhage, in Rowland LP (ed): *A Textbook of Neurology*, ed 7. Philadelphia, Lea & Febiger, 1984, pp 185-188.

79. Solomon S: Clinical neurology and neuropathology, in Kaplan HI, Sadock BJ (eds): *Comprehensive Textbook of Psychiatry*, ed 4. Baltimore, Williams & Wilkins Co, 1985, pp 452-453.

80. Solomon S: Application of neurology to psychiatry, in Kaplan HI, Sadock BJ (eds): *Comprehensive Textbook of Psychiatry*, ed 4. Baltimore, Williams & Wilkins Co, 1985, pp 149-150.

81. Rivlin RS: Disorders of vitamin metabolism, in Wyngaarden JB, Smith LH: *Cecil Textbook of Medicine*, ed 17. Philadelphia, WB Saunders Co, 1985, pp 1201-1202.

82. Emery EJ, Szymanski HV: Psychological symptoms preceding diagnosed myasthenia gravis. *Psychosomatics* 1981;22:993-995.

83. Tourian A: Wilson's disease, in Wyngaarden JB, Smith LH: *Cecil Textbook of Medicine*, ed 17. Philadelphia, WB Saunders Co, 1985, p 1159.

84. Rao SV, Greene CA, Ellinoff V: Recurrent abdominal colic as the sole symptom of Wilson's disease: case report. *Milit Med* 1981;146:584-585.

85. Peterson GC: Organic mental disorders induced by drugs or poisons, in Kaplan HI, Freedman AM, Sadock BJ (eds): *Comprehensive Textbook of Psychiatry*, ed 3. Baltimore, Williams & Wilkins Co, 1980, pp 1437-1451.

86. Osler W: Doctor and nurse, from *Aequanimitas and Other Addresses*, ed 2. Philadelphia, Blakiston, 1925, p 15.

87. Osler W: Nurse and patient, from *Aquenamitas and Other Addresses*, ed 2. Philadelphia, Blakiston, 1925, p 155.

88. Deutsch H: Some psychoanalytic observations in surgery. *Psychosom Med* 1942;4:105.

89. Hackett TP, Cassem NH, Wishnic HA: The coronary care unit: an appraisal of psychological hazards. *N Engl J Med* 1968;279:1365.

90. Cay EL, Vetter N, Philip AE, et al: Psychological reactions to a coronary care unit. *J Psychosom Res* 1972;16:437.

91. Vetter NJ, Cay EL, Philip AE, et al: Anxiety on admission to a coronary care unit. *J Psychosom Res* 1977;21:73-78.

92. Lansky S, Gendel M: Symbiotic regressive behavior patterns in childhood malignancy. *Clin Pediatr* 1978;17:133-138.

93. Janis IL: *Psychological Stress: Psychoanalytic and Behavioral Studies of Surgical Patients.* New York, John Wiley & Sons, Inc, 1959.

94. Goble REA, Gowers JI, Morgan DC, et al: Artificial pacemaker patients treatment outcome and IPAT anxiety scale. *J Psychosom Res* 1978;22:177-182.

95. Titchener JL: Psychiatry and surgery, in *Comprehensive Textbook of Psychiatry*, ed 1. Baltimore, Williams & Wilkins Co, 1967, pp 1131-1134.

96. Morse RM, Litin EM: Postoperative delirium: a study of etiologic factors. *Am J Psychiatry* 1969;126:388.

97. Weisman AD, Hackett TP: Psychosis after eye surgery: establishment of specific doctor-patient relationship in prevention and treatment of "black patch" delirium. *N Engl J Med* 1958;258:1284.

98. Blachly PH, Star A: A post-cardiotomy delirium. *Am J Psychiatry* 1964;121:371.

99. Peterson GC: Organic mental disorders associated with brain trauma, in Kaplan HI, Freedman AM, Sadock BJ (eds): *Comprehensive Textbook of Psychiatry*, ed 3. Baltimore, Williams & Wilkins Co, 1980, pp 1430-1431.

100. Goldstein K: The effect of brain damage on personality. *Psychiatry* 1952;15:245.

101. Lishman WA: Brain damage in relation to psychiatric disability after head injury. *Br J Psychiatry* 1968;114:377.

102. Sheehan DV: Panic attacks and phobias. *N Engl J Med* 1982;307:156-158.

103. Liebowitz MR, Klein DF: Assessment and treatment of phobic anxiety. *J Clin Psychiatry* 1979;40:486-492.

104. American Psychiatric Association: *Diagnostic and Statistical Manual of Mental Disorders*, ed 3. Washington, American Psychiatric Association, 1980, pp 232-233.

105. American Psychiatric Association: Diagnostic and Statistical Manual of Mental Disorders, ed 3. Washington, American Psychiatric Association, 1980, pp 299-301.

106. American Psychiatric Association: *Diagnostic and Statistical Manual of Mental Disorders*, ed 3. Washington, American Psychiatric Association, 1980, pp 225-230.

107. American Psychiatric Association: *Diagnostic and Statistical Manual of Mental Disorders*, ed 3. Washington, American Psychiatric Association, 1980, pp 226-227.
108. American Psychiatric Association: *Diagnostic and Statistical Manual of Mental Disorders*, ed 3. Washington, American Psychiatric Association, 1980, pp 227-228.
109. American Psychiatric Association: *Diagnostic and Statistical Manual of Mental Disorders*, ed 3. Washington, American Psychiatric Association, 1980, pp 228-230.
110. American Psychiatric Association: *Diagnostic and Statistical Manual of Mental Disorders*, ed 3. Washington, American Psychiatric Association, 1980, pp 234-235.
111. Blacker KH, Levitt M: The differential diagnosis of obsessive-compulsive symptoms. *Compr Psychiatry* 1979;20(6):532-546.
112. Pies R: Distinguishing obsessional from psychotic phenomena. *J Clin Psychopharmacol* 1984;4:345-347.
113. American Psychiatric Association: *Diagnostic and Statistical Manual of Mental Disorders*, ed 3. Washington, American Psychiatric Association, 1980, pp 241-244.
114. American Psychiatric Association: *Diagnostic and Statistical Manual of Mental Disorders*, ed 3. Washington, American Psychiatric Association, 1980, pp 247-249.
115. American Psychiatric Association: *Diagnostic and Statistical Manual of Mental Disorders*, ed 3. Washington, American Psychiatric Association, 1980, pp 249-251.
116. American Psychiatric Association: *Diagnostic and Statistical Manual of Mental Disorders*, ed 3. Washington, American Psychiatric Association, 1980, pp 244-247.
117. American Psychiatric Association: *Diagnostic and Statistical Manual of Mental Disorders*, ed 3. Washington, American Psychiatric Association, pp 259-260.
118. Hamilton M: The clinical distinction between anxiety and depression. *Br J Pharmacol* 1983;15:165s-169s.
119. American Psychiatric Association: *Diagnostic and Statistical Manual of Mental Disorders*, ed 3. Washington, American Psychiatric Association, pp 206-210.
120. American Psychiatric Association: *Diagnostic and Statistical Manual of Mental Disorders*, ed 3. Washington, American Psychiatric Association, p 189.
121. American Psychiatric Association: *Diagnostic and Statistical Manual of Mental Disorders*, ed 3. Washington, American Psychiatric Association, pp 199-200.
122. American Psychiatric Association: *Diagnostic and Statistical Manual of Mental Disorders*, ed 3. Washington, American Psychiatric Association, pp 195-198.
123. American Psychiatric Association: *Diagnostic and Statistical Manual of Mental Disorders*, ed 3. Washington, American Psychiatric Association, pp 200-202.

2 Depression

George N. McNeil

DEPRESSION A condition characterized by despondency and self-condemnation and, in the extreme, by disturbance in somatic functions such as sleep and appetite.

Depression may best be viewed as a spectrum. At its most benign it has come to describe a normal part of the human experience. At the other extreme it is an incapacitating disease warranting prompt medical attention.

FEATURES

Case report A 50-year-old married father of three was self-referred for "pressures over the last year." He related a number of misfortunes that had befallen his adult daughters and described a deepening sense of despair over his family's troubles. He had recently sold his home and already felt regret over this.

Further history showed sleep disturbance with awakening at 3 to 4 AM, poor appetite with loss of 10 lbs, and markedly decreased sex drive. He also noted diurnal variation in mood with mornings being most difficult. Suicide had occurred to him.

Mood

As might be expected, mood disturbance is a signal feature of depression, with a prevalence of 90% in depressed patients.[1] Sadness is most often described, although feelings of anger and guilt are commonly seen.

Affected patients are apt to relate feeling "blue," "down in the dumps," or given the growing public awareness of the disorder "depressed."

Frequently, anxiety is a concomitant to the depressed state, and in some cases the anxious or agitated mood dominates the clinical picture. Since it has major treatment implications the distinction between primary anxiety and depression is extremely important (see below).

Some depressed patients present without obvious disturbance of mood (a perplexing state of depression *sine* depression!) Common "depressive equivalents" seen in such cases are vague somatic complaints such as fatigue or ill-defined pain.

Thought

A general slowing of thought production is most characteristic of depression. This is often coupled with a slowing of physical activity yielding the descriptive term "psychomotor retardation." This slowing is usually quite apparent in the diagnostic interview where the patient's flow of speech is halting and at times painfully slow.

Some depressed patients do not manifest psychomotor retardation but show ample evidence of their disorder in the area of thought *content*. Ideas of self-reproach are virtually a *sine qua non* of depression (and serve to distinguish depressive disorders from *normal grief*, wherein self-esteem is largely unaltered). The patient described in the case above not only felt blameworthy for his troubles, he resisted supportive attempts to lighten his burden of guilt.

Hand in hand with feelings of "badness" and worthlessness, one often encounters hopelessness. The depressed patient may truly believe that it is his lot never to recover from his benighted state. In this setting it is not difficult to understand the emergence of ruminative thoughts about suicide, which the patient may see as the only solution to his dismal condition. Rumination about harming others, often loved ones, may also plague the depressed patient and serves as a further source of guilt.

Frankly psychotic thought marks some cases of major depression. Delusions that are "mood congruent" are fairly easily understood in the content of the illness. These delusions are often somatic and involve notions such as "my insides are rotting." More bizarre, less congruent delusions may also be seen and may raise difficulty in distinguishing major depression from other psychotic disorders such as schizophrenia.

Behavior

The patient with psychomotor retardation may be at pains to perform the simplest tasks. Job performance almost invariably suffers, and even basic self-care may become onerous. Family and friends usually note the reduction of activity and can help to document a decline in personal hygiene.

Paradoxically, depression may also be associated with agitated behavior. Pacing, hand wringing and frequent sighing may readily lead to the mistaken diagnosis of primary anxiety.

Close observers usually note progressive withdrawal on the part of the depressed patient. Feeling worthless at his core the patient often feels unworthy of human contact and may set out on an ominous course of alienation from human support (a course that may well culminate in suicide.)

The depressed patient's withdrawal may be facilitated by testiness, demanding behavior, or frank outbursts of anger. Even without these added noxious influences, the very state of depression has an enervating influence upon relationships. Even the physician who sees the patient but briefly can usually attest to this.

Sleep disturbance is a very common manifestation of depression. Patients most often complain of difficulty falling asleep or of early awakening. However, excessive sleep (hypersomnia) may also be reported.

Loss of appetite and poor eating are very commonly seen, as is associated weight loss. Less typically, overeating may be seen. A distinct lack of pleasure in such overeating characterizes the depressed patient. Indeed, guilt over weight gain may compound the depression.

Loss of sex drive (libido) often results in marked diminution of sexual activity. This information is often not volunteered by the patient, underscoring the importance of the physician's obtaining a sexual history.

For some depressed patients, pain or other somatic complaints are the major manifestation of the mood disorder. Such patients clearly pose a major diagnostic challenge to the physician. Blumer and Heilbronn have summarized an extensive clinical experience with patients suffering from chronic pain of obscure origin ("pain-prone disorder").[2] They point out that complaints of somatic pain "tend to be ubiquitous" in depressed patients. They argue further that chronic pain may mask clinical depression and may be seen in that light as an unconscious defense against depressed mood. The pain-prone patient, they say, is characterized by prominent guilt, by masochistic tendencies including avoidance of success, by unfulfilled strong aggressive drives, and by emergence of pain at the time of loss or threatened loss.

The same authors go on to describe the potentially harmful bond that the pain-prone patient may make with physicians. Such patients look to surgery and to medical intervention for cure and may suffer needless invasive procedures and escalating mutual frustration with their doctors. Analgesic abuse may also occur. While this tends to be a chronic disorder, most responsive to an ongoing relationship with a physician determined to "first, do no harm," the authors argue that some patients respond favorably to therapeutic doses of antidepressants.

Other somatic symptoms may also indicate underlying depression. While there is a burden of proof to rule out "organic" causes for vague physical complaints, depression should be considered in the face of ill-defined gastrointestinal (GI) complaints, fatigue, sexual dysfunction, shortness of breath, etc.[3-5]

Suicide is clearly the most serious behavioral correlate of depression. This is a symptom of such import that it will be dealt with in its own right (see chapter 10). In brief, it may be seen as a by-product of the hopelessness, despair, and alienation of the depressed patient. Given the impact of suicide upon those close to the patient, the act may also be seen as a product of profound anger.

The close association between suicide and depressive disorders mandates that the physician ask the depressed patient about suicidal thoughts (which are very common) or plans (less common). It is crucial for both doctor and patient to know that the suicidal state is ephemeral and that brief psychiatric hospitalization may be life-saving.

The depressed patient may behave in self-destructive ways considerably more subtle than attempting suicide. The patient described at the beginning of the chapter sold a home very dear to him before coming for treatment. After successful treatment of his depression he regretted this decision and could make no sense of it except as an unconscious means of punishing himself. Another patient abruptly gave up his job as a top executive for a thriving company. When his depression cleared he deeply regretted this, finding that his post had been filled and was no longer available to him.

If one recalls that the depressed patient typically feels deserving of punishment, then this pursuit of life at a lower level begins to make perverse sense. The phenomenon has perhaps been best described in the person of Herman Melville's Ishmael: "Whenever I find myself growing grim about the mouth; whenever it is a damp, drizzly November in my soul; whenever I find myself involuntarily pausing before coffin warehouses, and bringing up the rear of every funeral I meet; and especially whenever my hypos [hypochondria, which Melville insightfully links with the depressed state], get such an upper hand on me, that it requires a strong moral principle to prevent me from deliberately stepping into the street, and methodically knocking people's hats off [note the link between melancholy and anger], then, I account it high time to get to sea as soon as I can. This is my substitute for pistol and ball. With a philosophic flourish Cato throws himself upon his sword; I quietly take to the ship."[6]

This sort of *forme fruste* suicidal behavior also demands an active role of the physician. The patient should be warned against making major decisions while depressed, in the knowledge that such decisions often unwittingly court disaster. If such decisions must be made they should be made only after scrutiny by patient *and* physician. (In cases of complex legal or financial matters, obviously other expert opinion should be sought.) It can be argued that this sort of activity violates the highly sensible premise that doctors should avoid running their patients' lives. We believe such violation to be justifiable if it serves the end of preventing or attenuating suffering.

Physical Examination and Laboratory Findings

The depressed patient often *appears* depressed: worn, haggard, disheveled. His gaze is often downcast and his posture slumped. Personal hygiene often is neglected. Motor activity may be slowed.

In the agitated or apprehensive patient, autonomic activity may be altered, and dryness of mucous membranes, tachycardia, labile elevation of blood pressure, and moist palms may be noted.

Up to 90% of depressed patients exhibit weight loss.[7] This may at times be profound and its course quite fulminant. The appearance of such patients often (appropriately) prompts an investigation into the possibility of occult malignancy or other chronic disease.

Physical findings will be discussed in more detail in the section on differential diagnosis.

Until recently the laboratory assessment of depression was limited for all practical purposes to the administration of psychological tests. Despite newer developments in neurochemistry, such tests maintain an important place in the diagnosis of depression. Significant elevation of the two scales on the Minnesota Multiphasic Personality Inventory (MMPI) lends support to this diagnosis. The Hamilton Depression Scale is a widely used instrument for "quantifying" depression. Similarly, the Zung Self-Rating Depression Scale is designed to assess the degree of clinical depression. The Zung Scale has the advantage of being a self-administered test.

Best documented of the neurohumoral abnormalities seen in depression is the escape from normal control of adrenal cortisol secretion.[8-10] Not only are some depressed patients hypersecreters of cortisol, but they fail to suppress this hypersecretion after dexamethasone administration (Dexamethasone, a powerful glucocorticoid, normally causes feedback inhibition of the hypothalamic-pituitary-adrenal axis. Failure of this inhibition is classically seen in autonomously functioning adrenal neoplasms.)

Carroll et al initially suggested high specificity (on the order of 95%) of a positive dexamethasone suppression test (DST) in the diagnosis of major depression.[11] More recently, others have demonstrated nonsuppression in a broad array of psychiatric disorders and have thus questioned the test's utility.[12] It has been suggested that early papers that supported the use of DST had flawed methodology.[13] In truth, the abnormal DST may reflect factors as nonspecific as the level of stress affecting the patient. Perhaps the most sanguine view of the DST that seems reasonable at present is that of Kolsis et al.[14] Noting that the test's specificity is a matter of controversy these workers focused on the sensitivity of the test in a group of 132 hospitalized, depressed patients. They noted that a positive test identifies a subgroup of depressed patients. These patients tend to be anxious, to have disturbances in sleep and psychomotor function, to have recent weight loss, and to be older. We feel that, taken in the aggregate, the literature does not support routine clinical use of the DST.

In 1972, Prange et al described another endocrine "marker" in major depression.[15] They noted that some depressed patients had a blunted pituitary response (lower than expected levels of thyroid-stimulating hormone TSH) to the hypothalamic thyrotropin-releasing hormone (TRH). Here again, test sensitivity has been shown to approximate only 50%. It has been suggested, however, that the *combined* yield of the dexamethasone suppression test and the TRH test may approach 90%.[16]

Inasmuch as thyroid function, like adrenal function, may be influenced by factors as diverse and nonspecific as surgery, acute or chronic medical illness, and other stresses, it seems prudent to reserve judgment about TRH testing. We certainly do not advocate its routine use in diagnosing depression. Of even less certain significance are findings that major depression may be associated with a blunted growth hormone response to insulin or to an amphetamine.[17] Experience with this test is insufficient to predict its future clinical relevance.

Considerable interest has also been generated by the laboratory assay of neurotransmitters and their metabolites. This will be discussed further below.

Interviewer's Reaction

Insofar as the physician is treated like other important people in the depressed patient's life, he finds himself the object of petulance and finds his ability to help sharply questioned. In the face of increasingly desperate demands to "do something," he finds his patience tested to the limits.

The depressed patient's hopeless, benighted view of his world tends to be infectious. The interviewer is apt to feel sapped and mildly depressed in turn.

It is hardly surprising that the interviewer would want to escape the pall of depression and the noxious force of angry demands. In escaping, however, he joins the company of others who have been alienated by the patient. He accedes to the patient's pathologic drive to isolate himself, and he helps to confirm the patient's sense of worthlessness.

The physician's wish to avoid the depressed patient may be enhanced by his own feelings of despair. If not experienced in treating depression he may share the patient's hopelessness about the condition. He may feel annoyed at what seems to represent weakness of will and may admonish the patient to "snap out of it" noting that he has "no reason to be depressed." Even the physician skilled in treating depression is apt to be annoyed at the patient's rejection of reassurance and insistent pessimism.

Aversion to the depressed patient is thus extremely common. Like other less-than-laudable feelings that physicians have toward their patients, this need not be harmful. It is important, however, that the physician recognize such feelings and control any resultant behavior. The risk of failing to do this is an unwitting collaboration with the patient's self-punitive drives. This may be seen, for example, in the prescription of large supplies of antidepressant drugs to the potentially suicidal patient with the careless instruction to "come back in 3 months." Such behavior is compounded when a missed follow-up appointment is met with relief, unalloyed by concern for the depressed patient's welfare.

In summary, interviewing and treating the depressed patient is arduous. It demands a display of hope that may belie the physician's doubts. It demands perseverance and close clinical follow-up when avoidance of the patient feels most desirable. It demands a certain imperviousness to the hostility of the patient (something made far easier by viewing the anger as a product of illness rather than a personal insult.)

PATHOGENESIS

Psychodynamic Explanation

Loss is central to the psychodynamics of depression. To the extent that loss is an inevitable part of the human condition, we all harbor to some degree the potential for depression.

From earliest infancy we suffer the pangs of loss. Mother's disappearance from view may be indistinguishable by the infant from her annihilation. Hence, her absence is likely to elicit wails of protest. Not surprisingly, this behavior is not unique to the human species. Most any animal, separated from parental protection and sustenance when these commodities are necessary for its survival, will create a hue and cry sufficient to attract parental attention. Such behavior is clearly adaptive to the survival of the species.

The response of the child to the sustained loss has been well studied by Spitz[18], Bowlby[19], and others, and a well-documented syndrome of childhood, or "anaclitic" depression, has emerged (anaclitic: literally, "no one to lean on"). Children deprived of a consistent parental figure proceed from the sort of protest described above to a period of despair. Here crying abates and gives way to quiet sadness. The child in a hospital or other institutional setting is more manageable in this state, but the implications of this are ominous.[20] The stage of despair in turn is followed by detachment. The detached child becomes absorbed in solipsistic activity (rocking, head-banging) and turns away from human contact. Return of a "lost" parent at this stage is likely to be met with apathy.

If childhood losses are sustained or repeated, then protest, despair, and detachment may become a *modus vivendi*, extending into adult life and forming the basis for lifelong depression. Early deprivation and detachment are also commonly cited as a template for adult psychopathy, a disorder marked by inability to form social ties and a lack of concern for anyone but the self.

In the adult, the cycle of protest, despair, and detachment does not have the pathogenic significance that it carries for children. Indeed, the three stages describe a normal process of bereavement or grieving. Eric Lindemann's work, done in the aftermath of the Coconut Grove nightclub fire, stands as a landmark in the study of bereavement.[21] Lindemann, and others since, noted angry protest in the face of loss. Such protest is commonly directed at physicians and others, while its unconscious origins most likely lie in a sense of abandonment and rage at the one dead. Angry protest usually gives way to (or alternates with) the tears and sadness (despair) commonly associated with grief. This state, in turn, is superseded by a giving up or detachment from the lost loved one. Detachment in this case is the normal, *non*-pathogenic product of loss; and it allows the bereaved adult to resume the business of life.

Freud's view on the pathogenesis of depression is set forth in *Mourning and Melancholia*, originally published in 1917.[22] Freud, too, noted the central role of loss in depression, but reasoned that *introjection* was critical to the development of the disorder. This process involves an unconscious assimilation of the lost object into the self, thereby mitigating the loss. By this process, for instance, a bereaved widow might assume some of the tastes and habits of her deceased husband. Freud reasoned that it was *ambivalence* toward this introject that led to the syndrome of depression. Whatever hostile or aggressive feelings might have been directed at the lost object in life, became directed at the self, which (through introjection) has subsumed the lost object. Indeed, this turning against the self of angry feelings and impulses characterizes the depressed state.

Freud's observations were conceived not in a vacuum but through careful observation of patients in psychoanalysis. Though ancient by the standards of medical science and though a bit cumbersome, his psychodynamic theory of depression continues to be validated in the analytically oriented treatment of depressed patients.

Biochemical Model

There is a considerable body of evidence supporting a major role for biogenic amines (principally norepinephrine [NE] and serotonin or 5-hydroxytryptamine (5-HT)) in the genesis of some depression. Evidence for such a role stems largely from the clinical response of depressed patients to antidepressant drugs and, conversely, by the production of depressed states by amine-depleting drugs such as reserpine.

The clinical picture that best lends itself to biochemical explanation is that of major depression with "biologic" symptoms (see discussion of psychiatric differential diagnosis below). Affected patients usually note disturbance in sleep, appetite, and other biologic functions. Frequently, a diurnal variation in mood (worse in the morning) is noted. Such patients have long been noted to be most responsive to treatment with monoamine oxidase inhibitors (MAOIs) or tricyclic antidepressants (TCAs).

Monoamine oxidase is a major enzyme responsible for the degradation of NE and 5-HT. A central effect of MAOIs is therefore the inhibition of the breakdown of these monoamines. Such inhibition allows the monoamines a "longer life" and an increased opportunity to act as neurotransmitters. This neurotransmitter activity is believed to be responsible for the maintenance of normal mood and for clinical improvement from depression.

Tricyclic antidepressants block the reuptake of monoamines into presynaptic neurons and thus enhance the presence of these amines in the synaptic cleft. This, too, affords the monoamines an increased chance of binding to postsynaptic receptors, fulfilling their role as neurotransmitters.

The response of depressed patients to MAOIs and TCAs is supportive but not conclusive evidence for the role of monoamines in depression. Considerable attention has been paid to the measurement of NE and 5-HT metabolites, which are felt to give at least a crude reflection of brain concentrations of the monoamines.

Most clinicians are familiar with vanillylmandelic acid (VMA), a major urinary metabolite of NE. Urinary VMA assay has long been used to detect the presence of a monoamine- secreting pheochromocytoma. The measurement of urinary VMA in depression, however, has not been found to be useful, since the preponderance of urinary VMA has its source in the *peripheral* autonomic nervous system. *Central* or brain NE metabolism seems best reflected in urinary 3-methoxy-4-hydroxyphenylglycol (MHPG). It has been estimated that 63% of urinary MHPG is derived from brain NE[23].

The principal, readily measurable by-product of 5-HT metabolism is 5-hydroxyindoleacetic acid (5-HIAA). This, too, is excreted in the urine; and its use in the study of depression is flawed (like that of VMA measurement) by the fact that urinary 5-HIAA reflects, primarily, peripheral serotonin turnover. (Urinary 5-HIAA assays are useful, for example, in the detection of carcinoid syndrome.) At present, the most accurate reflection of brain 5-HT turnover is in measurement of cerebrospinal fluid 5-HIAA. Since transport of 5-HIAA from blood to CSF is virtually nil, this measurement should be unaffected by peripheral serotonin. While some brain 5-HIAA is transported into the blood, this transport can be impeded by administration of probenecid. Thus CSF 5-HIAA measured after probenecid is given is felt to reflect best the state of brain 5-HT turnover.[24]

In its simplest form, the amine hypothesis of depression would predict that depressed patients would have low urinary MHPG levels and/or low CSF 5-HIAA levels. While some early work supported this construct,[25-30] ongoing research has yielded inconsistent, confusing data on monoamine metabolites in depression. This might discourage the clinician from obtaining metabolite levels as aids to diagnosis.

Monoamine *receptors* have also attracted considerable research interest. It has long been noted that β-adrenergic receptor blockers, such as propranolol hydrochloride, may induce a syndrome indistinguishable from major depression.[31] This side effect seems to be fairly specific to lipophilic β-blockers (drugs avid to brain tissue) and may be relieved by substituting a hydrophilic β-blocker.[32] These findings make a reasonable case for dysfunction of central (brain) β-receptors in this form of iatrogenic depression.

Does β-receptor dysfunction play a role in other depressive disorders? Pandey et al have suggested that it may.[33] They studied lymphocytes (a readily accessible source of β_2-receptors) of depressed patients, measuring cyclic AMP response to stimulation with isoproteronol (a β-receptor agonist). Their depressed patients showed a significantly blunted response when compared with schizophrenic patients and controls. Was this blunted response secondary to a deficiency of β- receptors? Was it secondary to endogenous blockade of β-receptors?[34] These questions are unanswered at present.

The availability of radiolabeled chemicals that bind specifically (are specific ligands) to receptor sites has enabled researchers to study the number and affinity of receptors in various tissues and to study the influence of disease states and/or drugs upon receptors.[35] Such studies have consistently shown that antidepressant treatment (be it with electroshock therapy, any of the antidepressant drugs, or by rapid eye movement [REM] sleep deprivation) results in a decrease in measurable cerebral β-receptors (downregulation).[36]

One suspects that the down-regulation of β-receptors resulting from antidepressant treatment is a by-product of increased synaptic norepinephrine. (Down-regulation of receptors seems to be a normal, homeostatic response to increases in ligand concentration.) This has been supported by ablation of noradrenergic neurons which project to the forebrain.[36] Such ablation negates the effect of antidepressant treatment upon β-receptors. A synergistic role for serotonin is suggested by the finding that ablation of the 5-HT system also prevents β-receptor down-regulation in response to antidepressants.[36]

The role of another monoamine receptor also bears mention. The α_2-adrenergic receptor is a presynaptic, inhibitory receptor, stimulation of which *inhibits* release of NE into the synaptic cleft. The antihypertensive drug clonidine hydrochloride is the best known α_2-agonist, and this drug has been implicated in the genesis of depressive symptoms. Conversely, many antidepressants produce down-regulation of α_2- receptors.[36] The question arises: Is there a state of nature tnat corresponds to this clonidine-induced depression? Garcia-Sevilla et al studying radioligand binding of an α_2-agonist to the platelets of depressed patients, found 21% more α_2-binding sites in depressed patients than in controls[37] Others have not yet been able to reproduce these findings.[38]

A useful adjunct to the theory that some depression may result from underactivity of NE and 5-HT is the theory that overactivity of *cholinergic* neurons may predispose to depression. McCarley has proposed a unitary hypothesis of sorts, taking into account not only adrenergic and cholin--ergic activity but observable changes in REM sleep in depression.[39] He notes that patients with major depression tend to have an earlier onset of REM sleep (decreased REM latency) and a higher density of REM activity. Both these abnormalities are reversed by successful treatment with tricyclic antidepressants. (Indeed, the normalization of REM sleep precedes clinical antidepressant response.)

McCarley goes on to note that REM sleep is subject to both adrenergic and cholinergic control. Adrenergic neurons arising in the locus ceruleus and raphe nuclei of the brainstem exert an inhibitory effect on REM sleep, just as their activity has a mitigating effect on depression. Cholinergic neurons of the pontine reticular activating system seem to *promote* REM sleep. Cholinergic blockers then would be expected to normalize REM sleep in depression and to have antidepressant properties in their own right. To summarize this hypothesis, depression might result from adrenergic underactivity, cholinergic overactivity, or a relative imbalance of both systems.

Clearly, the amine hypothesis is gaining in complexity as brain research grows. One additional current theory that bears mention is the "dysregulation hypothesis." As elegantly described by Siever and Davis, this postulates that depression results not from a quantitative deficiency in synaptic monoamines but from poorly coordinated, erratic firing of noradrenergic neurons.[40] In the words of the electrophysiologist, this results in a decrease in "signal-to-noise ratio" of neuronal firing. This hypothesis reconciles the conflicting data on MHPG and 5-HIAA levels mentioned earlier. It is also compatible with research data on the effects of biological rhythms on mood (see "Environment," below).

Genetics

While depression and related affective disturbances (eg, manic-depressive illness or bipolar affective illness) cluster in certain families, a clear, mendelian pattern of inheritance is lacking. It has been demonstrated that relatives of patients with bipolar or unipolar illness are more likely to suffer from bipolar or unipolar depression than are relatives of controls.

Of the affective disorders, bipolar illness seems to lend itself best to the genetic hypothesis and has been most extensively studied.[41] Kallmann's study of families of affected patients showed a concordance of 100% in his limited sample of monozygotic twins.[42] Dizygotic twins and siblings showed a 25.5% concordance. Other workers have suggested linkage of a manic-depressive gene to the X-chromosome loci for color blindness and the XG_a blood subtype.[43,44] The occasional father-son transmission of bipolar illness argues against X-linked inheritance; and others have postulated autosomal dominant inheritance of a gene with variable penetrance. Perhaps more plausible is a polygenic type of inheritance. Recent study of families affected by both unipolar and bipolar illness suggests that a gene linked to the histocompatibility (HLA) locus on chromosome 6 may contribute to affective disorder.[45]

Genetic clustering of unipolar depression is less striking than that of bipolar illness. Relatives of unipolar depressed patients carry a risk of unipolar illness two to five times that of the general population. (Relatives of bipolar patients have an 8- to tenfold increase in risk of developing bipolar illness.)[46]

Environment

The finding of family clusters of affective illness raises the question not only of genetic influence but the role of environment. The review of psychodynamic factors in depression underscores the importance of environment. There is copious clinical evidence suggesting that the child subject to sustained early losses or privation is at risk for depression. Early separation from parents and inconsistent foster home rearing might, for example, produce this risk. Similarly, exposure to consistent abuse or denigration by one or both parents provides a solid substrate for later depression. On the other hand, "good-enough" parenting, as described by Winnicott can be seen as a hedge against future depression.[47]

Adult losses may be seen as a major contributor to depression. In a study of depressed British women, Brown and Harris suggested that virtually all depression could be explained by psychosocial factors.[48] They noted, in particular, several "vulnerability factors" including "the absence of close ties or employment, the presence of three or more children under fourteen, and the loss of mother before the age of eleven."

Others have noted that major life changes (be they financial, personal, work, or health-related) may predispose toward depression.[49,50] While psychiatry is not particularly receptive to notions of luck or accident, it seems reasonable to wonder if depression might be the product of the "slings and arrows of outrageous fortune."[51] A classic example of this is found in the Old Testament account of Job. Through no apparent personal fault or unconscious conniving, Job was visited with serious reversals in health and material wealth and with major loss of social support. The scriptural account of Job's response has been said to be a classic description of major depression.[52]

One cannot be in the business of medicine without seeing numerous latter-day Jobs, though rarely is their fall from prominence as striking. Some patients seem destined either by personal limitation or by forces of society and nature never to escape adversity. But their depression is every bit as keenly felt. (It is the oppressed, depressed state of this large segment of humanity which seems to have spurred psychiatry onto the slippery path of social change.)

There are those who view depression as a normative response to a world full of absurdity, a world that defies meaningful existence. This view led Camus to comment that, "There is but one serious philosophic problem, and that is suicide. The principal task of man is to respond to life's apparent meaninglessness, despair, and its absurd quality,"[53] and may have had a role in his death at an early age in an automobile accident.

One need not share the view of the existentialist Camus to appreciate the role of environment in causing psychiatric morbidity. For example, the specific effects of burglary and vandalism upon elderly victims have been studied.[54] "Catastrophic effects," including anxiety, paranoia, and severe depression are described in these patients.

Indeed, the elderly are particularly vulnerable to situational or environmental shocks. They are most likely to have suffered interpersonal losses by death or migration of the ever-mobile family. They have invariably suffered some loss of physical strength and vitality. Often they have been extruded from the workplace, signaling a further loss of vitality. Too often, financial adversity clouds the picture as reliable income gives way to less substantial and less dependable support from the government. They are apt to be more vulnerable to the depredations of swindlers, robbers, and other noxious individuals. This concatenation of factors would seem to be closely related to much depression in the elderly and to the trend toward ever- increasing suicide rates with increasing age.

Environmental factors may also play a part in the striking difference between the prevalence of depression in men and women.[55] Women have typically been undervalued in Western society. In addition, they have generally been limited in work and other creative pursuits — activities that may serve to mitigate depression. Recent movement toward parity between the sexes might have a very positive effect here. Yet even this movement is associated with some depressive casualty: the woman who feels she must excel both in the traditional feminine role and the modern role of the woman in the workplace. The compromise necessary to fulfill these diverse functions may be a source of guilt and depression.

One additional environmental factor bears mention in discussing the pathogenesis of depression: *disruption of circadian rhythm* or the normal sleep cycle. It has been noted that the period of recovery from rapid transit through several time zones (jet lag) may be accompanied by significant depression.[56] Frequent, irregular awakening, such as that encountered by medical personnel, has been similarly implicated.[57] One wonders if the recovery from these environmental insults might not be associated with REM sleep rebound, which as noted earlier (see "Biochemical Model") is in turn associated with depression.

The short days and long nights of northern winters are associated in popular lore with depression. "Cabin fever" is an extremely common malady in these climes. Folk remedies vary from southern vacations to the more economical *spiritus frumenti* . While this phenomenon has received little serious scientific attention, one wonders about its bearing on the prodigious rate of alcohol consumption in states such as Maine and Alaska.

Lewy et al have shed some light on the possible role of circadian shifts in producing depression.[58] They reported a 63-year-old man with recurrent winter depressions, refractory to conventional treatment. The patient was exposed to levels of artificial light equivalent to daylight for periods that approximated summer norms. His striking clinical improvement was paralleled by a drop in measurable melatonin, suggesting an alteration in function of the light-responsive pineal gland. The precise mechanism for this man's depression, and its improvement, remains unclear; but the case lends support to the importance of biologic rhythms in the regulation of mood. More recently this phenomenon has been demonstrated in a series of 13 patients with seasonal affective disorder.[59]

DIFFERENTIAL DIAGNOSIS

Drugs

While most physicians are aware of the oft-repeated association between reserpine and depression, there are a host of other chemical agents that may induce depression; and iatrogenic depression may go unrecognized. In a retrospective chart review of patients diagnosed as depressed at a family practice clinic, Katerndahl noted that 43% of these patients were taking at least one drug associated with depression.[60] Table 2-1 lists drugs and toxins that have been reported as precipitants to depression.

The *antihypertensives* (reserpine, α-methyldopa, propranolol, prazosin hydrochloride, clonidine and guanethidine) vary in their specific mode of action but share a common antagonism of norepinephrine-mediated receptor function. Such antagonism is clearly desirable in the peripheral autonomic nervous system where it results in a decrease in vascular tone and a resultant drop in blood pressure. It would appear, however, that there is a parallel interference with *brain* norepinephrine activity that in some patients leads to clinical depression. This is dramatically demonstrated in the clinical improvement that often follows withdrawal of one of the offending drugs (or, in the case of propranolol, substitution of a related drug such as atenolol, which is much less avid to brain tissue).

Digitalis glycosides have been in use for centuries. Their salutary effect in some cases of dropsy (edema) was noted long before their effect on the heart was known. Today the various digitalis preparations (primarily digoxin and digitoxin) are used principally to increase myocardial contractility in congestive heart failure. A common secondary use is to decrease atrioventricular (A-V) nodal conduction (and thus decrease ventricular rate) in cases of atrial flutter or fibrillation. Many patients are prescribed these drugs chronically, and anecdotal reports of associated depression (usually mild) abound.[63] (This reaction, which is seen at therapeutic drug levels, is to be distinguished from the organic brain syndrome that may be seen with digitalis toxicity.) One experienced cardiologist has noted that "so many of the old folks [on digitalis] just seem to lose their joie de vivre." (DS Dock, MD, personal communication, November 1984).

The pathogenesis of this reaction is unclear. It is known, however, that digitalis exerts its effect on heart muscle by impairing membrane permeability to sodium and potassium. It is at least tempting to surmise that similar alteration of neuronal membranes in the CNS could lead to impaired neuronal function and, in some cases, to clinical depression. While this is no more than conjecture, it is known that membrane permeability to sodium ion is crucial to normal neuronal electrical conduction.

Lidocaine is commonly used intravenously (IV) to terminate life-threatening ventricular arrhythmias. The drug's clinical effect is due to a subtle interplay of actions upon the myocardial membrane. That similar effects occur in neuronal tissue is suggested by the profusion of neurologic side effects sometimes caused by lidocaine (paresthesias, drowsiness, dissociative states).[63] The precise connection between lidocaine and depression remains speculative.

Disopyramide phosphate (Norpace) is an oral agent for treatment of ventricular dysrhythmia. There have been rare reports of depression and other mental disturbance seen early in the course of treatment with this drug.

Although an array of mental disturbances are seen in association with *corticosteroid* use (as for rheumatoid arthritis or other chronic inflammatory disease, for immunosuppression in organ transplant recipients, etc) depression is often described. Curiously, euphoria is also associated with corticosteroid excess. In fact, the euphoriant response is most typical of exogenous (drug-induced) steroid excess; while depression seems more typical of endogenous hypercorticism.[63] An explanation for these phenomena is, at present, lacking.

While there is strong anecdotal support for the hypothesis that *oral contraceptives* may cause depression, there has not been compelling documentation of this.[63] Depression has been specifically linked to relatively high progestin content in the contraceptive preparation, and newer preparations with lower progestin content seem to be less associated with mood disturbance.

Cimetidine is a histamine receptor antagonist that has revolutionized the treatment of peptic ulcer disease. Several related compounds are being pressed into production in view of the tremendous marketing suc-

Table 2-1
Drugs and Toxins Associated with Depression

I. Antihypertensives
Reserpine[60-62]
α-Methyldopa[61-63]
Propranolol hydrochloride (and other lipophilic β-adrenergic blockers)[32, 61-63]
Prazosin[63]
Clonidine hydrochloride[61,64]
Guanethidine[61]

II. Cardiotonic, antidysrhythmic, and antiangina preparations
Digitalis[63]
Lidocaine[63]
Disopyramide phosphate[62]
Propranolol[32, 61-63]
Metoprolol[32]

III. Corticosteroids[61-63]

IV. Oral contraceptives[61-63]

V. Cimetidine[62,63]

VI. Antiglaucoma treatment
Timolol maleate[32]

VII. Indomethacin[62,63,65]

VIII. Antimicrobials
Cycloserine[61,62,66]
Isoniazid (INH)[62,64]
Nalidixic acid[62]

IX. Disulfiram[62,63]

X. Antineoplastic drugs
   Vincristine sulfate[61,67,68]
   Vinblastine sulfate[61,62,67,68]

XI. Cholinergic agonists
   Physostigmine[39]
   Organophosphate insecticides[39]

XII. Organic solvents[69]

XIII. Levodopa[61-63,70]

XIV. Drug withdrawal
   Caffeine[71]
   Nicotine[72]
   Amphetamines, cocaine[62,63,73]
   Fenfluramine hydrochloride, other anorectics[62,63]
   Barbiturates[62]

XV. Psychotropic drugs
   Benzodiazepines[62,63]
   Chlorpromazine, other aliphatic phenothiazines[7,68]

XVI. Alcohol[64,74]

XVII. Others
   Halothane[62]
   Phenylephrine hydrochloride[62]
   Anticonvulsants[62]
   Baclofen[62]
   Pentazocine[62]
   Morphine, other opiates[73]

cess of the parent drug. As experience with cimetidine has increased, a number of associated mental disturbances, including depression, have been noted. It has been suggested that such problems may be caused by interference with a central neurotransmitter function of histamine.[63]

The use of ophthalmic drops is usually not associated with systemic side effects. However, systemic absorption may take place and has been reported with *timolol maleate* , a preparation used to treat certain cases of glaucoma.[32] A lipophilic β-adrenergic blocker, timolol might be expected to cause depression in some patients. While we have not found documented reports of depression induced by ophthalmic timolol use, we recently observed a young woman with atypical depression associated with timolol treatment for glaucoma.

Indomethacin has well established anti-inflammatory and antipyretic properties and is used in the treatment of acute arthritis and other inflammatory disorders. Drug side effects (largely gastrointestinal) militate against long-term use of the drug. Like aspirin, indomethacin acts as an inhibitor of prostaglandin formation. Whether this action is responsible for its CNS side effects is unknown, but major depressive reactions have been reported in association with its use.[62,63,65]

In view of the availability of other excellent antituberculous agents, *cycloserine* is seldom used today. Its use may be complicated by a broad array of CNS side effects, including seizures, psychotic states, and depression.[61,62,66]

Cycloserine is structurally similar to d-alanine and exerts its antibiotic effect by interfering with the incorporation of this amino acid into the protein component of bacterial cell walls. Given our growing understanding of the neurohumoral importance of small peptides, one might argue that a similar inhibition of psychoactive peptide synthesis might account for cycloserine's CNS side effects.

Isoniazid (INH) is a commonly used antituberculous drug. Its use has led to rare reports of CNS toxicity, including depression.[62]

Nalidixic acid is an antibiotic effective against most urinary pathogens and therefore used to treat urinary tract infections. In rare cases, its use has been associated with depression.[62]

Numerous other antibiotics have been at least weakly implicated in causing depression.[60] Many of these act by inhibition of bacterial peptide synthesis, leading us to wonder again if mood disturbance might be a product of drug action upon CNS peptide synthesis.

Disulfiram is commonly used as an adjunct to the treatment of chronic alcoholism. The drug interferes with the catabolism of ethanol, leading to accumulation of acetaldehyde and to a highly uncomfortable (and at rare times fatal) clinical syndrome. In the absence of interaction with alcohol, disulfiram side effects are few but include a symptom of fatigue, lassitude, and loss of sexual potency that resembles depression.[62,63]

Of the cytotoxic drugs used to treat cancer, the vinca alkaloids *vincristine* [61,67,68] and *vinblastine* [61,62,67,68] have been implicated as causing depression. Both compounds are complex dimers that contain indole rings. The same indole core is found in serotonin, reserpine, and LSD; and it is tempting to ascribe to this the psychoactive properties of these agents. It has also been suggested that the vinca alkaloids interfere with the function of dopamine β-hydroxylase, the terminal enzyme responsible for the conversion of dopamine to norepinephrine.[67]

The "cholinergic model" of depression has been discussed above. Support for this model has been drawn from observation of patients with *organophosphate insecticide* poisoning. This potent anticholinesterase has been clearly linked both to increases in REM sleep and to depressive reactions. Similarly, *physostigmine* has been observed to produce depressive signs and symptoms in experimental subjects.[39]

Levodopa has become a mainstay in the treatment of Parkinson's disease. Since the drug's therapeutic effect necessitates avidity to the brain, it is not surprising that it has diverse CNS side effects. Most common among these are involuntary movement disorders, euphoria, and psychosis. Since levodopa is a precursor of norepinephrine, it seems paradoxical that depression has been reported secondary to the drug.[61-63,70] It seems possible that this might be caused by minor metabolites of levodopa (such as 3-0-methyldopa, which has a long half-life and therefore accumulates in the CNS).

Withdrawal of various drugs may cause depression. *Amphetamines and cocaine* are sympathomimetics widely used as recreational drugs. The former may be legitimately prescribed for attention deficit disorder in children and narcolepsy in adults. Related agents, such as *fenluramine hydrochloride*, are extensively used as anorectics. Rapid withdrawal of these agents is associated with the clinical picture of "crashing." Affected patients experience intense somatic discomfort, including cramps of striated and GI musculature, chills, sweats, and extreme fatigue. There are likely to be terrifying nightmares, and depression of suicidal proportions may occur.[62,63,73]

Withdrawal from prolonged use of high-dose *barbiturates* is well known as a serious, potentially fatal phenomenon. Withdrawal from lower doses of barbiturates may be problematic in its own right. The hypnotic properties of these drugs are associated with suppression of REM sleep. Their cessation after chronic use is likely to be accompanied by a period of REM rebound, during which there is excessive REM sleep. In accord with certain biochemical models previously discussed, this period of REM rebound is commonly associated with depression.[39]

Some chemicals are so commonly injested as to escape notice as "drugs." *Caffeine* and *nicotine* are among these. Both are often ingested in prodigious amounts, and withdrawal from both has been suggested as a precipitant to depression.[71,72]

Of the "psychotropic drugs" (drugs whose therapeutic effect is to mitigate disorders of mood or thinking), the *benzodiazepines* have primarily been identified as causing depression.[62,63] While this should lead to caution in their use, it should not lead to blanket condemnation of these agents which on balance are remarkably safe. The use of diazepam or other benzodiazepines to treat the sleeplessness and anxiety that often accompany bereavement or adjustment disorder with depressed mood is often very helpful. On the other hand, unidentified major depression with agitated features might very well be made worse with these agents. Further complicating the case for (or against) benzodiazepines is the discovery of alprazolam, a benzodiazepine derivative with antidepressant properties.

Haloperidol is an extremely popular antipsychotic agent that is associated with anecdotal reports of depressive side effects (McNEILAB, Inc, Fort Washington, PA, personal communications, March 1983). These seem to be poorly documented, however. Use of *aliphatic phenothiazines* (chlorpromazine and others) has similarly been linked with occasional depression.[7,68]

Alcohol is clearly the most commonly used psychoactive drug, although such use is seldom by prescription. The interrelationship of alcohol with depression is complex. There are patients in whom alcohol abuse seems to stem from an attempt at self-medication for various uncomfortable feelings, including anxiety and depression. Indeed, the disinhibiting, euphoriant effect that soon follows the ingestion of ethanol is well known to most of us and would seem to lend support to this form of self-prescription. However, alcohol is a general CNS depressant[74] and it has been noted that after several days of alcohol ingestion, alcoholics often have *worsening* of anxiety and depression. In fact, the psychiatric morbidity of alcoholics is so protean that most agree with the wisdom of treating the substance abuse before making another psychiatric diagnosis. This is exemplified by a patient treated by one of the authors:

Case report   A 50-year-old thrice-married father of four sought "psychoanalysis" for symptoms of depression. He was suffering from appetite loss, sleep disturbance with early morning awakening, and vague thoughts of suicide. He had previously had over 3 years of analytic treatment for feelings of depression that were truly lifelong but which episodically became much worse. He had also been treated by various physicians with antidepressants and benzodiazepines, and he continued to take these daily.

Careful drug history showed that he had problems with alcohol abuse dating from his teens and that the level of abuse had recently increased. Treatment consisted primarily of gradually overcoming his denial of his alcoholism. With abstinence from alcohol his mood improved markedly, and vegetative symptoms of depression disappeared. He was also withdrawn from benzodiazepines but continued to take (and to claim benefit from) 25 mg/d of amitriptyline hydrochloride.

High doses, or high plasma levels, of *anticonvulsants* have been associated with various CNS side effects, including depression.[62] Drugs thus implicated include *phenobarbital, primidone, phenytoin, ethosuximid*, and *clonazepam*.

Postoperative depression has been reported with the use of *halothane*, a popular general anesthetic.[62]

Patients with nasal congestion may become quite habituated to nasal sprays. *Phenylephrine hydrochloride* (Neo-Synephrine Hydrochloride) is a popular decongestant spray that acts as an α-receptor sympathomimetic. Overuse of this agent has been associated with various mental symptoms, among them depression. It would seem most likely for depression to occur in the period of drug withdrawal (as with other sympathomimetics like the amphetamines).

Baclofen is a centrally active muscle relaxant commonly used in patients with disruption of upper motor neuron function and resultant spasticity. A derivative of γ-aminobutyric acid (GABA), baclofen is thought to function as a mimic of that inhibitory neurotransmitter. In view of this putative action, it is not surprising that depression has been reported as a drug side effect.[62] (It might be recalled that diazepam and other benzodiazepines are thought to be GABA-mimetic.)

Morphine and other opiates are not infrequently associated with dysphoric mood.[73] Similarly, *pentazocine*, an analgesic with mixed opiate agonist and antagonist action, has been implicated as causing depression.[62] Addiction to these agents is, of course, common and is associated with marked dysphoria.

Medical Disorders

A wide array of diseases may present with symptoms of depression. The clinician who avoids premature diagnostic closure and who makes full use of historical data, physical examination, and laboratory tests should be able to detect the majority of these diseases. However, the opportunity for misdiagnosis is considerable. In one series of 157 depressed patients seen in the primary care setting, roughly 40% had at least one undetected nonpsychiatric disorder known to be associated with depression.[60]

Medical Disease

Chronic medical illness of any sort is highly associated with depression. Different authors report an incidence of 25% or more of depression in the medically ill.[75-77] Such depression is presumably a product of the debility caused by the underlying disease and may be seen as a psychological reaction to loss of vitality.

In some medical illness, however, depression seems to be caused directly and is often an early symptom if not the only symptom. It is to this group of illnesses that we now turn our attention. Table 2-2 lists the medical disorders associated with depression.

Infectious diseases Depression may be seen as a sequela to virtually any severe infection.[81] However, the depressive syndrome is particularly apt to follow certain viral infections (influenza, infectious mononucleosis, viral hepatitis,[60] viral pneumonia,[60,81] and viral encephalitis[81]). The pathogenesis of postinfectious depression is unclear, although it is tempting to postulate a mechanism mediated through the immune system.

Influenza virus causes respiratory infection and a syndrome including headache, fever, myalgia, and prostration. Epidemics of "flu" are most likely to occur in winter, and emergence of new viral strains has been associated with worldwide (pandemic) outbreaks. The diagnosis of influenza infection is made largely on the basis of history. Fever should be present, but specific physical findings are not to be found. Laboratory confirmation of the diagnosis can be made by finding a rise in antiviral antibody titers drawn during the acute illness and during convalescence.

There have been numerous reports of postinfluenza depression.[78] At least some of these reports have not been supported by serologic evidence for influenze infection. Despite the general acceptance of this diagnostic entity, Sinanan and Hillary have questioned its legitimacy.[78] Studying 400 psychiatric clinic patients, 215 of whom were depressed, these authors found no significant difference in influenza antibody titers between depressed and nondepressed patients.

Infectious mononucleosis is usually a benign disease, showing a predilection for adolescents and presenting with fever, fatigue, lymphadenopathy, hepatosplenomegaly, and pharyngitis. Among less common symptoms are those involving the CNS. Meningoencephalitis has been reported, as has transverse myelitis. Hendler and Leahy report two cases of infectious mononucleosis with subsequent depression of suicidal proportions.[79] Both cases were documented with the physical findings noted above and by specific serologic tests ("mono spot" test or heterophile titer). Cadie et al have reported a somewhat larger series of patients with anxiety and depression subsequent to infectious mononucleosis.[80]

Viral hepatitis is a systemic illness whose major effect is upon the liver, where it produces inflammation and hepatocellular damage. It is often caused by serologically identifiable viruses (A and B virus), although "non-A, non-B" infections are commonly seen after blood transfusion. Transmission of the disorder may be by oral or parenteral routes. Sexual transmission has also been described.

The disease is often preceded by a period of nonspecific malaise which is followed by marked fatigue, anorexia, and fever. A sudden aversion to cigarettes may also be noted. Within a matter of days, jaundice appears, and on physical examination an enlarged and tender liver is found. Jaundice usually peaks within 2 weeks but the period of recovery (eg, residual liver enzyme abnormalities) usually takes up to 4 months. Hall has noted the fairly common occurrence of severe depression during this recovery phase.[81]

Viral pneumonia is a diagnosis usually made in the face of clinical evidence for pneumonia (fever, cough, abnormal auscultatory findings over the lung fields, infiltrate(s) on chest film) when a bacterial agent cannot be identified. The clinical diagnosis may be supported by serologic evidence of infection by adenovirus, parainfluenza virus, influenza virus, or other respiratory pathogen. Depression is a common feature of these pneumonias.[60,81]

It is not surprising that *viral encephalitis* is associated with a broad

Table 2-2
Medical Disorders Associated with Depression

I. Infectious disease
   Influenza[78]
   Infectious mononucleosis[79,80]
   Viral hepatitis[60,81]
   Brucellosis[60]
   Typhoid[82]
   Malaria[60]
   Viral pneumonia[60,81]
   Tuberculosis[60]
   Tertiary syphilis[7]
   Viral encephalitis[81]
   Amebiasis[83]
   Giardiasis[83]
   Strongyloidiasis

II. Neoplasm
   Pancreatic carcinoma[60]
   Bronchogenic carcinoma[85]
   Oat cell carcinoma[60,86]
   Brain tumor (primary or metastatic)[7,60]
   Lymphoma[60,87]

III. Cardiovascular/pulmonary disease
   Hypoxia[86,88]
   Mitral valve prolapse[89]
   Sleep apnea[90,91]
   Mesenteric artery occlusion[92]

IV. Endocrine disorder
   Hypothyroidism[7,81]
   Hyperthyroidism[81,93-95]
   Cushing's syndrome[96]
   Addison's disease[7]
   Primary aldosteronism (Conn's disease)[97]
   Menopause[7, 98-100]
   Postpartum depression[101]
   Diabetes mellitus[102]
   Hyperinsulinism[7]
   Hypoparathyroidism[60]
   Hyperparathyroidism[7]
   Hypopituitarism[60]
   Acromegaly[60]

V. Metabolic disturbance
    Uremia[60, 81]
    Hyponatremia[7]
    Hypokalemia[7]
    Elevated serum bicarbonate[7, 81]
    Gout[81]

VI. Nutritional deficiency
    Pellagra[7]
    Thiamine deficiency[7]
    Scurvy[7, 103]
    Vitamin B_{12} deficiency[7]
    Folate deficiency[7, 81]
    Pyridoxine deficiency[7, 81]
    Iron deficiency[7]
    Protein deficiency[7]

VII. Gastrointestinal disease
    Cirrhosis[60, 104]
    Inflammatory bowel disease[60]
    Celiac disease[105]
    Whipple's disease[60]
    Pancreatitis[60]

VIII. Collagen-vascular disease
    Systemic lupus erythematosus[60,106]
    Rheumatoid arthritis[60, 107]
    Polyarteritis nodosa[60]
    Giant cell arteritis[60]

IX. Central nervous system disease
    Multiple sclerosis[108-110]
    Parkinson's disease[109, 110]
    Dementia[7, 111]
    Brain tumor[7, 112, 113]
    Stroke[7, 114, 115]
    Huntington's disease[60]
    Chronic subdural hematoma[60, 116]
    Temporal lobe seizures[86, 117]
    Myasthenia gravis [118]

X. Miscellaneous
    Cranial irradiation[86, 119, 120]
    Amyloidosis[7, 81]
    Psoriasis[81]
    Sarcoidosis[60]
    Wilson's disease[81]
    Factitious depression[121]

spectrum of neurologic deficits and emotional changes, since the disease involves inflammation or possibly destruction of brain tissue. Many viruses may cause the typical clinical picture of fever, meningeal irritation, and neurologic deficit. Some very common viruses (measles, mumps, influenza) have a rare association with encephalitis. Other more unusual pathogens (eastern and western equine encephalitis virus, St Louis encephalitis virus, and others) are more avid to the CNS and thus more likely to be associated with encephalitis. These more common pathogens are carried by insect vectors (anthropod-borne or arboviruses), and thus the viral encephalitides are diseases of warm months. Furthermore, they are rarely encountered in the eastern United States.

The severity of viral encephalitis varies greatly. Eastern equine encephalitis has been noted to have a mortality of 60% or more, and its survivors commonly have permanent brain damage.[122] On the other hand, St Louis encephalitis infection may go undetected. Yet recovery from this relatively benign infection is commonly associated with depression.[81]

Diagnosis of viral encephalitis is supported by finding CSF pleocytosis without culture evidence of bacterial, fungal, or other organisms. Serologic diagnosis may be made by finding a rise in specific antiviral antibodies between acute and convalescent periods of the illness.

Though no longer endemic to the United States, *malaria* has a very high prevalence worldwide; and the patient recently returned from the tropics and complaining of relapsing fever, chills, muscle aches, and severe headache might be suspected of harboring *Plasmodia* (the protozoan responsible for malaria). Physical examination of the patient with malaria commonly shows fever and hepatosplenomegaly. Laboratory investigation may show anemia and should show parasitized red blood cells on a smear of peripheral blood.

In one particularly virulent form of malaria the parasites lead to thrombosis of small blood vessels. When cerebral vessels are involved, focal neurologic deficits may ensue as may a more diffuse organic brain syndrome.

Even in the absence of cerebral malaria, recovery from the disease may be accompanied by significant depression.[81] It has also been suggested that the antimalarial drugs chloroquine and quinacrine hydrochloride may produce depression, thus complicating differential diagnosis further.

Brucellosis is a disease caused by bacteria of the genus *Brucella*, organisms that are transmitted to man from animals such as cattle, sheep, goats, and pigs. It is thus a disease largely confined to rural areas and to people exposed to such animals. Both acute and chronic brucellosis are characterized by fever and a paucity of more specific signs and symptoms. Weakness, lassitude, and depression are commonly associated complaints, as are vague aches and pains.[60] Chronic infection may persist thus for months to years. Suspicion of this often subtle illness may be confirmed by positive blood cultures or by specific serologic tests.

A number of psychiatric syndromes have been noted as rare concomitants of *typhoid fever* .[82] These include psychosis, mania, catatonia, or depression, which in even rarer cases may be *principal* findings in this disease. This systemic illness is caused by ingestion of the bacterium Salmonella typhosa and is characterized by fever, headache, lassitude, abdominal pain, anorexia, and constipation. Characteristic physical findings include lymphadenopathy, splenomegaly, and pinkish skin papules ("rose spots," which though classic are relatively infrequent.) Laboratory investigation typically shows a relative neutropenia (4000-6000 WBC/υL). The causative bacterium may be cultured from blood or stool. Finally, serologic tests are available to detect disease-specific agglutinins.

Emotional lability and depression are also reported in association with *tuberculosis* even in the absence of direct CNS infection.[60] Isoniazid and cycloserine, both used to treat infection with *Mycobacterium tuberculosis* , have themselves been implicated in causing depression, which may further confuse attempts at diagnosis. At one time the scourge of Western civilization, tuberculosis remains common in the developing countries and poorer areas of western nations. While it is most often a pulmonary illness, presenting with low-grade fever, cough, and apical lung infiltrates on x-ray film, it may involve virtually any organ (as in miliary infection). Correct diagnosis is suggested by chest radiologic findings and confirmed by demonstration of *M. tuberculosis* by smear or culture of sputum (or less commonly of urine or gastric contents). Skin testing with antigens derived from the offending bacterium (PPD testing) may also aid in diagnosis, although positive testing does not distinguish between active and inactive disease, and false-negatives may occur.

While *syphilis* no longer enjoys the place of prominence it enjoyed in nineteenth century medicine, it is far from being a museum item. The disease is most commonly spread by sexual transmission of the bacterium *Treponema pallidum* . The earliest evidence of infection (primary stage) consists of an indurated ulcer (hard chancre) on the genitalia. If untreated, the illness is likely to give way in a matter of weeks to a secondary stage characterized by generalized rash, fever, malaise, headache, and myalgia. If still untreated, the disease may enter a stage of latency only to emerge with late involvement of virtually any organ system. Perhaps the most devastating feature of late syphilis is seen with nervous system involvement. Peripheral neuropathy is common, and focal neurologic deficits of any sort may be a result of syphilitic brain involvement. Extensive brain involvement is characteristically associated with manic behavior and intellectual deterioration ("general paresis of the insane"). Hall points out, however, that 25% of patients with general paresis present with moderate to severe depression, at times without focal neurologic deficits.[81]

Correct diagnosis of neurosyphilis depends on suspecting the disorder and drawing blood serologies (VDRL or rapid plama reagin [RPR] tests). Positive test results should be followed by a more specific flourescent treponemal antibody (FTA) test. Syphilitic disease of the CSF is confirmed by positive CNS serology.

Parasitic illness is not terribly common in the industrialized west. There has been brief mention, however, of depression as a concomitant of infestation with three of the more common protozoans: *Giardia lamblia, Strongyloides stercoralis* , and *Endamoeba hystolytica* . Parrish and Bueno estimate anecdotally that 10% of patients with giardiasis or amebiasis are depressed, and they note that depression may be the only symptom of infestation.[83] Correct diagnosis may require a high index of suspicion for parasitic disease and scrupulous examination of stool specimens for protozoans or cysts. *Giardia lamblia* is sometimes retrieved only from duodenal aspirates.

Neoplasm Depression in the patient with cancer may have diverse etiologies. Simply ascribing the mood disorder to the psychological impact of this dread disease may lead to important errors in diagnosis.[86] For example, the clinical course of some cancers may be complicated by metabolic disturbances such as hypoxia, hypercalcemia, and hypoglycemia, each of which may produce an array of emotional disturbances, including depression. (These disorders will be more fully discussed below.) Furthermore, nutrition may be markedly impaired in patients with cancer, leading to any number of vitamin or cofactor deficiencies, which in turn may predispose to depression (see below).

A number of anticancer therapies may in their own right cause symptoms of depression. Among common drug therapies, corticosteroids and vinca alkaloids (vincristine, vinblastine), have previously been discussed as agents of depression. *Radiation therapy* has also been suggested as a cause of depression. While serious doubt exists that this treatment *per se* causes mood disturbance, *cranial* irradiation seems to have a high correlation with depression.[119] Proctor et al reported a group of adults treated with cranial irradiation for acute lymphoblastic leukemia, all of whom experienced depression as a sequela to the treatment.[120] The same group found that pretreatment with imipramine tended to prevent these depressive sequelae.

Brain metastasis may also account for depression in the patient with cancer. As is the case in patients with primary brain tumors, such lesions may not initially produce focal neurologic deficits but may present with depression.[7] Temporal lobe tumors in particular may present with affective disturbance. Seizures caused by brain tumors may also produce depressive symptoms if they involve the temporal lobes.[86]

Detection of brain tumor in the absence of a discrete neurologic deficit may be very difficult. The onset of mood or personality change or of headache or other vague symptoms in a patient previously free of such troubles should raise the index of suspicion. Thorough neurologic examination is important but, again, may be negative. Funduscopic examination should be done to detect papilledema. Furthermore, EEG and radionuclide or CT scanning of the brain are important diagnostic tools.

Several non-CNS neoplasms have been noted to cause depression. *Pancreatic carcinoma* may be clinically silent until quite advanced, and depression has commonly been noted to precede other symptoms and signs. Tumors originating in the tail of the pancreas, in particular, must become quite large before impinging upon the common duct and causing "painless jaundice," a common presenting symptom of pancreatic neoplasm.

In the absence of jaundice, anorexia, weight loss, or other GI symptoms, the diagnosis of pancreatic cancer is extremely difficult, and metastasis may be extensive before the disorder is suspected. Severe pain (with or without jaundice) that "bores through" to the patient's back may suggest this disorder. Physical examination may be quite unrevealing early in the course of the disease unless jaundice is seen. Upper GI radiography may reveal distortion by tumor of contrast material in the duodenal sweep. Endoscopy, with retrograde contrast studies of the pancreatic duct system and of hepatic drainage, may be especially helpful in arriving at a correct diagnosis, as may CT scanning of the abdomen.

Lung cancer is not commonly associated with depressive symptoms, except as a psychological reaction to the gravity of the illness. One of the authors, however, recently experienced a case of *bronchogenic carcinoma* which presented as a first episode of major depression. Solomon and Solomon report a 51-year-old woman with manic-depressive illness who presented with symptoms of major depression, including 10.2 kg weight loss.[85] The patient was noted to be pale, and routine hemogram showed a hematocrit of 26%. Chest film then showed a bronchogenic carcinoma. Making diagnosis difficult was the fact that the patient had not complained of cough, hemoptysis, chest pain, or shortness of breath, symptoms that would have led to earlier chest films and diagnosis. Her weight loss and lassitude were readily ascribed to the concurrent depression.

Oat cell carcinoma is a less common pulmonary neoplasm that has also been associated with depression. These tumors often have endocrine activity, and depression may ensue from tumor secretion of parathormone or ACTH (see below).

Depression may be seen as a rare presenting feature of *lymphoma.* In a series of 229 patients with this cancerous condition of the lymphoid tissue, Hutchinson et al reported but one case in which depression was the presenting sign.[87] In other cases, depression was seen as a feature of exacerbation of the disease.

Lymphoma may be quite advanced before generalized swelling of lymphoid tissue is found on physical examination. This is most apt to be the case when the disease is confined to the retroperitoneum. In such cases, lassitude and weight loss may be incorrectly attributed to simple depression. The presence of fever or pruritis should be a warning of the presence of the underlying disease.

In some cases, lymphoma may be associated with the production of a parathormonelike substance, which in theory could lead to depression.[81] In addition, one may see direct involvement of the brain in lymphoma. In such cases depression might be caused as it may be by any other brain neoplasm.

Cardiovascular/pulmonary disease The brain has a large oxygen requirement and is thus exquisitely sensitive to oxygen deprivation or *hypoxia..* Hypoxia may result from several pathophysiologic mechanisms: (1) A reduction in cardiac output, as seen in *congestive heart failure* , will cause decreased cerebral perfusion and, hence, some degree of cerebral hypoxia. (2) Since the lungs are responsible for oxygenation of the blood, *lung disease* of myriad causes may cause hypoxia. (3) Lowered oxygen tension in ambient air (as seen in *high altitude*) results in hypoxia. (4) Impairment of hemoglobin transport of oxygen, such as that seen in *carbon monoxide poisoning* or in *methemoglobinemia* may cause hypoxic insult to tissues with high O_2 dependence. *Severe anemia* can produce the same picture. (5) Some poisons (eg, *arsenic, cyanide**) inhibit cellular utilization of oxygen and thus may lead to hypoxic tissue damage.

---

*Cyanide poisoning is likely to produce death within minutes, so does not represent a serious diagnostic consideration in the depressed patient.

Acute hypoxia is likely to be associated with symptoms akin to anxiety: air hunger, rapid pulse, and a sense of foreboding. Chronic hypoxia, on the other hand, may present with lassitude, apathy and psychomotor retardation, symptoms readily confused with depression.[122] The medical history and physical examination are usually sufficient to detect significant cardiopulmonary disease. Obviously, special attention should be paid to signs of congestive heart failure (tachycardia, an enlarged area of cardiac dullness, an S3 gallop, evidence of pulmonary congestion, peripheral venous congestion, etc). Chronic lung disease may be indicated by use of accessory muscles of respiration, by increase in the anteroposterior chest diameter, by clubbing of the fingers, by cyanosis, and other more specific signs.

If cardiopulmonary disease is suspected, the chest film may confirm intrinsic lung disease or cardiomegaly with congestive heart failure. If other forms of hypoxia are suspected, a hemoglobin determination should be done. Arterial blood gases are the definitive test in diagnosing hypoxemia. If carbon monoxide poisoning is suspected, carboxyhemoglobin levels should be determined. A rare cause of a depressive syndrome, *chronic arsenic poisoning* , may be detected by urinary assay or by analysis of hair or nails.[123]

When hypoxia is severe enough and of sufficient duration neuronal death may occur with permanent behavioral sequelae. Patients with *postanoxic encephalopathy* commonly show the clinical picture of dementia. Confusion and memory disturbance are usually salient. Focal neurologic deficits may be seen. In addition, severe depression has been described.[88]

Mitral valve prolapse has been previously described (see Anxiety) and is perhaps most likely to be misdiagnosed as "acute anxiety." Szmuilowicz and Flannery, however, have described a significant coincidence of depression with this disorder.[89] Correct diagnosis depends upon careful auscultation of the heart with the finding of a systolic click with (or without) the systolic murmur of mitral regurgitation.

Sleep apnea is a disorder characterized by frequent, prolonged apneic periods occurring during sleep.[90] Recognition of the disorder has grown with the proliferation of sleep laboratories where the definitive diagnosis may be made. The disorder should be suspected, however, in the patient with sleep disturbance and daytime somnolence.

Emotional disturbance, particularly depression, is commonly associated with the sleep apnea syndrome. Since sleep disturbance is a major feature of "functional" depressive disorders, sleep apnea may readily be mistaken for simple depression. For example, Sandblom et al recently reported a 36-year-old man treated with amoxapine for depression before the diagnosis of sleep apnea was made.[91]

Sleep apnea may occur as a result of brainstem dysfunction with disturbance of medullary respiratory drive centers (this is most likely the genesis of sleep apnea as seen in the premature infant). On the other hand, *obstructive* sleep apnea seems to be produced by upper airway obstruction during sleep. It is most common in men who give (or whose bed partners give) a long history of loud snoring. If the disorder remains undetected and untreated, chronic nocturnal hypoxia may lead to pulmonary hypertension and cor pulmonale.

Dvoredsky has reported the highly unusual case of a 46-year-old woman with 3 years of weight loss, inability to eat, and abdominal pain.[92] Exhaustive evaluation (including exploratory laparotomy) failed to show any organic disease, and a presumptive diagnosis of depression was made. Only persistent medical evaluation yielded first an abnormal upper GI series and in response to this, an arteriogram that showed high-grade obstruction of both celiac and superior mesenteric arteries. Vascular surgery resulted in complete clearing of depressive symptoms.

Endocrine disease   Extremes of endocrine function (either hyper or hypofunction) are commonly associated with emotional symptoms, including depression.

Hypothyroidism is marked by a generalized slowing of bodily function. Not only does the hypothyroid patient manifest specific findings such as a slowed pulse and a delay in relaxation of deep tendon reflexes, but gross motor and cognitive function are also slowed. The patient commonly complains of fatigue, weight gain, and constipation. He may in addition feel depressed. ("Myxedema madness," on the other hand, is an uncommon psychotic disturbance predicated on prolonged, severe hypothyroidism.)

The medical history is important in diagnosing hypothyroidism. Most cases are probably a result of autoimmune thyroiditis (Hashimoto's disease), and a history of thyroid enlargement and/or tenderness may then be elicited. Less commonly, hypothyroidism is iatrogenic. Thyroidectomy or radioactive iodine treatment ("chemical thyroidectomy") may be responsible, as may treatment with antithyroid drugs such as propylthiouracil. Lithium carbonate, which inhibits the thyroid's response to pituitary stimulation, may also induce hypothyroidism.

In addition to the clinical signs and symptoms noted above, cold intolerance may be noted, as may a thickening of skin and hair and a generalized nonpitting edema. Patients suspected of being hypothyroid should have thyroid hormone levels tested, low levels confirming the diagnosis.

Thyrotoxicosis is generally associated with symptoms akin to anxiety. However, "apathetic hyperthyroidism" has been well described and may be associated with symptoms of major depression which clears with restoration of hormonal balance. Typically, the patient so affected is elderly and shows weight loss but few of the other "classic" signs of hyperthyroidism (fine tremor, agitation, increased sweating, exophthalmos). Kronfol et al, for example, report a 67-year-old woman with symptoms of major depression.[95] Routine thyroid function testing showed her to be markedly hyperthyroid, and her depression resolved completely to antithyroid treatment alone (propylthiouracil followed by radioactive iodine). Younger patients have also been reported with this disorder.[93,94] Thyrotoxicosis is usually associated with goiter, or at least by a "toxic" thyroid nodule; and physical examination should include careful palpation of the neck. In the laboratory, increased levels of circulating thyroid hormone confirm the diagnosis.

Adrenal hypofunction (*Addison's disease*) is often associated with symptoms of depression. Addison's original description described a patient who "... becomes languid and weak, indisposed to either bodily or mental exertion; the appetite is impaired or entirely lost ...."[124] Weight loss and vague abdominal discomfort are also commonly noted. On physical examination, hypotension and hyperpigmentation (particularly in scars, in creases of the palms and soles) may be noted. Since impaired adrenal function may be secondary to tuberculosis or other systemic illness, there may be physical signs of these related illnesses. In the laboratory, hyponatremia and hyperkalemia may be seen. The diagnosis is confirmed by showing a blunted cortisol response to the administration of ACTH.

Somewhat paradoxically, *excessive* circulating cortisol may also cause depression. Iatrogenic *Cushing's syndrome* has already been discussed. Spontaneous Cushing's syndrome may arise from primary hyperplasia of the adrenal cortex (less commonly, from adrenal carcinoma) or from an ACTH-secreting tumor. Cushing's original clinical descriptions were of patients with pituitary basophilic adenomas—Cushing's *disease*. Other tumors, such as oat cell carcinoma of the lung, may also secrete ACTH. In any case, the syndrome is marked by truncal obesity, hypertension, easy bruising, and cutaneous striae. Puffy ("cushingoid") facies are common and a dorsal fat pad ("buffalo hump") may be seen. Affected women may show hirsutism secondary to hypersecretion of adrenal androgens.

Emotional disturbances may predate other signs of Cushing's syndrome.[78] Most common among these is depression. Kelly et al evaluated a small cohort of patients with Cushing's syndrome and reported that 8 of

12 (60%) were depressed.[96] Other estimates cite a 33% incidence.[81] The diagnosis should be suspected in anyone receiving corticosteroid treatment or in anyone displaying any of the above physical signs. In the laboratory over 90% of patients with Cushing's syndrome will show glucose intolerance (usually elicited only by glucose tolerance testing, but in roughly 20% of cases presenting as frank diabetes).[96] More specific laboratory indicators include elevated serum cortisol levels and elevated urinary 17-hydroxycorticosteroid levels.

Depression is also associated with aldosterone secreting tumors of the adrenal (*Conn's disease*). Affected patients typically present with weakness (which may be profound if hypokalemia is severe enough), apathy, anorexia, and constipation. Physical examination usually shows muscle weakness and hypertension, although the latter may well be the solitary finding. In the laboratory, hypokalemia should raise the index of suspicion for this disorder. (Diagnosis may be confirmed by doing split renal vein aldosterone assays.) Malinow and Lion report a young woman with hypertension, weakness, and a serum potassium of 1.4 mEq/L whose depression promptly abated with careful IV potassium replacement.[97]

The role of *estrogen deficiency* in the induction of depression is a point of debate. Winokur has suggested that the menopause does not pose an increased risk of depression.[98] Others have studied gynecology clinic patients and found them to be at increased risk for both anxiety and depression during menopause.[99] Estrogen replacement therapy has been reported to cause relief of these symptoms.[7,100]

Postpartum depression has been felt by some to be related to a drop in the relatively high levels of estrogen circulating during pregnancy. It is important to distinguish this disorder from the more common and considerably more benign *postpartum blues* . The latter occur frequently within the first few days after parturition and usually remit spontaneously within a few days. The patient with postpartum blues tends to be irritable, easily slighted, and prone to tears. Full-blown postpartum depression is rarer (estimates range from 0.1% to 12.0% depending on inclusion criteria).[101] It may occur any time within 6 months of parturition, and its symptoms are indistinguishable from major depression. Indeed, some argue that postpartum depression shares not only clinical features but pathogenesis with major depression and that a separate diagnostic category is not warranted.

Premenstrual syndrome (PMS) has received tremendous attention in the lay literature. While its inclusion as an endocrine disorder is arguable, its association with depressive changes in some women has been noted.[125]

By definition, this is a self-limited disorder although many affected women meet criteria for a lifetime diagnosis of major depression.[125]

The symptoms of *diabetes mellitus* are a product of underactivity of insulin and resultant underutilization of glucose at the cellular level. Since neuronal tissue has high glucose demands, it is not surprising that unrecognized or poorly controlled diabetes is associated with changes in mentation. Diabetes often presents with the insidious development of weight loss and lassitude, symptoms, if taken alone, suggesting depression.[102] Additional history, however, should reveal polydipsia, polyuria, and polyphagia—symptoms all directly attributable to cellular underutilization of glucose. Early in the course of the disease, physical findings may be few. Proper diagnosis at this stage depends upon obtaining fasting and postprandial blood glucose levels. More nascent disease may require glucose tolerance testing for detection. Later on, diabetes affects virtually every organ system. Salient features are found in examining the eyes, where cataracts and retinal hemorrhages, exudates, and microaneurysms are common. A diffuse peripheral neuropathy is also a common late sequela.

At times diabetes may present with hyperosmolar or ketoacidotic coma, neither of which is likely to be mistaken for depression. The routine screening of blood glucose levels in the comatose patient leads to proper diagnosis. Recurrent ketoacidosis or hyperosmolar coma may combine with the ravages of premature atherosclerosis to produce an organic mental syndrome, which may resemble either depression or schizophrenia.[81]

Hyperinsulinism is a somewhat controversial disorder that has been invoked to explain a wide array of psychopathology (see chapter 1). Quite simply, excessive levels of circulating insulin cause a drop in blood glucose levels, creating a "fuel shortage" in all cells, most notably the highly glucose-dependent brain cells. Part of the body's homeostatic response to this is an outpouring of epinephrine, which causes a liberation of glucose from liver glycogen stores. The high levels of circulating epinephrine also tend to cause a state of sympathetic autonomic arousal which can closely mimic acute anxiety. Altschule reports the considerably rarer occurrence of depression in affected patients.[7]

Hyperinsulinism most clearly occurs in the relatively rare cases of pancreatic β-islet cell tumors. More controversial is the occurrence of "reactive hypoglycemia," which happens in the absence of insulin-secreting tumors and presumably represents a response to large dietary loads of carbohydrate. These two entities should be distinguishable by the fact that insulin-secreting tumors result in *fasting* hypoglycemia (blood glucose levels of 30-40 mg/dL or less). If low blood glucose levels lead to the suspicion of hyperinsulinism, insulin radioimmunoassays should be performed. Suspected insulinomas may require arteriography for positive identification.

In cases of untreated hyperinsulinism, frank neuronal damage may occur as a result of recurrent hypoglycemia. Affected patients may develop dementia, whose major features may resemble depression or schizophrenia.[81]

Parathormone is normally produced by the parathyroid glands and, in opposition to the hormone calcitonin, helps to maintain normal serum calcium levels by freeing calcium from bone. *Hyperparathyroidism* is a state usually arising *de novo* from an adenoma of one of the parathyroid glands. Less commonly, nonparathyroid tumors (eg, *oat cell carcinoma* of the lung) may elaborate high levels of parathormone. In addition, *chronic renal disease* with resultant hyperphosphatemia may stimulate excess parathyroid activity and may even result in secondary formation of parathyroid adenomas.

Hyperparathyroidism is quite apt to develop insidiously, and emotional symptoms may predate the classic symptoms of bone pain and renal colic by months or even years. With multichannel autoanalyzers routinely determining serum calcium levels, the disorder is often diagnosed when asymptomatic.

Emotional symptoms associated with hypercalcemia (serum calcium greater than 10.5 mg/dL) include lassitude, anorexia, weakness, constipation, and depressed mood. With marked hypercalcemia (serum calcium greater than 12 mg/dL) a psychotic delirium may occur.[81] Since physical findings are quite likely to be absent, correct diagnosis depends on finding an elevation of serum calcium. This may be followed by radioimmunoassay of parathormone levels. Radiographs of the hands may reveal typical resorptive changes in the terminal phalanges.

Hypoparathyroidism is almost always seen as a sequel to surgical removal of the parathyroid glands. Thus the patient with hypocalcemia and a history of neck surgery should raise high suspicion of this disorder. The mental changes associated with hypoparathyroidism may mimic acute anxiety. The disorder is discussed more fully in chapter 1. The disorder may also produce fatigue and frank depression. If it is left untreated, an organic brain syndrome with frank cognitive impairment may supervene.

Panhypopituitarism may occur as a result of invasion of the pituitary by tumor. It is also seen in the postpartum setting, particularly as a sequela to uterine hemorrhage and hypotension. Affected patients have secondary hypofunction of the thyroid, adrenal cortical, and gonadal hormones. Associated symptoms may develop insidiously and be quite vague. Fatigue, apathy, and loss of libido may easily be mistaken for depression. The alert physician will detect a loss of pubic or axillary hair or other loss of secondary sex characteristics. Signs of thyroid and adrenal hypofunction may also be seen. If hypopituitarism is secondary to tumor, the optic chiasm may be impinged upon with resultant bitemporal visual field loss. The diagnosis may be confirmed by CT scanning (showing tumor or recent hemorrhage) or by assay of pituitary hormones (ACTH, TSH, FSH are readily measured).

Acromegaly is a condition arising from an adenomatous tumor of pituitary acidophilic cells, cells that produce growth hormone. Its onset is usually insidious, with subtle changes in facial features and increase in the size of hands, feet, and head. It may take years, however, for the classic picture of mandibular overgrowth with prognathism to develop. Meanwhile, emotional lability may be a dominant feature of the disorder, and depression may be seen. Correct diagnosis is suggested by the changes in body habitus. Radiologic evidence of pituitary enlargement may be seen, and bitemporal visual field cuts may be detected.

Metabolic disturbances Kidney failure may ensue from any of a multitude of diseases. It is beyond the scope of this chapter to list these, but it will suffice to say that the syndrome of *uremia* , which is the final common pathway of these diseases, may feature prominent depression. Uremia is associated clinically with fatigue, apathy, and distractability. Loss of libido and of appetite are commonly seen. It is crucial that associated physical findings be sought. Arterial hypertension should be seen, and may be quite marked. The skin may show a "uremic frost." A pericardial friction rub may be detected. Peripheral neuropathy is common. If the syndrome be advanced, the more subtle emotional changes noted above may give way to delirium or coma. The diagnosis is confirmed by finding elevations of blood urea nitrogen (BUN) and serum creatinine, signifying decreased renal clearance of these substances.

There may be a host of associated metabolic disturbances resulting from decreased renal function. Hyperkalemia may be seen (see below). Elevations in serum phosphate may result in secondary hyperparathyroidism (see above). Retention of hydrogen ion with metabolic acidosis may give lowered levels of serum bicarbonate. Each of these metabolic disturbances may in itself be associated with emotional symptoms.

Sodium ion is crucial to the propagation of neuronal action potentials, so it is not surprising that significant sodium depletion (*hyponatremia*) causes disturbances of brain function. Hyponatremia may result from overzealous treatment with diuretics (particularly if fluid replacement favors free water over sodium). Although less common, severe hyponatremia may be seen in cases of *inappropriate antidiuretic hormone (ADH) secretion*. (Inappropriate ADH may be produced by some tumors, such as oat cell carcinoma. It may also be seen with disease of the lungs or the CNS.) Early symptoms may include apathy and depression. If the disorder is untreated, frank delirium, seizures, and coma may supervene. Diagnosis is made by finding a markedly low serum sodium.

Potassium ion is also a crucial factor in neuronal firing, and either excess or deficiency of serum potassium may produce depression. Conversely, correction of the potassium imbalance relieves the depressive symptoms. *Hyperkalemia* may be seen in kidney failure or in patients treated with aldosterone inhibitors (eg, spironolactone). Adrenal insufficiency may also produce hyperkalemia. The diagnosis is made by finding elevation of serum potassium. The ECG may show the typical peaked T wave of hyperkalemia.

Hypokalemia is a common byproduct of diuretic treatment. It may also be seen with severe diarrhea, with chronic steroid therapy, and cases of mineralocorticoid (aldosterone) excess (see *Conn's disease* above). Proper diagnosis is made by determining the serum potassium level. Hypokalemia may be suggested by ECG findings of QT interval prolongation, a broad T wave, and subsequent prominent U wave.

Calcium seems to play an important role in regulating neuronal membrane permeability to sodium and potassium, as well as in the release of neurotransmitters. Perturbation in calcium concentration might then be expected to affect neuronal function, and this expectation is borne out clinically, as has been discussed above. *Hypercalcemia* of the sort seen with hyperparathyroidism may also be seen with some neoplasms, particularly where there is lytic involvement of bone (eg, multiple myeloma). Excessive intake of milk and antacids (milk-alkali syndrome) may also produce hypercalcemia. Sarcoidosis and steroid therapy are also associated with elevated serum calcium. The diagnosis of depression due to hypercalcemia is suggested by finding elevation of serum calcium levels.

Elevation of serum bicarbonate has also been known to produce depressive symptoms. Such elevation may commonly result from excessive ingestion of antacids, from loss of gastric acid (metabolic alkalosis) secondary to vomiting or gastric suction, or as a compensatory response to respiratory acidosis. Anxiety, paranoia, and, in the extreme, stupor may also result from abnormally elevated bicarbonate. The diagnosis may be made from serum bicarbonate levels which have become a routine part of serum electrolyte determinations.

Gout is a poorly documented cause of depression, and it is not clear whether mood disturbance may accompany acute gout or only chronic (and potentially debilitating) disease.[81] The essence of the disease is a serum concentration of uric acid that is supersaturated. This may result in spontaneous precipitation of uric acid crystals in joints (acute gouty arthritis) or in the kidneys (gout nephropathy). Acute monoarticular arthritis (classically involving the metatarsophalangeal joint of the great toe) may suggest the disorder, as may a history of ureteral stones. Patients with leukemia or other blood dyscrasias may overproduce uric acid, which is a byproduct of nucleic acid degradation. Alcoholics may also have elevated serum uric acid levels (most likely due to increased urate synthesis).[126] Thiazide diuretics may interfere with renal tubular secretion of uric acid and may thus cause hyperuricemia.

Nutritional deficiency Serious dietary deficiencies are unusual in modern western societies. Yet they are still seen, particularly in the poor and the elderly, and they may produce striking mental symptoms, including depression.

Pellagra is a condition resulting from inadequate intake of nicotinic acid or its precursor, tryptophan. Diets markedly poor in protein are most often responsible for this disorder, whose major clinical features include stomatitis, dermatitis, diarrhea, dementia, and (in the extreme) death. Before the full-blown clinical picture develops, emotional changes may predominate. These may consist of nervousness (pellagra has been discussed in chapter 1) or of agitated depression. Lassitude, anorexia, and insomnia may further lead to the impression of primary depression. Laboratory findings in pellagra are quite nonspecific, and correct diagnosis depends upon detecting the systemic signs and symptoms of the disorder in a patient with inadequate nutrition.

In Western societies *thiamine deficiency* is most often seen in chronic alcoholics, in whom it is associated with the Wernicke-Korsakoff syndrome (see chapter 1). Worldwide, the disorder has been most often seen in people whose major dietary staple is polished rice. In the latter setting, the Wernicke-Korsakoff syndrome is not seen, but insidious neurologic impairment does occur. This is apt to be heralded by lethargy and a heavy feeling in the extremities—symptoms readily confused with depression. (Anorexia and weight loss are also usually present.) As the disorder progresses, weakness, muscular pain and atrophy, paresthesias, and decreased deep tendon reflexes supervene. Some patients also develop cardiac enlargement and congestive heart failure (beriberi heart disease). Correct diagnosis depends upon obtaining an abnormal dietary history and upon finding evidence of neurologic and/or cardiac impairment. It may be confirmed by 24-hour urine assays for thiamine.

Depression has been reported as a salient feature of *scurvy* , and the affective disturbance has been shown to clear after treatment with ascorbic acid. Scurvy is now uncommon but may be seen in persons with diets bereft of fruits and fresh vegetables. The disorder is classically marked by swollen, bleeding gums, hemorrhagic skin lesions, and painful weakness of the legs. Clinical suspicion of scurvy may be confirmed by determining plasma levels of ascorbic acid.

The clinical features of *vitamin B_{12} deficiency* have previously been discussed (see chapter 1). A spectrum of emotional disturbance may accompany this disorder, with depression occurring at the milder end and full-blown psychosis marking the other extreme. The presence of neurologic abnormalities of corticospinal tract and/or posterior column function help to make the diagnosis. In the laboratory, macrocytic anemia may be noted, with hypersegmentation of neutrophils. Serum B_{12} levels should be low.

Folic acid deficiency can produce anemia that is indistinguishable on peripheral blood smear from B_{12} deficiency anemia. Like B_{12} deficiency, folate deficiency may present a spectrum from depressive disorder to psychosis. Unlike B_{12} deficiency, folate deficiency is not associated with corticospinal tract and posterior column dysfunction. Folate deficiency is usually seen in the setting of generalized intestinal malabsorption (as in sprue). It may also be associated with pregnancy, alcoholism, and with use of oral contraceptives, some anticancer drugs, and anticonvulsant drugs such as phenytoin and primidone. Correct diagnosis is established by determining the serum folic acid level.

Deficiency of pyridoxine (vitamin B_6) is most likely to be seen in alcoholics or in patients taking oral contraceptives or isoniazid. The disorder is suggested by the development of peripheral neuropathy (with either hypesthesia or hyperesthesia) in patients at risk. Loss of position and vibratory sensation may also be seen. Depression has also been described in affected patients.

Depression is also reported in association with *iron deficiency* . The anemia associated with this disorder, like other anemias, commonly produces lassitude and fatigue. More specific symptoms of depression may be attributable to the fact that iron is a component not just of hemoglobin but of numerous enzymes. Cytochrome oxidases, for example, are iron-containing enzymes found in mitochondria where they are crucial to cellular respiration. It seems reasonable to speculate that dysfunction of this enzyme system might cause protean symptoms, including depression.

The diagnosis of iron deficiency is suggested by a history of excessive blood loss (dietary deficiency is unusual but is seen in patients with bizarre diets, most notably in compulsive consumers of laundry starch or ice). Physical findings include conjunctival pallor, tachycardia, and, often, a systolic cardiac flow murmur. The hemogram and peripheral blood smear show a hypochromic, microcytic anemia. The ratio of serum iron to iron binding capacity is markedly low. And special staining of the bone marrow aspirate shows depleted iron stores.

Dietary *protein deficiency* , while rare in the developed world, is not uncommon in underdeveloped countries. Its manifestations in children (most notably in the child weaned prematurely from the breast or fed dilute commercial formula) are striking and include musclewasting, edema, diarrhea, lassitude, and growth retardation. Symptoms in the adult may be a bit more insidious, but again weight loss and wasting are prominent features. Weakness, edema, impotence, amenorrhea, and diarrhea are also common as is depression. The latter may be due in part to deficiency of the essential amino acids phenylalanine and tryptophan, precursors to the important neurotransmitters norepinephrine and serotonin (see above). (Essential amino acids cannot be synthesized in humans and must be supplied by dietary protein.)

Gastrointestinal disease

Cirrhosis is a nonspecific term that describes chronic fibrotic changes in the liver from any etiology. Chronic alcoholism is a common cause of the disorder. Cirrhosis may also be a sequela to severe infectious or drug-induced hepatitis (postnecrotic cirrhosis), and there are numerous less common etiologies.[104]

The clinical onset of cirrhosis is likely to be insidious and may be marked by complaints of fatigue, weakness and poor appetite—symptoms readily confused with depression. As the disorder progresses, more striking evidence of liver dysfunction appears, such as jaundice, edema, ascites, and spider telangiectasias. Physical examination may reveal liver enlargement, but as the disorder progresses the liver is apt to become scarred and shrunken. Splenomegaly may be seen secondary to an increase in portal venous pressure. Portal hypertension may also cause visible venous collaterals over the abdomen ("caput medusae") and may cause esophageal varices, which may bleed with disastrous results. Still further progression of the disorder is likely to result in hepatic encephalopathy, a delirious state unlikely to be confused with depression.

Early in the course of cirrhosis proper diagnosis may be very dependent upon obtaining a history of alcoholism or other insult to the liver. Physical findings may include any of those described above or may simply include stigmata of chronic alcoholism. In the laboratory, hepatocellular damage is likely to be reflected by elevation of serum lactic dehydrogenase (LDH) and SGOT. Hepatic insufficiency may be indicated by low serum albumin or by low BUN. Bilirubin may be elevated even in the absence of jaundice. Needle biopsy of the liver may be desirable for definitive diagnosis.

In the patient with depressive symptoms and evidence of cirrhosis it is important that *Wilson's disease* be considered. Early treatment is extremely important in this disorder, which will be more fully discussed below.

Much has been made of the psychological profile of the patient with *inflammatory bowel* disease. Classically, affected patients are somewhat perjoratively described as hostile, dependent, and depressed. It is generally agreed, however, that a great many affected patients fit no character profile; and it is arguable that hostility, dependence, and depression could very well be a result of this serious chronic illness.

The diagnosis of inflammatory bowel disease is suggested by episodic, severe, bloody diarrhea which often results in anemia and weight loss. Associated arthritis may be present, suggesting a generalized autoimmune process which may play a part in the genesis of depression. In the laboratory, examination of the stool for amebae and culture for enteric pathogens should rule out infectious colitis. Sigmoidoscopy and barium enema usually have features characteristic of either ulcerative colitis or regional (granulomatous) enteritis. (Small intestinal contrast studies are helpful to distinguish the latter, given its propensity for the small intestine). The erythrocyte sedimentation rate is usually elevated, with active disease, and antinuclear antibodies may be detected in the serum.

Malabsorption of protein and other essential nutrients may result from a host of small intestinal diseases and other disorders.[127] These disorders are commonly associated with long-standing diarrhea; and they may result in secondary deficiencies of protein, iron, vitamin B_{12} or folate— states discussed above as associated with depressive symptoms.

Celiac disease (nontropical sprue, gluten enteropathy) is a disorder associated with sensitivity of the small intestinal mucosa to gluten, a protein component of flour ground from wheat, barley, or rye. Affected patients develop blunting of intestinal villi, and malabsorption leads clinically to chronic diarrhea. Hallert et al have reported ten patients with adult celiac disease in whom depression was quantified by Minnesota Multiphasic Personality Inventory (MMPI) testing and in whom determinations of spinal fluid monoamine metabolites was made.[105] The group showed significant reductions in CSF 5-HIAA, MHPG, and homovanillic acid (HVA), a major dopamine metabolite. They also found that MHPG concentrations bore a significant inverse relationship to elevation of the MMPI depression scale. The authors speculate that malabsorption of monoamine precursors may account for these findings.

Katerndahl singled out *Whipple's disease* from among the malabsorption syndromes for special mention in connection with depression.[60] This rare type of malabsorption is associated with skin pigmentation and arthritis (again raising the question of a systemic autoimmune phenomonon). Diagnosis is made by small intestinal biopsy which shows "foamladen" macrophages in the lamina propria of the gut mucosa.[128]

Chronic pancreatitis is also associated with malabsorption, although fat malabsorption seems to be most prominent due to inadequate lipase activity. The disorder is usually a late sequela to chronic alcoholism. It may also occur in patients with gallstones (presumably secondary to obstruction of pancreatic drainage). The disease is usually characterized by bouts of acute upper abdominal pain associated with elevation of serum amylase levels. Abdominal films may reveal pancreatic calcification. Depression has been noted as a concomitant of chronic pancreatitis. Whether this is a specific response or a nonspecific response to chronic disease is not clear. *Acute* pancreatitis, on the other hand, is known to produce a toxic psychosis which is probably directly related to perturbations in fluid and electrolyte balance.

Collagen-vascular disease   This group of diseases is obscure in origin and protean in expression. These disorders seem to have in common a disturbance in immune function, with an allergic type of reaction being mounted against the body's own tissues. It is tempting to speculate that autoantibodies may be formed which are specific to CNS monoamine receptors and act as blockers at these receptor sites, a situation analogous to that seen in patients with myasthenia gravis who have demonstrable antibodies to cholinergic receptors at the myoneural junction. Whether by this or by some more complex mechanism, the collagen vascular diseases often present with depression.

Systemic lupus erythematosus (SLE) is a disorder most commonly seen in females from 13 to 40 years of age.[106] It is a chronic disease marked by episodic relapses and remissions and affecting every organ system. The disease is likely to present with nonspecific symptoms such as fatigue, malaise, anorexia, and weight loss. Unless fever is detected these symptoms may well be ascribed to simple depression.

As the disease progresses its systemic nature becomes apparent. Skin lesions of various sorts may be seen (although the classic malar "butterfly rash" is relatively uncommon). The joints are commonly involved, and such involvement ranges from vague arthralgias without objective findings to acute or at times chronic and deforming arthritis. Nephritic changes may lead to renal failure.

Lupus vasculitis may cause circulatory impairment to any organ, although the brain is perhaps the most dramatically affected. Depending upon the vessels involved, neurologic deficits of virtually any type may be seen. Organic psychosis is not uncommon in this setting and may be confused with steroid-induced psychosis, since these drugs are central to the treatment of active SLE.

In the laboratory, SLE is characterized by elevation of the ESR and by the presence of antinuclear antibodies. More diagnostic is a positive LE cell preparation. Biopsy of skin, muscle, or lymph nodes may yield diagnostic microscopical findings.

Rheumatoid arthritis is also a systemic disease, whose major feature is a hypertrophic, inflammatory reaction in the synovial lining of joints. Due to its chronic nature the disorder often produces crippling joint abnormalities. The onset of illness is likely to be insidious, however, and fatigue, anorexia, and weight loss may dominate the picture. Again, depression may well be the mistaken diagnosis. The onset of fever and frank polyarthritis (redness, swelling, and joint tenderness) should raise a suspicion of rheumatoid arthritis. The presence of subcutaneous (rheumatoid) nodules should increase that suspicion. In the laboratory, an elevated sedimentation rate serves as a nonspecific indicator of ongoing inflammation. Serologic tests for rheumatoid factor are considerably more specific and are positive in roughly 80% of adults with rheumatoid arthritis.[107]

Nonspecific complaints may also herald the onset of *polyarteritis nodosa*, a relatively uncommon disorder marked by inflammation and thrombosis of small arteries. Fatigue, anorexia, weight loss, headache, and aching muscles may be readily ascribed to depression. Fever should alert the physician to something beyond uncomplicated depression. Nodules in the skin or subcutaneous tissues may be an aid to proper diagnosis. Joint soreness and aching, tender muscles are often seen. Abdominal pain is a common feature. Arteritis may affect virtually any organ; and infarction of myocardium, liver, kidneys, *or brain* may be seen. The latter obviously may result in a wide array of focal neurologic deficits. Peripheral neuritis is a fairly common feature and is presumably due to involvement of the vasa nervorum. Hypertension may be present.

In the laboratory, polyarteritis nodosa is characterized by elevation of the white blood count with a predominance of neutrophils. Eosinophilia may also be seen. The sedimentation rate is high. A wide array of serum protein abnormalities may be seen (eg, hyperglobulinemia). Skin or muscle biopsy may confirm the diagnosis.

Temporal or giant cell arteritis is a rare disorder that is felt by some to represent a variant of polyarteritis nodosa. The dominant feature of the disease is a vasculitis that shows a predilection for the temporal and occipital arteries. In its classic form, temporal arteritis presents in a patient over 50 years of age with throbbing headache and swollen, nodular, tender temporal or occipital arteries. If the disease involves carotid, ophthalmic or retinal arteries, serious visual impairment may occur. As with the other collagen vascular diseases, however, the onset of temporal arteritis may be insidious and fatigue, anorexia, and weight loss may suggest depression.

Polymyalgia rheumatica is a condition that is often a prodrome to temporal arteritis, presenting with weakness, sore muscles, and other vague constitutional symptoms. Elevation of the sedimentation rate may be the only clear objective datum suggesting serious illness. Since treatment with corticosteriods may be crucial to saving the patient's sight, a high index of suspicion is important in the elderly patient with headache and constitutional symptoms. The temporal and occipital arteries should be palpated. Nodular, tender segments may be biopsied to confirm the diagnosis.

Central nervous system disease   Since the brain is the putative seat of emotion (the liver having long since lost favor in this regard), it is not surprising that some CNS diseases may mimic depression. Among these is *multiple sclerosis* (MS), a chronic demyelinating disease with a highly variable course usually marked by periods of remission. Since any part of the nervous system's white matter may be affected by the disease, MS is associated with protean neurologic deficits. The diagnosis should be suspected in the younger patient with symptoms pointing to lesions in disparate parts of the CNS. Such deficits may remit at least partially, usually to be followed by exacerbation of the illness. The clinical suspicion of MS may be supported by finding elevation of CSF γ-globulin. Measuring visual, auditory, or somatosensory evoked potentials may reveal even subclinical demyelination.

The ravages of multiple sclerosis may in time lead to secondary depression (yet some patients show mild euphoria, their frontal lobe involvement presumably sparing them from the gravity of their disability). This should not be difficult to diagnose in the face of well-established neurologic deficits. Some patients with MS, on the other hand, will *present* with depression; and this may precede other localizing signs. Goodstein and Ferrell report three such patients, two of whom received multiple courses of antidepressant treatment (including electroshock) to no avail before "hard" neurologic signs supervened and proper diagnosis was made.[108]

Depression has long been noted as a concomitant of *Parkinson's disease* , with estimates of incidence ranging from 40% to 90%.[109] Given the chronic, disabling nature of the disease, one must suspect that much of this depression is reactive in nature (secondary depression). Asnis has suggested, however, that Parkinson's disease and primary depression may share a common pathogenesis.[109] He reports a patient with Parkinson's disease and depression whose extrapyramidal symptoms (resting tremor, bradykinesia, masklike facies, festinating gait, decreased arm swing, micrographia) responded favorably to electroconvulsive therapy (ECT) even before his depression responded. Asnis goes on to cite postmortem studies showing not only decreased dopamine but decreased norepinephrine and serotonin in the brains of patients with Parkinson's disease. He points to ECT increases of brain tyrosine hydroxylase activity and posits that this could be responsible for increased synthesis of dopamine and its metabolite norepinephrine, thus explaining improvement of both extrapyramidal symptoms and depression.

The distinction between primary depression and *dementia* can represent a challenge even to the geriatrician. Symptoms of depression in the elderly are often comingled with signs of cognitive disturbance (impairment of memory, ability to calculate, of judgment and orientation). Improvement of cognitive loss with antidepressant treatment has led to the concept of "depressive pseudodementia."[111] Often, however, even successful use of antidepressants yields but partial improvement in symptoms of dementia, supporting the notion that dementia and depression commonly coexist. Drawing upon his large experience at the interface between psychiatry and internal medicine, Altschule points out that it is not uncommon for symptoms of agitated depression to herald the onset of idiopathic dementia (Alzheimer's disease).[7] The differential diagnosis of dementia will be discussed separately (see chapter 3).

Brain tumors usually cause discrete loss of neurologic function before attaining great size. Tumors of the frontal and temporal lobes often present exceptions to this rule and may grow undetected for months or even years. Depression may be the only associated symptom in such cases. As such tumors become advanced, impaired judgment and memory may supervene, and severe headache may reflect intracranial hypertension. In such cases examination of the optic discs commonly shows papilledema. The occurrence of seizures should lead to a prompt search for structural brain disease. More specific signs may occur, depending upon the location and spread of the tumor. Frontal lobe tumors involving the inferior surface may impair olfactory nerve function leading to anosmia. Deep temporal lobe tumors may impinge upon optic radiations causing a contralateral, homonymous superior quadrant visual field defect. Posterior extension of frontal lobe tumors may lead to involvement of the motor cortex, while posterior and superior spread of temporal lobe tumors may produce fluent aphasia.

It should be remembered, of course, that the term "brain tumor" is generic and is used to describe an intracerebral mass of *any* kind. Such tumor may represent primary neoplasm (eg, glioma); metastatic cancer (the brain is a common site of blood-borne metastasis; lung cancer is a particularly common primary source), abscess, granuloma, or other less common processes (*Echinococcus* cyst, etc).

The sequelae of *stroke* are such that depression may be seen as a logical reaction to this disorder. However, Robinson et al suggest that depression may be a product of stroke that is *independent* of the severity of neurologic loss.[7,114] Following a group of 103 patients attending a stroke clinic, Robinson and Price found that depression was more likely to ensue from a left hemispheric stroke than from right hemispheric injury and that injury to the left frontal area seemed to confer particular vulnerability to depression.[115] Depression arising from such injury was described as often severe, with suicide occurring at times. Without treatment, such depression was noted to last an average of 7 or 8 months. Treatment with antidepressants and psychotherapy seemed to have a beneficial effect.

All of these findings may be seen as supporting the hypothesis that depression may be a *direct* result of some strokes, particularly those affecting the left frontal area. Neurologic findings in stroke affecting the frontal lobes may be less than striking unless cortical damage has extended caudally to involve the motor cortex (with resultant hemiparesis). Cognitive and behavioral change may dominate the clinical picture. Physical findings may be limited to pathologic reflexes (eg, grasp, suck, rooting reflexes). The CT scan may be extremely helpful in localizing an area of infarcted cerebral cortex.

Huntington's disease (chronic chorea) is a devastating disorder characterized by progressive dementia and variable disturbances in movement (generally a writhing, choreoathetoid movement). The disease is inherited in autosomal dominant fashion. Gene penetrance seems to be quite high, and the disorder usually begins insidiously in middle age. Diagnosis is made on the basis of family history and the findings of dementia and choreoathetosis (these symptoms usually develop concomitantly). Since the movement disorder is felt to reflect hypersensitivity of the basal ganglia to dopamine, dopamine challenge has become a controversial means of early diagnosis of the disease. CT scanning may reveal brain atrophy, particularly in the area of the basal ganglia.

While depression may be seen as a reaction to any chronic, disabling disease, severe depression seems to be particularly common in this disorder. Suicide is described as a frequent occurrence.[129,130] Whether or not such depression is in part a direct product of the disease process is arguable. Given the extensive neuronal loss that occurs with this disorder it is not unreasonable to suspect impairment of monoamine pathways that are crucial to mood.

Subdural hematoma is a result of traumatic disruption of small veins and leaking of blood into the subdural space. The blood clots, and the organized clot may, in time, become calcified. The subdural collection's effect upon the brain is a mass effect, and in that regard subdural hematomas may be considered a "special case" of brain tumor (see above). Depending upon the function of the underlying cortex, varying neurologic deficits may be seen. Headache, papilledema, and generalized convulsions are not uncommon. The history of trauma may not be evident (and should be suspected in those prone to falls, such as the elderly, and the alcoholic). And the onset of clinical signs may be insidious. Lethargy, irritability. and forgetfulness may suggest a functional disturbance such as depression. Progressive clouding of consciousness should alert the clinician to the more emergent situation, and the CT scan should reveal the mass effect of the subdural. (The collection of blood in the acute subdural is usually readily seen on the CT scan. The anemic patient may pose a problem here since blood with a Hct in the low 30s is radiographically isodense with brain tissue.)

Temporal lobe epilepsy (complex partial seizure disorder) has been previously discussed (see chapter 1). The *inter*ictal personality of the temporal lobe epileptic is apt to be marked by affective lability, and depressive mood swings may be pronounced. Correct diagnosis depends upon eliciting a history suggesting psychomotor seizures (episodic, self-limited alterations in perception and thought ... stereotyped, "automatic" behavior may also be seen along with clouding or loss of consciousness).[131] Major motor seizures are often seen as a concomitant of temporal lobe epilepsy and so may turn up in the review of systems. Diagnosis may be confirmed by finding temporal lobe dysrhythmia on the EEG.

Myasthenia gravis is a disorder of the neuromuscular junction, characterized clinically by easy fatigability. Any muscle group may be affected, but the muscles of the head (facial, oculomotor, laryngeal, and pharyngeal muscles) and the respiratory muscles are most commonly affected. The examiner may be able to demonstrate rapid fatigue with exercise of involved muscles (ptosis of the eyelids is often demonstrable). Intravenous injection of edrophonium chloride (Tensilon) produces instant dramatic reversal of myasthenic weakness and is an important diagnostic tool.

The course of myasthenia gravis is highly variable. The disease may be progressive or may remain stable for long periods. In cases of progressive illness, secondary depression may be seen, just as it might be in any other chronic, debilitating disease. On the other hand, Emery and Szymanski have reported a 17-year-old patient in whom vague somatic complaints were accompanied by mixed symptoms of anxiety and depression.[118] Indeed, major depression was diagnosed before the definitive diagnosis of myasthenia gravis was made during an episode of acute respiratory failure.

Miscellaneous disorders associated with depression

Sarcoidosis is a systemic disease of unknown etiology characterized by granuloma formation which may involve virtually any organ system. The clinical presentation of the illness, of course, depends upon the organs involved. At times, sarcoidosis may present with only vague constitutional symptoms (low-grade fever, fatigue, malaise, weakness, weight loss). But for the presence of fever, which may be slight, this picture might be mistaken for depression. The meninges and cerebral cortex itself may become involved in granuloma formation, in which case discrete neurologic deficits may occur. Frontal or temporal lobe involvement might create a picture with prominent affective changes, including depression.

Patients with sarcoidosis commonly exhibit lymphadenopathy. Enlargement of pulmonary hilar lymph nodes is usually noted on chest film. In addition, the lung parenchyma may be involved, and respiratory symptoms such as cough and dyspnea are common. Proper diagnosis depends upon demonstrating the clinical and radiologic picture of sarcoid. Biopsy of involved tissues (eg, lymph node, liver, skin) may be confirmatory. Skin testing (the Kveim test) is positive in 50% to 80% of affected patients.[132]

Wilson's disease, a familial disorder of copper homeostasis which results in pathologic deposition of copper in both brain and liver, has been discussed previously (see chapter 1). The disease is characterized classically by cirrhosis, a brownish corneal ring of pigment (the Kayser-Fleischer ring), and by evidence of basal ganglion dysfunction. It is not uncommon, however, for psychiatric symptoms to precede these findings. A wide range of premonitory symptoms have been described, including major affective disturbances.[81]

The appearance of tremor, rigidity, or other dyskinesia in the young patient with recent change in affect or personality should raise the suspicion of Wilson's disease. Similarly, derangement of liver function studies, even in the absence of clinical liver disease, should prompt further investigation. Abnormal corneal pigment should be looked for. Depressed levels of serum copper and its carrier protein ceruloplasmin should also be sought.

Depression associated with *cranial irradiation* has been discussed above. Depression has also been described as a concomitant of amyloidosis and psoriasis.[81] Documentation of this association is not strong, and it is difficult to rule out secondary or reactive depression in these chronic diseases.

Finally, Leonidas has reported three cases of *factitious depression* which underscore the perils of cross-cultural psychiatry.[121] All three patients were Haitian immigrants who presented to physicians complaining of fatigue. In Haitian dialect, "depression" is the word used to describe physical exhaustion, having no connotation whatever of affective disturbance. As it turned out, all three patients had ample reason to be overtired (two from overwork, one from sexual heroics), and all three had unnecessary psychiatric referrals.

Trauma

Depression may be seen as a sequela to any serious trauma and as such may be seen as a reaction to loss of physical function or bodily integrity. The patient with *spinal cord injury* stands as a poignant example of this sort of loss. Often associated with devastating loss of function, spinal cord injury has an ironic proclivity for the young and the active, people for whom the loss is only more dramatic.

It has commonly been assumed that most, if not all, patients with permanent disability from spinal cord injury become depressed.[133,134] Fullerton et al have taken a careful look at diagnosis in a series of 30 patients with spinal cord injury, finding but nine patients (30%) who met research diagnostic criteria for depression following their injury.[135] Depression seemed to be equally distributed between paraplegics and quadriplegics in this series. However, complete cord transection had a higher association with depression than did partial transection. While this study still shows depression to be a common sequela to spinal cord injury, it shows it to be far from universal and suggests that careful diagnostic scrutiny might lead to confusion between despondency (which must approach 100%) and depression.

Any mutilating injury may give rise to clinical depression. This is exemplified by the most visible form of disfigurement: *facial injury* . Nordlicht has summarized his experience with patients suffering from serious facial trauma.[136] He points out that mutilating injury may signify to the unconscious a fulfillment of the threat underlying "castration anxiety." And he goes on to assert that facial disfigurement is virtually always followed by a period of mourning and that such mourning may give way to frank depression.

While depression following trauma that is mutilating or debilitating seems to be psychological in origin and related to feelings of loss, depression following certain brain injuries may have a more direct, biologic basis. Temporal lobe epilepsy has been associated with depression, and frontotemporal brain tumors have been known to produce depressive states.[137,138] Hambert and Willen, however, have reported two patients with prolonged, treatment-resistant, severe depressions (culminating in suicide), both of which were associated with old frontotemporal lobe trauma.[139]

Robinson and Szetela have studied depression in a group of patients with left hemispheric strokes or trauma.[140] Controlling for the degree of clinical neurologic impairment and of lesion size (indicated by CT scanning), they found that severity of depression could be correlated to proximity of the lesion to the frontal pole. They suggest that these more anterior lesions may cause depression by interrupting critical neuronal pathways (eg, catecholamine-rich pathways) in the frontal cortex.

Ross and Rush report several cases of depression in brain damaged patients and underscore some of the difficulties in establishing the diagnosis.[141] *Right hemispheric damage* , they point out, may lead to disturbance in the reporting of feelings, and the resultant flat affect may be misconstrued as depression. (On the other hand the flat, matter-of-fact reporting of severe dysphoria may lead the clinician to an *under* estimation of the patient's depression.)

Bilateral brain damage may be associated with the affective dyscontrol seen in *pseudobulbar palsy* . Patients with this disturbance show marked lability of affect, with episodic laughter or crying that is unprovoked and seems to come from "out of the blue."

Major depression may coexist with the confusing picture of pseudobulbar palsy or right hemispheric injury. Its detection may be difficult, however.[141] Vegetative symptoms (eg, sleep or appetite disturbance) should also be looked for, their presence suggesting *bona fide* depression regardless of the confounding presence of brain damage.

Surgical Complications

Inasmuch as surgery is often associated with loss of function or of bodily integrity, it is not surprising that depression is a common sequel. (In fact, acute depression has been reported in anticipation of surgery.)[142] Titchener reported on a series of 200 surgical patients randomly selected over the course of 1 year.[143] Of these, roughly 4% suffered from major depression during the postoperative course. In the series of Stengel et al, 80 postoperative patients were referred for psychiatric consultation over 5 years; 45% had depressive illness.[144]

Certain surgical procedures have been particularly associated with depressive sequelae. *Mastectomy* is one such procedure. Maguire et al followed a group of 75 women for 1 year following mastectomy, finding that 21% suffered from moderate or severe depression after 1 year (compared with 8% of controls with benign breast disease).[145]

Worden and Weisman studied 40 patients with newly diagnosed breast cancer, finding 20% who reported frank depression.[146] In a comparison group of women with other malignancy, 18% reported depression, leading these authors to question the special significance of breast cancer surgery in the pathogenesis of depression.

Hysterectomy also represents, for some, an important symbolic loss; and depression is reported in association with this operation. Reports on the frequency of posthysterectomy depression vary widely. Melody reported an incidence of roughly 4% in the first 3 months postoperatively.[147] Richards cited a 36.5% incidence over the course of 5 years, later revising this figure to 70%.[148] This wide disparity suggests that these data are flawed. Among the other factors that confound a pure analysis of the effect of hysterectomy is the premorbid mental condition of the women under study. It has been suggested, for instance, that women with *pre* -existing depression may be more likely to undergo hysterectomy than their emotionally stable peers. Ananth has written a thorough review of the complex interplay between depression and hysterectomy.[149]

While not associated with the depressive morbidity for which hysterectomy is noted, *sterilization* by tubal ligation may have a similar emotional outcome. Elison reported two relatively small series of patients in which there was a 30% incidence of posttubal ligation depression, compared to an 80% incidence after hysterectomy.[150]

Abortion may also be associated with depression although the literature on this is surprisingly scant. Cavenar et al, for example, report two women who suffered depressions after therapeutic abortions.[151] In both cases depression occurred at the anniversary of what would have been birth had the pregnancies been carried to term. The authors surmise that these depressions represent incomplete or pathologic mourning for the loss of the fetus.

Psychiatrists have become well-integrated into many organ transplant teams, and there has been considerable experience in observing the sequelae of *kidney transplantation* . McCabe and Corry, for example, report 20 kidney recipients, followed over 18 months.[152] Eight of these (40%) met research diagnostic criteria for depression. The authors caution that these data may reflect the common association of depression with any severe or chronic medical illness. They also note the virtually universal use of corticosteroids in these patients to manage graft rejection. In addition, antihypertensive medicines are very commonly required by these patients. The association of depression with use of these drugs has been previously discussed.

Psychiatric Illness

Depression forms at least a facet of many psychiatric illnesses. (Again, the term "psychiatric illness" is used advisedly. It is only slightly preferable to "functional illness." In either case an absence of biologic determinants is implied. As our understanding of these disorders grows, such assumption is likely to be found wanting.) Distinguishing among these takes on special importance in view of the specificity of various biologic treatments (lithium, antidepressant drugs, electroshock). Recent trends in psychiatric diagnosis, which are typified in the third edition of the American Psychiatric Association's *Diagnostic and Statistical Manual* (DSM-III),[153] have shown movement toward greater diagnostic rigor. This, in turn, should lead to more selective and rational use of antidepressant treatments.

Major depression represents the paradigm of depressive disorders, and as perhaps the most treatable of these disorders it should be strongly considered. It is a common malady affecting as much as 15% of the population at some time during their life (lifetime prevalence rates for women [20% to 26%] are considerably higher than those for men [8% to 12%]).[154] The causes of this disorder may be genetic, biochemical, psychological, or a mixture of these (see above). Previously, depression seen in the setting of high psychosocial stress ("reactive" depression) was distinguished from other severe, "endogenous" depression. This distinction does not seem particularly useful clinically, since major depression may have both reactive and endogenous features.

The clinical picture of major depression was described earlier in this chapter. Central to the diagnosis is the presence of persistent "dysphoric mood"[153] (Table 2-3). Affected patients describe sadness, fearfulness, and loss of pleasure in life. They may also be noted to be irritable.

In addition to the mood disturbance, DSM-III requries documentation of at least four cardinal symptoms of depression, seen consistently for at least 2 weeks. These symptoms include: (1) *appetite disturbance* (either decrease, or, less typically, increase); (2) *sleep disturbance* (insomnia, or, less typically, hypersomnia); (3) slowing of speech, thought, and action (*psychomotor retardation* ; less typically, agitation may be seen); (4) *reduced sex drive* or loss of interest in other pleasurable activity; (5) *loss of physical energy* ; (6) feelings of *worthlessness and guilt* ; (7) impaired ability to concentrate; (8) preoccupation with *death or suicide*.

Almost invariably, a thorough history and mental status examination will provide data enough to strongly suspect major depression. Past medi-

Table 2-3
Psychiatric Differential Diagnosis of the Depressed Patient

I. Major depression
II. Manic depressive illness (bipolar disorder, depressed)
III. Dysthymic disorder (depressive neurosis)
IV. Cyclothymic disorder
V. Personality disorder, particularly borderline personality disorder
VI. Normal bereavement
VII. Adjustment disorder with depressed mood
VIII. Depression secondary to schizophrenia, anxiety disorder, somatoform disorder

---

cal history should be explored and review of systems done (including current drug use) in view of the numerous organic states that may mimic major depression. Physical examination of the patient with uncomplicated major depression may show nothing beyond psychomotor retardation and, frequently, an ill-kempt appearance.

Laboratory findings in major depression are of somewhat limited help due to the low sensitivity of currently available tests (see above). Instead, having established rigorous clinical criteria for the disorder, the physician will usually prescribe either electroshock or antidepressant drug therapy. Both of these treatments are highly effective if done correctly.

Depression seen in the context of *manic-depressive illness* (bipolar disorder) is likely to be indistinguishable from major depression as described above. Indeed, the detection of bipolar disorder is not of great consequence in the treatment of the acutely depressed patient. (On the other hand, the *long-term* management of bipolar illness is the highest indication for lithium therapy, a treatment with unquestionable benefit for this disorder.) Antidepressant drugs or electroshock are usually effective in treating either unipolar depression or bipolar depressed patients. (The latter group, however, may shift from depression into mania as a result of antidepressant treatment.)

The history of a manic episode is what separates bipolar from unipolar depressive illness. Mania is characterized by DSM-III as a period of "elevated, expansive, or irritable mood."[153] This is seen in concert with at least three of the following symptoms, lasting for a week or more:

1. Increase in activity, restlessness
2. Increased talking, pressured speech

3. Flight of ideas or "racing thoughts"
4. Grandiosity
5. Decreased need for sleep
6. Distractibility
7. Poor judgment, indiscretion in sexual, financial and other activity[153]

Some patients with bipolar illness will not have a clear history of manic episodes, and only longitudinal follow-up may reveal the true nature of the illness. Yet others will manifest clear depressed episodes, and *forme fruste* manic episodes (bipolar-II disorder).

Dysthmic disorder may initially be mistaken for major depression. Indeed, the two disorders have many symptoms in common, including dysphoric mood, fatigue, sleep disturbance, loss of interest in pleasurable activities, and suicidal thoughts.[153] Confronted with these symptoms, the clinician is often moved to prescribe antidepressant medicine. Poor or partial response to multiple antidepressants often leads to a reassessment of diagnosis and a retrospective finding of dysthmic disorder.

Two features serve to distinguish dysthymic disorder from major depression. One is its chronicity. Depression is shown to have been fairly persistent for at least 2 years. Some patients recall persistent depression since childhood. This is in clear distinction from major depression which can be seen as much more of an intercurrent illness. Second, the depressive symptoms of dysthymic disorder are of insufficient severity to meet the criteria for major depression.[153] Severity of symptoms may be difficult to quantify, however. It is our experience that the strident complaints of the dysthymic patient may well lead to a diagnosis of major depression (perhaps by activating a sense of distress and despair within the clinician). It is only after one learns that the stridency is chronic, as is the psychic pain, that dysthymia comes to be considered. The question "When was the last time you did not feel depressed?" may be extremely useful in identifying this common disorder.

Cyclothymic disorder is to manic-depressive illness what dysthymic disorder is to major depression. It is a chronic (at least 2 years duration) disorder marked by depressive and hypomanic mood swings, neither of which is sufficient in severity to meet criteria for major depression or mania.[153] In keeping with these severity criteria, there are no associated psychotic features (delusions, hallucinations, major derangement of thought), such as one might see in major affective illness. It should be noted that the patient with cyclothymic disorder may suffer from an intercurrent episode of major depression or mania. Treatment and recovery from such an episode should be expected to lead to a return to the cyclothymic baseline.

Personality disorders represent chronic, fixed, maladaptive ways of dealing with life. They have their onset in childhood or adolescence and dominate adult behavior. The patient with a personality (or character) disorder is likely to be impaired at work and unhappy in his relationships. As a result of this, depression is a common secondary feature of character disorder.

It is beyond the scope of this chapter to describe the diversity of character disorder. Such a problem should be suspected when depression is an outgrowth of chronic disturbance in relationships and effectiveness. Such depression is itself likely to be chronic. It should also be of insufficient severity to qualify as major depression. (Major depression may be superimposed upon personality disorder, however. So, the two diagnoses are not at all mutually exclusive.)

Among the personality disorders, one is particularly marked by its depressive features, as well as by the ferment almost invariably raised in its treatment. *Borderline personality disorder* is marked by intense, labile affect with depression and anger dominating the clinical picture.[155] The disorder is also characterized by impulsive behavior which often is self-destructive. Suicide gestures and self-mutilation are common. The borderline patient's relationships are marked by instability and by unreasonable idealization and equally unreasonable hatred and deprecation. It is in the tangled web of these relationships that the physician becomes involved, and he, too, becomes manipulated and alternately lionized or devalued. Complicating the picture further, the borderline patient may suffer brief periods of psychosis.

The pain of the borderline patient is likely to be well transmitted to the physician, and the mistaken diagnosis of major depression may be made, in part out of a wish to "do something." The therapeutic trial with antidepressant drugs is unlikely to meet with success and may simply culminate in impulsive drug overdose.

Normal bereavement may be mistaken for major depression, with resultant unnecessary use of antidepressants. The patient who has recently suffered a major loss, such as the death of a spouse, may be despondent and tearful. He may complain of difficulty sleeping and of poor appetite and loss of energy and interest. He may feel that life is no longer worth living. What sets him apart from the patient with depression is preservation of his self-esteem.[153,156,157] As bad as he feels, he does not feel worthless and does not feel the heavy burden of guilt. Furthermore, he does not suffer major impairment of his function. He is likely to view his sadness as normal. His physicians should see it likewise and need offer treatment no more aggressive than understanding and support.

While normal bereavement is likely to follow the death of a loved one, *adjustment disorder with depressed mood* may be seen as a response to other situational stressors.[153] These might include job loss or other financial mishaps, physical illness, natural disaster, etc. In any case the depressive response will be noted to be in excess of that expected from the given stressor, or it will be noted to impair the patient's level of function. (In the absence of such severity, one would simply diagnose a "problem in living" or "life circumstance problem." [153]) At the same time the depressive symptoms will not be of sufficient severity and duration to diagnose major depression. The natural history of adjustment disorder is such that the symptoms remit after resolution of the stressful precipitant.

Finally, depression may be seen as a secondary feature of a number of psychiatric disorders. Usually the primary disorder will be apparent, and depression may be seen as a reaction to this.

For example, depression is commonly seen in the course of *schizophrenia* . Roy reports a 6-year study of 100 paranoid schizophrenics, of whom 30% experienced symptoms of major depression superimposed upon their illness.[158] Others have suggested that the "flat affect" of the schizophrenic bespeaks depression. Ager and Milstein studied a group of 96 schizophrenic patients with flat affect using a self-rating depression scale.[159] While none of the patients appeared depressed or complained of depression, *all* gave test results suggesting moderate to severe depression.

The genesis of depression in the schizophrenic patient is not clear. Some have suggested that it is a result of damaged self-esteem.[160] MacKinnon, on the other hand, reported a case where control of grandiose psychotic symptoms resulted in a profound sense of loss.[161] Attempts to treat "postpsychotic depression" as a variant of major depression have generally been unsuccessful, suggesting a basic biologic difference between the disorders. Response to antidepressant drugs is generally disappointing, and treatment of the underlying schizophrenia remains the treatment of choice.[162]

The patient with *catatonic schizophrenia* may be difficult to distinguish from the depressed patient with profound psychomotor retardation. Here a past history of either schizophrenia or of affective illness may be extremely helpful in making the distinction. Also a positive family history for affective illness makes depression the more likely choice.

It is not unusual for the patient with an *anxiety disorder* to develop secondary depression. The impairment of function often attendant upon these disorders is likely to lead to a strong sense of loss and to impairment of self-esteem. This phenomenon seems to be particularly common in agoraphobia but may be seen in the course of other anxiety disorders as well. The clinical picture is usually dominated by the anxiety disorder, so that the secondary nature of the depression is clear.

The *somatizing patient* (see chapter 5) commonly complains of depression. Depression in such patients, who are characterized by chronic physical complaints or concerns, may be seen as similar to depression secondary to any other chronic illness. It matters little that there can usually be found no physiologic basis for the patient's symptoms. His dysfunction is every bit as real to him as if it had the clearest pathophysiology.

It is often suggested that psychogenic pain and other somatoform symptoms represent an unconscious defense against depression (that they are "depressive equivalents."[163,164] To the degree that depression is seen in the somatizing patient, this defense may be seen as unsuccessful. The depression seen by the clinician in this setting may then be the "tip of the iceberg," and some argue for empirical treatment of the somatizing patient with antidepressant measures.[163,164] In any event, the diagnostic primacy of the somatoform disorder is not likely to be missed by the clinician, whose skill and patience are put to the test by these patients.

In summary, depression may be a feature of a number of psychiatric disorders. It is an important task for the clinician to identify from among these the patient with major depression (or bipolar disorder, depressed). Such patients have a high likelihood of responding to treatment with antidepressant drugs or electroshock. Patients with other depressive disorders are much less likely to respond to these biologic treatments.

REFERENCES

1. Plutzky M: Identifying the depressed patient. *Primary Care* 1980;7:585-594.
2. Blumer D, Heilbronn M: Chronic pain as a variant of depressive disease. *J Nerv Ment Dis* 1982;170:381-408.
3. Drucker J, Heetner J, Wilder R: Depression in a medical setting. *Minn Med* 1980;June:399-404.
4. Anstett R, Poole S: Depressive equivalents in adults. *Am Fam Physician* 1982;25:151-156.
5. The polysymptomatic melancholic as patient in the internist's office, editorial. *Acta Med Scand* 1981;209:433-436.

118

6. Melville H: *Moby Dick*. New York, WW Norton, 1976, p 1.

7. Altschule M: Depression as seen by the internist. *DM* 1977;24:1-47.

8. Schlesser M, Winokur G, Sherman BM: Hypothalamic-pituitary-adrenal axis activity in depressive illness. *Arch Gen Psychiatry* 1980;37:737-743.

9. Sachar EJ, Asnis G, Nathan RS, et al: Dextroamphetamine and cortisol in depression. *Arch Gen Psychiatry* 1980;37:755-757.

10. Carroll BJ, Curtis GC, Mendels J: Neuroendocrine regulation in depression. *Arch Gen Psychiatry* 1976;33:1039-1044.

11. Carroll BJ, Feinberg M, Greden JF, et al: A specific laboratory test for the diagnosis of melancholia. *Arch Gen Psychiatry* 1981;38:15-22.

12. Aguilar MT, Lemaire M, Castro ML, et al: Study of the diagnostic value of the dexamethasone suppression test in endogenous depression. *J Affective Disord* 1984;6:33-42.

13. Davies J, Hall J, McFarlane A: Methodological standards in studies evaluating the dexamethasone suppression test. *Aust NZ J Psychiatry* 1984;18:273-276.

14. Kocsis JH, Davis JM, Katz MM: Depressive behavior and hyperactive adrenocortical function. *Am J Psychiatry* 1985;142:1291-1298.

15. Prange AJ, Wilson IC, Lara PP, et al: Effects of thyrotropin releasing hormone in depression. *Lancet* 1972;2:999-1002.

16. Gold MS, Pottash ALC, Extein I, et al: Diagnosis of depression in the 1980's. *JAMA* 1981;245:1562-1564.

17. van Praag HM: The significance of biological factors in the diagnosis of depressions: II hormonal variables. *Compr Psychiatry* 1982;23:216-226.

18. Spitz RA: Anaclitic depression. *Psychoanal Study Child* 1946;2:213 ff.

19. Bowlby J: *Attachment and Loss* . New York, Basic Books, 1969.

20. Spitz R: Hospitalism, in *The Psychoanalytic Study of the Child* . New York, International Universities Press, 1945, Vol 1, pp 53-74; 1946, Vol 2, pp 113-117.

21. Lindemann E: Symptomatology and management of acute grief. *Am J Psychiatry* 1944;101:141 ff.

22. Freud S: Mourning and melancholia, *Standard Edition of the Complete Psychological Works of Sigmund Freud* , Strachey J (trans). London, Hogarth Press, 1953-1966.

23. Maas JW, Hattox SE, Green NM, et al: 3-Methoxy-4-hydroxyphenylglycol (MHPG) excretion in depressive patients. *Arch Gen Psychiatry* 1968;19:129-134.

24. van Praag HM: The significance of biological factors in the diagnosis of depressions: I Biochemical variables. *Compr Psychiatry* 1982;23:124-235.

25. Goodwin FK, Potter WZ: Norepinephrine metabolite studies in affective illness, in Usdin E, Kopin IJ, Barchas J (eds):*Catecholamines: Basic and Clinical Frontiers* , ed 2. New York, Pergamon, 1979.

26. Maas JW, Fawcett JA, Dekirmenjien H: Catecholamine metabolism, depressive illness, and drug response. *Arch Gen Psychiatry* 1972;26:252-262.

27. Schildkraut JJ: Norepinephrine metabolism as biochemical criteria for classifying depressive disorders and predicting responses to treatment. *Am J Psychiatry* 1973;130:695-699.

28. van Praag HM, Korf J: Endogenous depressions with and without disturbances in the 5-hydroxytrypamine metabolism: a biochemical classification? *Psychopharmacol* 1971;19:148-152.

29. Asbert M, Thoren P, Traskman L, et al: "Serotonin depression": a biochemical subgroup within the affective disorders? *Science* 1976;191:478-480.

30. van Praag HM: Evidence of serotonin-deficient depression. *Neuropsychobiol* 1977;3:56-63.

31. Petrie WM, Maffucci RJ, Woosley RL: Propranolol and depression. *Am J Psychiatry* 1982;139:92-94.

32. McNeil GN, Shaw PK, Dock DS: Substitution of atenolol for propranolol in a case of propranolol-related depression. *Am J Psychiatry* 1982;139:1187-1188.

33. Pandey GN, Dysken MW, Garver DL, et al: Beta adrenergic receptor function in affective illness. *Am J Psychiatry* 1979;136:675-678.

34. Pert CB: A request for serum samples from psychiatric patients with associated autoimmune disease: is some psychosis caused by an autoimmune response to neurotransmitter receptors? *Comm, Psychopharmacol* 1977;1:307-309.

35. Motulsky HJ, Insel PA: Adrenergic receptors in man: direct identification, physiologic regulation, and clinical alterations. *N Engl J Med* 1982;307:18-29.

36. Paul SM, Janowsky A, Skolnick P: Monoaminergic neurotransmitters and antidepressant drugs, in Hales RE, Frances AS (eds): *Annual Review of the American Psychiatric Association* 1985, Vol 4, pp 37-48.

37. Garcia-Sevilla JA, Zis AP, Hollingsworth PJ, et al: Platelet alpha 2--adrenergic receptors in major depressive disorder: binding of tritiated clonidine before and after tricyclic antidepressant drug treatment. *Arch Gen Psychiatry* 1981;38:1327-1333.

38. Daiguji M, Meltzer HY, Tong C, et al: Alpha 2 adrenergic receptors in platelet membranes of depressed patients: no change in number of ^{3}H-Yohimbine affinity. *Life Sci* 1981;29:2059-2064.

39. McCarley RW: REM sleep and depression: common neurobiological control mechanisms. *Am J Psychiatry* 1982;139:565-570.

40. Siever L, Davis KL: Overview: toward a dysregulation hypothesis of depression. *Am J Psychiatry* 1985;142:1017-1031.

41. Gershon ES, Nurnberger JI, Berrettine WH, et al: Affective disorders: genetics, in Kaplan HI, Sadock BJ (eds): *Comprehensive Textbook of Psychiatry* , ed. 4, Baltimore, Williams & Wilkins Co. 1985. p 778.

42. Kallmann FJ: *Heredity in health and mental disorder* . New York, WW Norton, 1953.
43. Reich T, Clayton RS, Winokur G: Family history studies, V: the genetics of mania. *Am J Psychiatry* 1969;125:1358-1369.
44. Winokur G, Tanna V: Possible role of x-linked dominant factor in manic depressive disease. *Dis Nerv Syst* 1969;30:89-94.
45. Weitcamp LR, Stancer HC, Persad E, et al: Depressive disorders and HLA: a gene on chromosome 6 that can affect behavior. *N Engl J Med* 1981;305:1301-1306.
46. Drucker J, Heetner J, Wilder R: Depression in a medical setting. *Minn Med* 1980;June:399-404.
47. Meissner WW: Theories of personality and psychopathology: classic psychoanalysis, in Kaplan HI, Sadock BJ (eds): *Comprehensive Textbook of Psychiatry*, ed 3. Baltimore, Williams & Wilkins Co. 1980, p 394.
48. Social causes of depression, editorial. *Lancet* 1978;1:1343-1344.
49. Rahe RH: Recent life change stress and psychological depression. *RI Med J* 1980;63:98-100.
50. Paykel ES, Myers JK, Diendt MN, et al: Life events and depression. *Arch Gen Psychiatry* 1969;21:753-760.
51. Shakespeare W: *Hamlet* act III, scene I, line 58.
52. Kapusta MA, Frank S: The book of Job and the modern view of depression. *Ann Intern Med* 1977;86:667-672.
53. Camus A: *The Myth of Sisyphus and Other Essays*. New York, Random House, 1959.
54. Coakley D, Woodford-Williams E: The effects of burglary and vandalism on the health of old people. *Lancet* 1979;2:1066-1067.
55. Weissman MM, Klerman G: Sex differences and the epidemiology of depression. *Arch Gen Psychiatry* 1977;34:98-111.
56. Tec L: Depression and jet lag (letter). *Am J Psychiatry* 1981;138:858.
57. Pollitt J: The depressed patient. *Practitioner* 1978;220:205-212.
58. Lewy AJ, Kern HA, Rosenthal NE, et al: Bright artificial light treatment of a manic-depressive patient with a seasonal mood cycle. *Am J Psychiatry* 1982;139:1496-1498.
59. Rosenthal NE, Sack DA, Carpenter CJ, et al: Antidepressant effects of light in seasonal affective disorder. *Am J Psychiatry* 1985;142:163-170.
60. Katerndahl DA: Nonpsychiatric disorders associated with depression. *J Fam Pract* 1981;13:619-624.
61. Klerman GL: Depression in the medically ill. *Psychiatr Clin North Am* 1981;4:301-317.
62. Drugs that cause psychiatric symptoms. *Med Lett Drugs Ther* 1981;23(3):9-12.
63. Erman MK, Guggenheim FG: Psychiatric side effects of commonly used drugs. *Drug Ther Hosp* 1981;6:55-64.
64. Zisook S, Hall RCW, Gammon E: Drug treatment of depression. *Postgrad Med* 1980;67:153-161.

65. Flower RJ, Moncada S, Vane JR: Analgesic - antipyretics and anti-inflammatory agents, in Gilman AG, Goodman LS, Rall TW, et al (eds): *The Pharmacological Basis of Therapeutics* , ed 7. New York, MacMillan Publishing Co, 1985, p 696.

66. Mandell GL, Sande MA: Drugs used in the chemotherapy of tuberculosis and leprosy, in Gilman AG, Goodman GS, Rall TW, et al (eds): *The Pharmacological Basis of Therapeutics* , ed 7. New York, MacMillan Publishing Co, 1985, p 1209.

67. Calabresi P, Parks RE: Antiproliferative agents and drugs used for immunosuppression, in Gilman AG, Goodman GS, Rall TW, et al (eds): *The Pharmacological Basis of Therapeutics* , ed 6. New York, MacMillan Publishing Co, 1980, pp 1210-1211.

68. Silberfarb PM, Holland JCB, Anbar D, et al: Psychological response of patients receiving two drug regimens for lung carcinoma. *Am J Psychiatry* 1982;140:110-111.

69. Capurro PV, Capurro C: Solvent exposure and mental depression. *Clin Toxicology* 1979;15:193-195.

70. Bianchine JR: Drugs for Parkinson's disease, spasticity, and acute muscle spasms, in Gilman AG, Goodman LS, Rall TW, et al (eds): *The Pharmacological Basis of Therapeutics*, ed 6. New York, MacMillan Publishing Co, 1980, pp 1210-1211.

71. Neil JF, Himmelhoch JM, Mallinger AG, et al: Caffeinism complicating hypersomnic depressive episodes. *Compr Psychiatry* 1978;19:377-385.

72. Flanagan J, Maany I: Smoking and depression, letter. *Am J Psychiatry* 1982;139:541.

73. Jaffe JH: Drug addiction and drug abuse, in Gilman AG, Goodman LS, Rall TW, et al (eds): *The Pharmacological Basis of Therapeutics*, ed 6. New York, MacMillan Publishing Co, 1980, p 554.

74. Ritchie JM: The aliphatic alcohols, in Gilman AG, Goodman LS, Gilman A (eds): *The Pharmacological Basis of Therapeutics*, ed 6. New York, MacMillan Publishing Co, 1980, p 372.

75. Stewart MA, Drake F, Winokur G: Depression among medically ill patients. *Dis Nerv Syst* 1965;26:479-484.

76. Schwab J, Clemons RS, Bialow M, et al: A study of the somatic symptomatology of depression in medical patients. *Psychosomatics* 1965;6:273-27.

77. Ban T: Chronic disease and depression in the geriatric population. *J Clin Psychiatry* 1984;45:18-24.

78. Sinanan K, Hilary I: Post-influenzal depression. *Br J Psychiatry* 1981;138:131-133.

79. Hendler N, Leahy W: Psychiatric and neurologic sequelae of infectious mononucleosis. *Am J Psychiatry* 1978;135:842-844.

80. Cadie M, Nye FJ, Storey P: Anxiety and depression after infectious mononucleosis. *Br J Psychiatry* 1976;128:559-564.

81. Hall RCW (ed): *Psychiatric Presentations of Medical Illness*. New York, Spectrum, 1980.

82. Braude AI (ed): *Medical Microbiology and Infectious Disease.* Philadelphia, WB Saunders Co, 1981.
83. Parrish L, Bueno H: Depression with amebiasis and giardiosis, letter. *J Fam Pract* 1982;15:616.
84. Haggerty JJ, Sandler R: Strangyloidiasis presenting as depression: a case report. *J Clin Psychiatry* 1982;43:340-341.
85. Solomon JG, Solomon S: Psychotic depression and bronchogenic carcinoma. *Am J Psychiatry* 1978;135:859-860.
86. Goldberg RJ: Management of depression in the patient with advanced cancer. *JAMA* 1981;246:373-376.
87. Hutchinson EC, Leonard BJ, Mavolsley C, et al: Neurological complications of the reticuloses. *Brain* 1958;81:75-92.
88. Sandok BA: Organic mental disorders associated with circulatory disturbances, in Kaplan HI, Freedman AM, Sadock BJ (eds): *Comprehensive Textbook of Psychiatry*, ed 3. Baltimore, Williams & Wilkins Co, 1980, p 1401.
89. Szmuilowicz J, Flannery JG: Mitral valve prolapse syndrome and psychological disturbance. *Psychosomatics* 1980;21:419-421.
90. Guilleminault C, Tilkian A, Dement WC: The sleep apnea syndromes. *Annu Rev Med* 1976;27:465-484.
91. Sandblom RE, Matsumote AM, Schoene RB: Obstructive sleep apnea syndrome induced by testosterone administration. *N Engl J Med* 1983;308:508-510.
92. Dvoredsky AE: An atypical depression. *Hosp Pract* 1980;15:25-32.
93. King D: Failure to suppress dexamethasone in depression secondary to thyrotoxicosis, letter. *Am J Psychiatry* 1981;138:1514-1515.
94. Folks DG, Petrie WM: Thyrotoxicosis presenting as depression, letter. *Br J Psychiatry* 1982;140:432-433.
95. Kronfol Z, Greden JF, Condon M, et al: Application of biological markers in depression secondary to thyrotoxicosis. *Am J Psychiatry* 1982;139:1319-1322.
96. Kelly WF, Checkley SA, Bender DA: Cushing's syndrome, tryptophan and depression. *Br J Psychiatry* 1980;136:125-132.
97. Malinow KC, Lion JR: Hyperaldosteronism (Conn's disease) presenting as depression. *J Clin Psychiatry* 1979;40: 358-359.
98. Winokur G: Depression in the menopause. *Am J Psychiatry* 1973;130:92-93.
99. Ballinger CB: Psychiatric morbidity and the menopause: survey of a gynecological outpatient clinic. *Br J Psychiatry* 1977;131:83-89.
100. Cambell S: Double blind psychometric studies on the effects of natural estrogens on post-menopausal women, in Cambell S (ed): *The Management of Menopause and Post-Menopausal Years* . London, University Park Press, 1978, p 149-158.
101. Vandenbergh RL: Postpartum depression. *Clin Obstet Gynecol* 1980;23:1105-1111.
102. Olefsky JM: Diabetes mellitus, in Wyngaarden JB, Smith LH (eds): *Cecil Textbook of Medicine*, ed 15. Philadelphia, WB Saunders Co, 1979, p 1776.

103. Dixit VM: Cause of depression in chronic scurvy. *Lancet* 1979;2:1077-1078.
104. Boyer TD: Cirrhosis of the liver, in Wyngaarden JB, Smith LH (eds): *Cecil Textbook of Medicine*, ed 15. Philadelphia, WB Saunders Co, 1979, p 835.
105. Hallert C, Astrom J, Seduall G: Psychic disturbances in adult coeliac disease. *Scand J Gastroenterol* 1982;17:25-28.
106. Steinberg AD: Systemic lupus erythematosus, in Wyngaarden JB, Smith LH (eds): *Cecil Textbook of Medicine*, ed 15. Philadelphia, WB Saunders Co, 1979, p 1924.
107. Bennett JC: Rheumatoid arthritis, in Wyngaarden JB, Smith LH (eds): *Cecil Textbook of Medicine*, ed 15. Philadelphia, WB Saunders Co, 1979, p 1913.
108. Goodstein RK, Ferrell RB: Multiple sclerosis-presenting as depressive illness. *Dis Nerv Syst* 1977;38:127-131.
109. Asnis G: Parkinson's disease, depression and ECT: a review and case study. *Am J Psychiatry* 1977;134:191-195.
110. Mayeux R, Williams JBN, Stern Y et al: Depression and Parkinson's disease. *Adv Neurol* 1984;40:241-250.
111. Shraberg D: The myth of pseudodementia: depression and the aging brain. *Am J Psychiatry* 1978;135:601-603.
112. Maurice-Williams RS, Sinar EJ: Depression caused by an intracranial meningioma relieved by leukotomy prior to diagnosis of the tumor, letter. *J Neurol Neurosurg Psychiatry* 1984;47:884-885.
113. Raboy JM, Arrahami E: Unmasking of cerebellar tumors by amitriptyline in depressive patients, letter. *J Neurol Neurosurg Psychiatry* 1985;48:291.
114. Robinson RG, Starr LB, Lipsey JR, et al: A two year longitudinal study of poststroke mood disorders. *J Nerv Ment Dis* 1985;173:221-226.
115. Robinson RG, Price TR: post-stroke depressive disorders: a follow-up study of 103 patients. *Stroke* 1982;13:635-640.
116. Alarcon RD, Thweatt RW: A case of subdural hematoma mimicking severe depression with conversion-like symptoms. *Am J Psychiatry* 1983;140:1360-1361.
117. Perini G, Mendius R: Depression and anxiety in complex partial seizures. *J Nerv Ment Dis* 1984;172:287-290.
118. Emery EJ, Szymanski HV: Psychological symptoms preceding diagnosed myasthenia gravis. *Psychosomatics* 1981;22:993-995.
119. Forester BM, Kornfeld DS, Fleiss J: Psychiatric aspects of radiotherapy. *Am J Psychiatry* 1978;135:960-963.
120. Proctor SJ, Kernahan J, Taylor P: Depression as a component of post cranial irradiation somnolence syndrome, letter. *Lancet* 1981;l:1215-1216.
121. Leonidas JR: Depression a la Haitian. *NY State J Med* 1982;82:754-755.
122. Wyngaarden JB, Smith LH (eds): *Cecil Textbook of Medicine*, ed 17. Philadelphia, WB Saunders Co, 1985, p 1745.

123. Klaassen CD: Heavy metals and heavy mental antagonists, in Gilman AF, Goodman LS, Rall TW et al (eds): *The Pharmacological Basis of Therapeutics* , ed 7. New York, MacMillan Publishing Co, 1985, p 1617.

124. Liddle SW: The adrenal cortex, in Beeson PB, McDermott W, Wyngaardaen VB (eds): *Cecil Textbook of Medicine*, ed 15. Philadelphia, WB Saunders Co, 1979, p 2148.

125. Holbreich V, Endicott J, Nee J: Premenstrual depressive changes. *Arch Gen Psychiatry* 1983;40:535-542.

126. Faller J, Fox IH: Ethanol-induced hyperuricemia: evidence for increased urate production by activation of adenine nucleotide turnover. *N Engl J Med* 1982;307:1598-1602.

127. Glickman RM: Malabsorption, pathophysiology and diagnosis, in Wyngaarden JB, Smith LH (eds): *Cecil Textbook of Medicine*, ed 15. Philadelphia, WB Saunders Co, 1979, p 722.

128. Sleisenger MH: Malabsorption, management, in Wyngaarden JB, Smith LH (eds): *Cecil Textbook of Medicine*, ed 15. Philadelphia, WB Saunders Co, 1979, p 734.

129. Solomon SS: Clinical neurology and neuropathology, in Kaplan HI, Sadock BJ (eds): *Comprehensive Textbook of Psychiatry*, ed 3. Baltimore, Williams & Wilkins Co, 1980, p 117.

130. Fahn S: The extrapyramidal disorders, in Wyngaarden VB, Smith LH: *Cecil Textbook of Medicine*, ed 17. Philadelphia, WB Saunders Co, 1985:2074.

131. Wells CE: Other organic brain syndromes, in Kaplan HI, Sadock BJ (eds): *Comprehensive Textbook of Psychiatry*, ed 3. Baltimore, Williams & Wilkins Co, 1980 p 879.

132. Jones DG: Sarcoidosis, in Wyngaarden VB, Smith LH (eds): *Cecil Textbook of Medicine*, ed 15. Philadelphia, WB Saunders Co, 1979, p 214.

133. Bracken MB, Shepard MJ: Coping and adaptation following acute spinal cord injury: a theoretical analysis. *Paraplegia* 1980;18:74-85.

134. Steward TD: Spinal cord injury: a role for the psychiatrist. *Am J Psychiatry* 1977;134:538-541.

135. Fullerton DT, Harvey RF, Klein MH, et al: Psychiatric disorders in patients with spinal cord injuries. *Arch Gen Psychiatry* 1981;38:1369-1371.

136. Nordlicht S: Facial disfigurement and psychiatric sequelae. *NY State J Med* 1979;79:1382-1384.

137. Weil AA: Ictal depression and anxiety in temporal lobe disorders. *Am J Psychiatry* 1956;113:149-157.

138. Slater E, Roth M: *Clinical Psychiatry*. London, Bailliere, Tindall and Cassell, 1969, p 527.

139. Hambert G, Willen R: Emotional disturbance and temporal lobe injury. *Compr Psychiatry* 1978;19:441-527.

140. Robinson RG, Szetala B: Mood change following left hemispheric brain injury. *Annu Neurol* 1981;9:447-453.

141. Ross ED, Rush AJ: Diagnosis and neuroanatomical correlates of depression in brain-damaged patients. *Arch Gen Psychiatry* 1981;38:1344-1354.

142. Sutherland AM: The psychological impact of postoperative cancer. *Bull NY Acad Med* 1957;33:428 ff.

143. Titchener JL: Psychiatry and surgery, in Freidman AM, Kaplan HI (eds): *Comprehensive Textbook of Psychiatry*, ed 1. Baltimore, Williams & Wilkins Co, 1967, pp 1331-1334.

144. Stengel E, Zeitlyn BB, Rayner EH: Postoperative psychosis. *J Ment Sci* 1958;104:389 ff.

145. Maguire GP, Lee EG, Bovington DJ, et al: Psychiatric problems in the first year after mastectomy. *Br Med J* 1978;1:963-965.

146. Worden JW, Weisman AD: The fallacy in postmastectomy depression. *Am J Med Sci* 1977;273:169-175.

147. Melody GF: Depressive reactions following hysterectomy. *Am J Obstet Gynecol* 1962;83:410-413.

148. Richards DN: Depression after hysterectomy. *Lancet* 1973;2:430-432.

149. Ananth J: Hysterectomy and depression. *Obstet Gynecol* 1978;52:724-729.

150. Ellison RM: Psychiatric complications following sterilization of women. *Med J Aust* 1965;2:625-628.

151. Cavenar JO, Maltbie AA, Sullivan JL: Aftermath of abortion: anniversary depression and abdominal pain. *Bull Menninger Clin* 1978;42:433-444.

152. McCabe MS, Corry RJ: Psychiatric illness and human renal transplantation. *J Clin Psychiatry* 1978;39:393-400.

153. *Diagnostic and Statistical Manual of Mental Disorders*, ed 3. Washington, American Psychiatric Association, 1980.

154. Cancro R: Overview of affective disorders, in Kaplan HI, Sadock BJ (eds): *Comprehensive Textbook of Psychiatry*, ed 3. Baltimore, Williams & Wilkins Co, 1980, p 762.

155. Gunderson JG, Singer MT: Defining borderline patients: an overview. *Am J Psychiatry* 1975;132:1-9.

156. Freud: Mourning and melancholia. *Standard Edition of the Complete Psychological Works of Sigmund Freud*, Strachey J (trans). London, Hogarth Press, 1953-1966.

157. Lindemann E: Symptomatology and management of acute grief. *Am J Psychiatry* 1944;101:141.

158. Roy A: Depression in chronic paranoid schizophrenia. *Br J Psychiatry* 1980;137:138-139.

159. Ager H, Milstein LN: Depression in chronic schizophrenia, letter. *Am J Psychiatry* 1978;135:870-871.

160. Stern MJ, Pillsbury JA, Sonnenberg SM: Postpsychotic depression in schizophrenia. *Compr Psychiatry* 1972;13:519-598.

161. MacKinnon BL: Postpsychotic depression and the need for personal significance. *Am J Psychiatry* 1977;134:427-429.

162. Becker RE: Implications of the efficacy of thiothixene and a chlorpromazine-imipramine combination for depression in schizophrenia. *Am J Psychiatry* 1983;140:208-211.
163. Blumer D, Heilbronn M: Chronic pain as a variant of depressive disease. *J Nerv Ment Dis* 1982;170:381-408.
164. Anstett R, Poole S: Depressive equivalents in adults. *Am Fam Physician* 1982;25:151-156.

3 Psychosis

George N. McNeil
Stephen M. Soreff

PSYCHOSIS: A major disturbance in perceiving and dealing with reality characterized by disordered thinking, bizarre behavior, extremes of affect, delusions, and hallucinations. The psychotic patient best approximates the lay concept of "madness."

Case report   A 22-year-old college student was brought to the emergency room by friends who noted several days of withdrawn, unusual behavior, and speech that did not make sense. The patient had previously been well but had recently been sleeping less and had felt tense. His friends thought that he may have ingested drug(s). During the interview he vacillated from tears to laughter to blank staring for no apparent reason. He admitted to hearing voices commenting upon his actions and occasionally telling him what to do.

ORGANIC VERSUS FUNCTIONAL PSYCHOSIS: PROBLEMS OF DEFINITION

As we have seen in an earlier chapter, mental illness may be ascribed to psychosocial causes (functional illness) or to derangement of the body's physiologic function (organic illness). We have also noted that increasing understanding of the biologic underpinnings of "functional" illness (and conversely the effect of psychosocial factors upon physical illness) has led to a blurring of the functional/organic dichotomy. Nevertheless, it remains critically important to distinguish the known causes of organic illness, since correct diagnosis has major implications for both prognosis and treatment. For example, the patient described above was suffering from an amphetamine psychosis. He might easily have been diagnosed as acutely schizophrenic, setting in motion a broad range of inappropriate assumptions.

The correct diagnosis of organic psychosis is particularly critical since, as Lipowski has pointed out, it may be a manifestation of life-threatening illness.[1] There are a number of syndromes subsumed under the heading of organic psychosis. *Organic hallucinosis* is marked by the presence of hallucinations in an otherwise unremarkable mental status (see chapter 4). Similarly, *organic delusional syndrome* involves the finding of a delusion in an otherwise undisturbed mental state. Both these disorders may be confused with schizophrenia unless the diagnostic criteria for that disorder are rigorously applied.

Delirium

Delirium, formerly called "acute organic brain sydrome," may also be associated with delusions and hallucinations and with disordered thinking. Thus, at first blush it, too, might be mistaken for functional psychosis. A signal feature of deliriuim, however, is a clouding of consciousness. The patient's level of awareness may wax and wane even within the span of a brief interview. Frequently, there is a history of marked disturbance in the cycle of sleep and waking. The delirious patient may be disoriented as to date and place (rarely is the patient unable to recall his name). Memory is likely to be impaired. While the patient with functional psychosis usually shows unimpaired orientation and memory, the profoundly disorganized schizophrenic or manic patient may be unable to answer questions pertaining to these functions. Thus disruption of orientation or memory is not pathognomonic for organicity. The patient may be unable to answer simple questions or perform simple tasks. Delirium develops rapidly and tends to run a fulminant course. If an underlying cause is not detected and treated, this course may culminate in death.

Dementia

Dementia, or chronic organic brain syndrome, may also be accompanied by delusional thinking and by impairment of abstract thinking. Judgment is apt to be impaired, and bizarre behavior may result. What usually distinguishes this syndrome from functional psychosis are impairment of memory and loss of intellectual function. Since schizophrenia, too, may be associated with progressive intellectual deterioration, the differential diagnosis may be difficult and may hinge upon the detection of underlying organic disease.*

FEATURES

Mood

The mood of the psychotic patient may be most notable for its extremes. *Mania* is characterized by elevation of mood that is typified by euphoria, giddiness, jocularity, or even a mystical sense of cosmic contentment. *Psychotic depression* is marked by profound despondency as described in the chapter on depression. In contrast to these extremes, the mood of the schizophrenic may appear inscrutable, if not absent (flatness of affect). It may be argued, however, that this outward manifestation may belie inner feelings ranging from terror to rage to nihilistic despair.

Lability of mood may also be seen and is felt by some to be a "soft" sign of organic psychosis. The patient described in the case above showed such rapid fluctuation of mood. Such lability is not at all pathognomonic of organicity, however. The manic patient, for instance, may rapidly shift from giddiness to anger and irritability.

Mood that is *bizarre* and *inappropriate* to the patient's train of thought is a hallmark of psychosis. The patient who describes tragic circumstances while unexplainably laughing should be suspected of having a psychotic disorder. Unfortunately, such findings are of little help in distinguishing organic from functional psychosis.

Thought

There is apt to be major disruption in the thinking of the psychotic patient. Logical thought and speech are likely to give way to what seems to be nonsense. Psychoanalytic theory posits that such nonsense represents the emergence of unconscious, "primary process" thinking. The patient may be unable to sustain an understandable flow of ideas but may flit from thought to apparently unrelated thought (*looseness of associations*). This disturbance is particularly associated with schizophrenia. In other instances the flow of thought may be abruptly cut off (*thought blocking*). While

---

*Schizophrenia was formerly called "dementia praecox," and it is quite possible that some forms of this illness may again be viewed as chronic organic brain syndromes as our understanding of the disorder improves.

this occasionally occurs in all people, it is particularly characteristic of schizophrenia. In the extreme, psychotic language may degenerate to an incomprehensible babble spiced with "made up" words or *neologisms* .

Aside from such qualitative disturbances in thought production, there may be quantitative changes in the thought and speech of the psychotic. The manic patient may note an overabundance of thoughts which "come too fast" and which are manifest in rapid, pressured speech and *tangential* thinking.* The psychotically depressed patient, on the other hand, is likely to have slow, impoverished thought and speech.

The *thought content* of the psychotic patient is also likely to be deranged. *Hallucinations* are common (see chapter 4). *Delusional thinking* is also commonly seen. Delusions may be defined as beliefs that are unshakably held by the patient but which fly in the face of reality. Such beliefs may have grandiose qualities ("I am the Christ"), paranoid qualities ("there is a plot against me") or other bizarre content. The diagnosis of delusions should be made with careful attention to the patient's life circumstances (might there, in fact, be a plot against him?). Special cultural and religious beliefs might also lead to a false impression of delusional thinking.

While *ambivalance* is to be found in all of us, it is particularly prominent in the thinking of the schizophrenic. Such patients may be virtually paralyzed by conflicting sentiments and wishes and may thus be kept from making the most basic or mundane decisions, instead becoming mired in inactivity.

Behavior

Bizarre behavior is apt to be the most tangible feature of psychosis. It is what sets the psychotic apart from the nonpsychotic world and what makes him frightening or otherwise objectionable. While the unobtrusive patient may languish in a psychotic state without coming to professional attention, socially unacceptable behavior tends rapidly to deliver him to psychiatric care.

The unusual behavior of the psychotic is often a response to his disordered thinking and may, in that light, make a certain amount of sense. The patient with delusions of being the Messiah may feel justified in pros-

---

*The distinction between tangential thinking and looseness of association may be the subtle, but the interviewer should be able to follow the associative links of tangential thinking.

elytizing in the city square. More ominously, the patient experiencing command hallucinations to kill may feel compelled to do just that. Fortunately such occurrences, while they receive tremendous public attention, are rare. While the behavior of the nonpsychotic is fettered by social convention and the restraints of the ego and superego, such checks are dissolved in psychosis. Thus may be seen chaotic behavior stemming from equally chaotic thought.

Conversely, the psychotic patient may retreat, perhaps in defense against such chaos, into a state of immobility and inaction (*catatonia*). In this state he shuns human interaction, dealing instead only with solipsistic (or *autistic*) concerns. The boundaries of his world shrink to the dimensions of his delusions.

Physical Examination and Laboratory Findings

Given the importance of detecting treatable causes of organic psychosis, a thorough physical examination (preceded, of course, by a complete medical history) is warranted. Physical findings specific to the various organic psychoses will be noted under differential diagnosis. Nonspecific findings in the psychotic patient include signs of autonomic arousal, eg, increased heart rate and blood pressure.

As an adjunct to physical examination the following routine laboratory data are useful in the differential diagnosis of psychosis. (These will be discussed further below.)

1. Complete blood count, with attention to cell morphology
2. Serum electrolytes, including calcium
3. Serum glucose
4. Liver and kidney function studies
5. Thyroid function studies
6. Syphilis serology
7. Urine drug screen
8. Electroencephalogram
9. CT scanning of the brain

Interviewer's Reaction

It seems that the psychotic state has always inspired a mixture of fear and awe. Ancient cultures (and primitive contemporary cultures) have attributed psychotic states to either demonic or divine possession. Psychotic people have thus tended either to be spurned or exalted. Though the modern clinician is capable of approaching psychosis from a far more enlightened position, he is likely to carry vestiges of the feelings of his forebears.

Despite our enlightenment the psychotic patient is apt to remain frightening. He may threaten the interviewer physically, in which case fear serves a healthy, self-preservative function. (The wise clinician will choose retreat over physical heroics with the violent patient!) The paranoid, delusional patient is perhaps most likely to pose such a threat, particularly when he, in turn, feels threatened by an aggressive interviewer or by excessive physical closeness on the part of the interviewer.

Aside from such realistic fear, the psychotic patient may evoke fear from a source more difficult to define. Spilling out as he does the unmodified contents of his unconscious (unchaining demons that are normally encountered largely in the controlled arena of sleep and dreaming), the psychotic may elicit in the interviewer a fear (entirely justified) that he, too, harbors such madness. In other words, an uneasy sense of identification with the psychotic patient may lead to a need to avoid or, worse, to make a scapegoat of the patient. A keen observer of human nature, Robert Frost[2] identified this primitive, oft unconscious fear:"They cannot scare me with their empty spaces/Between stars--on stars where no human race is/I have it in me so much nearer home/To scare myself with my own desert places.*

A less common response to psychosis is the exaltation of madness. The ancients' notion of divine madness seems to have taken root with some modern thinkers who see psychosis as a transcendent state, one to be more envied than treated. In Peter Shaffer's enormously popular contemporary play *Equus* , this theme is graphically put forth.[3] The play is, in fact, an account of the psychotic decompensation of a boy and about a psychiatrist who comes to glorify his madness.

It is our view that this latter-day worship of madness is born, at least in part, out of antipathy toward psychiatry. We are further convinced that those who would advocate the psychotic state have spent too little time living with psychotic people and observing the terrible disruption caused by madness. Without being craven apologists for psychiatric "business as

---

*From *The Poetry of Robert Frost* edited by Edward Connery Lathem. Copyright 1936 by Robert Frost, 1964 by Lesley Frost Ballantine, 1969 by Holt, Rinehart and Winston.

usual," we advocate a commitment to relieving, if not curing, the ravages of psychosis. Among other reactions elicited by the psychotic patient is the wish to help, and help we should.

PATHOGENESIS

Psychodynamic Explanation

Given our growth in understanding the biology of mental illness, few would attempt to explain psychosis in purely psychological terms. At the same time the psychodynamic model helps to enhance our understanding of psychosis.

It might be said that all of us share a psychotic heritage—that of our infancy. The human infant is born not just physically helpless but emotionally helpless. He is beset by the strongest of feelings (blind rage, abject terror of annihilation) and needs (principally the need for nurturance). And he has not yet developed the psychological equipment (ego defenses) with which to stem these emotional tides. His rudimentary defenses may consist of psychotic denial ("This cannot be my real mother who is treating me with such anger"), projection ("It is the world, not I, that is full of rage"), and psychotic distortion (eg, the solipsistic belief that "I am at the center of the universe, and all events are related to me").

The psychotic patient suffers at least a partial regression to this level of psychological organization. Why? It may be argued that the psychotic state represents a developmental arrest or "fixation." The infant who is the victim of chaotic parenting may never develop the basic trust upon which later psychological growth depends.[4] Under stress in later life, the fragile ego defenses of such a person may tumble like a house of cards, exposing the infantile psychotic core of the individual.

On the other hand, psychosis may be seen in patients without evidence of developmental trauma. In the face of stress of sufficient proportions, theoretically anyone has the potential for a psychotic regression. Such phenomena have been described, for instance, in psychologically healthy victims of disaster (see "Differential Diagnosis" below).

Psychosis in this setting presumably serves a protective function, allowing the affected patient surcease from an intolerable psychological assault—allowing him to say, in essence. "This is not really happening to me."

Genetics

There are fairly compelling data supporting a genetic component in the pathogenesis of both schizophrenia and manic-depressive psychosis. While the prevalence of schizophrenia in the general population is roughly 1%, it has been shown that the prevalence in first degree relatives of schizophrenic patients is between 10% and 15%.[5] Perhaps more compelling are studies of twins which have shown a concordance rate of schizophrenia of 15% in dizygotic twins and 47% in monozygotes.[6] (A concordance rate of less than 100% in monozygotes makes it clear that factors other than genetics have a role in disease causation.)

The "nature versus nurture" debate over the pathogenesis of schizophrenia is perhaps best addressed by studying schizophrenic parents and their offspring who have been adopted away from their biologic family of origin. This has been done by Rosenthal and Kety, who reported a significant increase in prevalence of schizophrenia in these offspring.[7]

Despite this evidence, no gene locus has been identified for schizophrenia. In fact, this illness probably has a polygenic form of inheritance, and its clinical expression is clearly affected by nongenetic factors.

The genetic basis for manic-depressive illness appears to be even stronger than that for schizophrenia. This has been discussed in the chapter 2. Again, the phenotypic expression of this illness seems to depend upon other factors as well as genetics.

Biologic Explanation

Brain function is exquisitely sensitive to chemical changes in neuronal milieu, and psychosis is but one of the gross manifestations of such change. The nature of such change is as varied as the differential diagnosis which will be discussed below. Suffice it to say that drugs, toxins, metabolic disturbances, endocrine imbalance, and local inflammatory processes may all cause sufficient changes in brain function to produce psychosis.

Although the "functional psychoses" (eg, schizophrenia, manic-depressive psychosis) are traditionally categorized separately from organic brain disease, there is mounting evidence for biologic factors in these disorders as well.

Numerous studies have focused upon *structural abnormalities* in functional psychosis. Taylor et al have demonstrated bilateral hemispheric abnormalities in neuropsychological testing of schizophrenic patients, while showing abnormality of nondominant hemisphere function in manic-depressives.[8] Flor-Henry, on the other hand, has suggested left hemispheric dysfunction in schizophrenia.[9]

Computed tomography (CT) has led to a number of studies of gross brain morphology. Cortical atrophy and ventricular enlargement have been noted by numerous observers in chronic schizophrenics.[10-12] Golden et al have correlated such changes with measurable disturbances in expression, reading, and arithmetic.[13] It has been suggested that pronounced ventricular enlargement is associated with "negative" symptoms of schizophrenia (anhedonia, flattened affect, alogia), while less marked enlargement is associated with "positive" symptoms (hallucinations, delusions). Heath et al, on the other hand, found CT scan abnormalities of the cerebellar vermis in 34 of 85 (40%) schizophrenic patients studied.[14] (These findings were not specific to schizophrenia and were seen in nine of 31 (29%) patients with "other" functional psychosis.) Others have noted a reversal of the normal occipital asymmetry in some schizophrenic patients.[15]

Newer imaging techniques include positron emission tomography (PET scanning), a technique that allows observation of brain metabolism. Using this technique, Buchsbaum et al found decreased frontal cortical activity and decreased activity in the left central gray matter in eight drug-free schizophrenic patients.[16] Others have confirmed the finding of "hypo-frontality" in both treated and untreated schizophrenics.[17]

The most widely accepted biochemical explanation for schizophrenia holds that excess dopamine activity is related to the illness.[18] Supporting this theory is the vast clinical experience with antipsychotic drugs which share the ability to block dopamine receptors. (Unfortunately this ability is a two-edged sword. Dopamine blockade in mesolimbic neuronal pathways is felt to mediate antipsychotic activity. Dopamine blockade in nigro-striatal neurons, on the other hand, may be associated with symptoms akin to Parkinson's disease [drug induced parkinsonism] or other involuntary movement disorders. And blockade of dopamine at the level of the pituitary is associated with increased circulating prolactin.)

The advent of radioligand binding techniques has allowed extensive study of brain dopamine receptors. Thus far, two receptor subtypes (D-1 and D-2) have been identified. D-2 receptors seem to be responsible for mediating the therapeutic activity of the antipsychotic drugs; the function of D-1 receptors remains unknown.

It is tempting to postulate that schizophrenia is a product of D-2 receptor supersensitivity (or "up-regulation"). Attempts to demonstrate this in postmortem brains of schizophrenics are confounded by the fact that most of these patients take antipsychotic drugs, whose receptor blockade might be expected to "up-regulate" D-2 receptors in itself. In a series reported by Crow et al, however, five of 20 patients had not been exposed to antipsychotic drugs in the year preceding death. These five still demonstrated some D-2 up-regulation.[19]

Other workers have not demonstrated D-2 up-regulation in schizophrenics. Still more conflicting data emerge from studies of spinal fluid homovanillic acid (HVA, a major metabolite of dopamine). Some schizophrenic patients seem to have high dopamine turnover (high CSF HVA); others do not.

Crow and others [20,21] have attempted to reconcile these conflicting data by proposing two subgroups of schizophrenia. Type I schizophrenia is characterized by prominent "positive symptoms" (hallucinations, delusions, psychic activation) and by a relatively good prognosis. This is the same subgroup that we know clinically to be responsive to antipsychotic drugs. It is suggested that this group of patients has an increase in D-2 receptors and relatively low HVA levels.

Crow's type II schizophrenia is marked by "negative symptoms" (flattening of affect, withdrawal, anhedonia), tends to be relatively refractory to antipsychotic drugs, and carries a poor prognosis. This subgroup has been associated with increased ventricular size on CT scanning of the brain. This group may also show no increase in D-2 receptors and normal levels of HVA.

An increase in norepinephrine has been suggested as the factor responsible for the "switch" from depression to mania in bipolar affective illness.[22,23] Supporting this theory is the observation that drugs, such as tricyclic antidepressants, which enhance norepinephrine activity, may also induce mania. (The "amine hypothesis" is discussed further in chapter 2.)

The search for other neurohumoral factors in psychosis continues. Considerable attention has been paid recently to the role of peptides with endogenous opiate activity. Terenius and coworkers first postulated that there was *excessive* activity of these peptides in schizophrenia and mania, and they showed some support for this by giving naloxone hydrochloride to schizophrenic patients in an open study and producing symptomatic improvement.[24,25] Unfortunately, these findings have not been convincingly borne out in double-blind studies. Kline et al, on the other hand, administered β-endorphin to schizophrenic and depressed patients, showed clinical improvement, and suggested that *deficiency* of that peptide may have a role in the pathogenesis of these disorders.[26]

Other brain peptides that have attracted attention include neurotensin, a 13–amino acid peptide with antipsychotic properties. Widerlov et al have shown low spinal fluid levels of neurotensin in a subgroup of schizo-phrenic patients, with normalization of levels after antipsychotic drug treatment.[27]

There are numerous other brain peptides whose role in psychotic or other behavior is unclear.[28] There are, no doubt, many other neuro-transmitter or neuromodulator substances awaiting discovery.

Finally, there is growing attention to the possibility that *immune dysfunction* plays a part in some psychotic disorders. For example, Gowdy has demonstrated increased immunoglobulin levels in schizophrenic patients.[29] Pandey et al have gone one step further and demonstrated antibrain antibodies in sera and spinal fluid of 48.1% of a group of schizophrenic patients (no control patients showed this abnormality).[30] Jankovic has suggested a role for cellular immunity by showing significant delayed hypersensitivity reactions to intradermal S-100 human brain protein in schizophrenic, depressed, and demented patients, with few reactions in controls.[31]

Knight has proposed a unified theory of sorts, which remains to be tested.[32] He notes the genetic predisposition for both schizophrenia and autoimmune disease and notes parallels in the variable age of onset of both types of disease as well as their variable course, marked by relapse and re-mission. He theorized that autoimmunity may be triggered in genetically vulnerable people by viral infection and postulates that antibodies to the dopamine receptor which stimulate that receptor site (analogous to the anti-thyroid antibodies of Graves' disease) might account for the symptoms of schizophrenia.

Environmental Factors

It is generally accepted that environmental stresses may play a role both in the genesis of some psychotic disorders and in the course of chron-ic psychosis.

Much attention has focused, for example, on the role of distorted family interaction in schizophrenia. Lidz has argued that schizophrenia is born out of continual covert and overt fighting between parents.[33] The children of such families are in an untenable position in the midst of the marital schism. Arieti, on the other hand, sees schizophrenia as a reaction to an intense, overbearing mother coupled with a weak, ineffective father.[34] (Others have wondered whether "overbearing," controlling parental behavior might not be a *response* to the empty, ambivalent schizophrenic child, rather than a factor in disease pathogenesis.) Bateson has suggested that schizophrenia arises out of "double bind" communication patterns. Such patterns involve a highly significant figure in the child's life (again, mothers seem to receive more than their share of calumny) who gives the child impossible, conflicting directives. By way of example, the double-binding mother gives her son two neckties for his birthday. When he arrives at the breakfast table wearing one, she asks why he did not wear the other. Haley has also noted faulty communication in the families of schizophrenics and has found a tendency for members to talk *past* one another, not *to* one another.[35] Taken either singly or together, these family patterns can be seen as undermining basic trust, individual security, and self-esteem—scarce commodities in the schizophrenic patient.

The family may also be critical in determining relapse in schizophrenia.[36,37] Specifically, it has been suggested that critical, hostile, "overinvolved" families increase the likelihood of relapse.

Beyond the family lies a broader network of social supports, which for many includes work, friends, neighbors, and the church. Chronic mental illness often leads to erosion of this network, and the loss of these supports in itself leaves the patient vulnerable to relapse.[38]

Epidemiologic studies have led to yet broader observations on the role of environment in mental illness. Faris and Dunham studied hospital admissions for schizophrenia and found that these increased with increasing proximity to the inner city.[39] Similarly, Hollingshead and Redlich found an inverse relationship between social class and severity of mental illness.[40] Both studies might be cited as evidence that poverty and other privation cause psychotic illness. However, they might also support the argument that the mentally ill tend to become poor and to drift toward the inner city.

It is sometimes said that our complex modern society in itself spawns psychosis ("a sane response to an insane world"). To keep such observations in perspective, it should be noted that earlier cultures have been seen as no less mad and that there are far more adaptive responses to societal insanity. For example, in the opening lines of *Scaramouche*, Rafael Sabatini describes his eighteenth century hero. "He was born with the gift of laughter and a sense that the world was mad."[41]

Goldhamer and Marshall render a more scientific argument against impugning modern society as a cause of psychosis.[42] Using the archives of asylums and almshouses they determined the incidence of functional psychosis in 1850 and compared this with figures for 1950. They found no significant difference despite the obvious sweeping societal changes that had occurred over the course of the century.

The role of overwhelming stress in causing psychosis is not clear. *Brief reactive psychosis* (see below) may be attributable to the stress of combat, natural disaster, or other unusual circumstances. On the other hand, more permanent psychotic sequelae do not seem predictably to follow such stress. Ursano et al did a 5-year follow-up study of 253 US Air Force prisoners of the Vietnam War.[43] None were psychotic at the time of their repatriation, and 1.1% developed a psychotic disorder in the 5-year period of follow-up (contrasted with a 7.3% incidence of neurosis and a 7.9% incidence of marital or work-related problems).

Finally, environmental factors may play a role in the development of *organic psychosis* . It is not unusual for the elderly patient removed from familiar surroundings to the strange environs of a hospital to become quite psychotic. In the absence of orienting stimuli (clocks, calendars, familiar faces, a window through which to see beyond the microcosm of illness), such a psychotic state may only become worse. The role of *sensory deprivation* in the genesis of psychosis will be discussed further below.

DIFFERENTIAL DIAGNOSIS

Drugs

Table 3-1 lists drugs that have been associated with symptoms of psychosis. Many of these have been discussed in earlier chapters, so they will not be belabored here.

Obviously the diagnosis of drug-induced psychosis depends crucially upon eliciting a history of drug use or exposure. In the case of the uncooperative patient, family, friends, and old medical records may be helpful. Physical examination may offer some clues. Anticholinergic psychosis is accompanied by dry skin, mydriasis, and other signs of parasympathetic blockade. Rapid pulse and other signs of sympathetic autonomic arousal may be secondary to sympathomimetics or to insulin-induced hypoglycemia. Steroid psychosis may be accompanied by stigmata of Cushing's syndrome. In the laboratory, chromatographic analysis of urine or serum may detect some of the more common drugs (eg, amphetamines).

Alcohol

Alcohol-related psychosis bears special mention if for no other reason than the enormous prevalence of abuse of this agent. While uncomplicated alcoholic intoxication is associated with some clouding of consciousness,

Table 3-1
Drugs and Toxins Associated with Psychosis

Drug	Reaction	Comment
1. Antihypertensives		
Propranolol hydro-chloride[44]	Confusion, hallucinations, paranoia	Similar reactions to other lipophilic β-adrenergic blockers
Methyldopa[44]	Paranoia, hallucinations	
2. Other cardiovascular agents		
digitalis glyco-side[44-46]	Delusions, hallucinations, delirium	Usually associated with excessive dose
Lidocaine hydro-chloride[44, 45]	Delirium	
Disopyramide[44]	Paranoia, hallucinations	
Phenytoin[44]	Halluciantions, paranoia, delirium	
Procainamide hydro-chloride[44]	Paranoia, hallucinations	
Quinidine[47]	Paranoia, dementia	
3. Corticosteroids[44,45,48]	Hallucinations, paranoia, confusion	Usually associated with high doses
4. Cimetidine[44,45,50]	Hallucinations, paranoia, delirium	
5. Antimicrobials		
Amphotericin B[44]	Delirium	
Cycloserine[44]	Hallucinations, paranoia, delirium	
Isoniazid[44,48]	Hallucinations, paranoia	
Nalidixic acid[44]	Hallucinations, confusion	Rare
Thiabendazole[44]	Hallucinations	
Niridazole[44]	Hallucinations, mania, confusion	
Quinacrine hydro-chloride	Hallucination, delirium	Usually dose-related
Chloroquine[44]	Confusion, delusions, hallucinations	
Dapsone[44]	Acute psychosis	
Procaine penicil-lin G[40]	Hallucinations, delirium	Felt to be due to procaine
6. Anticonvulsants[44] (phenytoin, etho-suximide, primidone)	Hallucinations, paranoia, delirium	Usually associated with high doses

7. Antidepressants[44,45]		
tricyclics (amitriptyline hydrochloride, imipramine hydrochloride, etc)	Anticholinergic psychosis	May also induce acute mania in susceptible patients
Monoamine oxidase inhibitors [48, 49] (phenelzine sulfate and others)	Hypomania, hallucinations, confusion	Rare
8. Anticholinergics[44,45,48]	Hallucinations, delusions,	Some antiparkinsonian
(atropine, scopolamine, benztropine mesylate, trihexyphenidyl hydrochloride, etc)	delirium, fever, dry skin mydriasis	drugs, tricyclic antidepressants are potent anticholinergic agents
9. Dopamine agonists		
Levodopa[44,45,48]	Hypomania, hallucinations, paranoia, delirium	Elderly more susceptible; chronic use increases risk
Bromocriptine[44]	Mania, hallucinations, paranoia	Symptoms may persist for weeks after stopping drug
Amantadine hydrochloride[44,48]	Hallucinations	
10. Sympathomimetics		
Amphetamines[44,48]	Hallucinations, paranoia, schizophrenialike psychosis, mania	Usually in the setting of of overdose: abuse
Cocaine[48,51,52]	Amphetaminelike psychosis	May be associated with small dose after repeated use (kindling)
Ephedrine[44,48]	Hallucinations, paranoia	Overdose
Methylphenidate hydrochloride[44]	Hallucinations	
Phenylephrine[44]	Hallucinations, paranoia	Associated with nasal spray overdose
11. Analgesics		
Pentazocine[44]	Hallucinations, paranoia	
Propoxyphene[44]	Hallucinations, paranoia, confusion	
12. Cytotoxic agents		
Asparaginase[44]	Confusion, paranoia	Common
Vincristine Sulfate[44]	Hallucinations	Uncommon, high dose

continued

Table 3-1
continued

Drug	Reaction	Comment
13. Anti-inflammatory agents		
Chloroquine[44]	See Antimicrobials	
Indomethacin[44]	Confusion, paranoia, hallucinations	Elderly more at risk
Sulindac[44]	Paranoia	Rare
14. Anihistamines[44]	Hallucinations, delirium	Usually with overdose
15. Others		
Aminocaproic acid	Delirium	Immediately after injection for antifibrinolysis
Baclofen[44]	Hallucinations, paranoia, mania	Seen during treatment or withdrawal
Bromides[48,52]	Mania, schizophreni-form psychosis	Present in some over-the-counter tranquilizers; symptoms dose-related
Diazepam[44]	Rage, hallucinations	With drug use or withdrawal
Disulfiram[44,48]	Hallucinations, delirium	Unrelated to alcohol re-action
Ethchlorvynal[44]	Hallucinations, paranoia, delirium	With drug use or with-drawal
Ketamine hydro-chloride[44]	Hallucinations, delirium	Common
Methysergide[44]	Hallucinations	
16. Drug withdrawal		
Alcohol[54]	Hallucinations, delirium	
Barbiturates[44]	Hallucinations, delirium tremens—like syndrome	
Diazepam[44]	Hallucinations, agitation	
Other sedatives, hypnotics[45]	Hallucinations, agitation, confusion	
Opiates[55]	Paranoia, agitation	
Antipsychotics	Recurrent psychosis	Hypersensitivity psychosis a possible phenome-non[56,57]
Lithium carbonate	Recurrent mania	

17. Drugs of abuse

Amphetamines	See Sympathomimetic agents	
Alcohol[58]	Hallucinations, paranoia, delirium, dementia	See text
Phencyclidine hydrochloride[48,59]	Schizophrenialike psychosis: bizarre sometimes dangerous behavior	Hypertension, seizures
LSD and other hallucinogens[48,60]	Hallucinations, derealization, impaired judgment	
Marijuana[55]	Hallucinations, bizarre behavior	Rare
Organic hydrocarbons[55]	Hallucinations, paranoia, delirium	Gasoline, glue sniffing paint thinner
AntiParkinsonian drugs[61]	See Anticholinergics	
Caffeine[62]	GI upset, tachycardia, tremor, delirium	In overdose

18. Toxins, heavy metals

Lead[63]	Mania, paranoia, delirium	Rare: massive lead exposure
Mercury[63]	Impaired judgement, emotional lability, memory impairment	Chronic industrial exposure
Manganese[63]	Hallucinations, confusion, emotional lability, parkinsonian symptoms	Mining exposure
Thallium[48,63]	Hallucinations, delirium, alopecia	Rat poison, depillatory agents
Organophosphate insecticides[64]	Delirium; schizophreniclike syndrome with chronic exposure	Cholinesterase inhibition

19. Hormones

Thyroid hormone[64,65]	Delusions, hallucinations, delirium, mania	Overdose; associated symptoms of hyperthyroidism
Insulin[64]	Delirium(acute hypoglycemia), dementia(chronic hypoglycemia)	

it is not accompanied by symptoms of psychosis. On the other hand, *pathologic intoxication* is a fulminant state produced in some people by minimal amounts of alcohol and marked by belligerence and at times paranoid delusions.[66] Violent behavior may accompany this and may at times be turned against the self in the form of suicide attempts. Episodes of pathologic intoxication may last moments to a day or more and are followed by prolonged sleep and amnesia for the episode.

Alcoholic paranoia is a syndrome usually involving delusions of marital infidelity or other themes of jealousy. These occur in chronic alcoholics in the setting of a clear sensorium and an otherwise unremarkable mental status. They also occur in the face of ongoing alcohol consumption and are thus to be distinguished from various withdrawal phenomena.

Wernicke's encephalopathy is a state of delirium seen in chronic alcoholics and attributable to a dietary deficiency of thiamine.[58] Affected patients usually show marked clouding of consciousness, disorientation, and confusion. These signs are typically accompanied by nystagmus and ocular palsies. Ataxic gait is also common. Detection of Wernicke's encephalopathy by history, mental status, and physical examination should be followed by prompt administration of thiamine. Failure to do this leads to the natural progression of the disorder to a state of dementia (*Korsakoff's psychosis*).

Korsakoff's psychosis is marked by a pronounced loss of recent memory.[58] Consonant with this impairment of new learning, affected patients tend to use confabulation to obscure their memory deficit. Insight into the deficit tends to be poor, and patients are apt to be quite convinced of the truth of their confabulation. This clinical picture is often complicated by a peripheral neuropathy, also secondary to thiamine deficiency.

Withdrawal from alcohol (or a relative withdrawal produced by reduction in intake) may result in *alcoholic hallucinosis*[54]. This syndrome usually occurs within 24 hours of a drop in blood alcohol level. The hallucinations may be auditory, visual, tactile, olfactory, or mixed, and are associated with the tremulousness and anxiety that mark early withdrawal. The sensorium is clear inasmuch as this syndrome is but a prelude to more advanced stages of alcohol withdrawal: generalized seizures and, finally, delirium tremens.

Delirium tremens (DTs) usually supervene three to five days after alcohol withdrawal but may occur as late as 14 days.[54] The syndrome is typified by global confusion, hallucinations, fever, and sympathetic autonomic arousal.

Medical Illnesses

Organic illness tends to be rather strikingly underdiagnosed in patients presenting with "psychiatric" symptoms (including psychosis). There have been numerous studies that underscore the prevalence of previously undetected medical disorders in patients referred for psychiatric treatment. Koranyi has summarized 14 of these studies, which encompass roughly 4500 psychiatric patients, more than 50% of whom suffered from significant, undetected organic illness.[67] In 22% of the total study population, such illness was directly related to psychiatric symptoms.

Psychotic symptoms are a fairly nonspecific response by the brain to a host of physical disorders (see Table 3-2). Indeed, virtually any serious medical disorder in its agonal phase is likely to produce delirium, which yields to coma, then death. This bespeaks the profound importance of differential diagnosis in the delirioius patient. Correct diagnosis of a treatable disorder may be life-saving.

Delirium may not be readily distinguishable from functional psychosis. Pro and Wells point out that the acutely disorganized psychotic patient is frequently unable to cooperate with the mental status examination.[111] Reliable assessment of memory, orientation, and other crucial functions may be impossible, and such a patient presents a diagnostic choice between delirium and acute schizophrenia.

Early dementia may similarly be confused with functional psychosis. Smith and Kiloh, reporting 200 consecutive hospital admissions with a provisional diagnosis of dementia, pointed out that cognitive loss may not be apparent early in the course of dementing illness.[112] The clinical picture may then be one of anxiety, depression, or of a schizophrenialike psychosis.

Clearly, a careful medical history may be enormously helpful in distinguishing early organicity from functional psychosis. A first psychotic episode in a patient over 40 years old with no apparent situational stresses is strongly suggestive of an organic process. Similarly a history of (or suggestive of) medical illness should bias the clinician toward organicity. As previously noted, a careful drug history is crucial.

A positive past history of schizophrenia or other functional psychosis should be treated advisedly. Schizophrenic patients are, if anything, more likely to fall prey to medical illness than is the population at large.[67] So their psychiatric diagnosis poses the peril of premature diagnostic closure.

Thorough physical and neurologic examinations are an absolute

Table 3-2
Illnesses Associated with Psychotic Symptoms

Disease	Symptoms	Comment
1. Endocrine		
Hypoglycemia[46,68,69]	Hallucinations, delirium	Convulsions; coma may supervene rapidly; trial of IV glucose; check blood glucose
Diabetic ketoacidosis[68,70]	Delirium	Check blood glucose
Hypothyroidism[67,68,71,72]	Delusions, hallucinations, delirium	"Myxedema madness," physical stigmata; check thyroid hormone levels
Thyrotoxicosis[67,68,71,73]	Mania or schizophrenialike syndrome, delirium, dementia	Check thyroid hormone levels
Hyperparathyroidism[68,71,73]	Delusions, delirium	Check serum calcium
Hypoparathyroidism[68,71]	Hallucinations, delirium	Tetany; check serum calcium
Hyperadrenocorticism[48,68,71,74]	Euphoria, schizophrenia-or manialike syndrome	Signs of Cushing's syndrome
Adrenal insufficiency[68,71]	Delirium, dementia	Check serum electrolytes
Pre-menstrual syndrome[75—77]	Agitation, delusions, hallucinations	Cyclical psychosis
2. Metabolic		
Hypoxia[68,71]	Delirium	Tachypnea, cyanosis; check arterial blood gases
Hepatic failure[48,68,71,78]	Delirium	Jaundice and other stigmata; check liver enzymes, serum NH_4^+
Renal failure[48,68,71]	Delirium	Hypertension and other stigmata; check serum creatinine

Electrolyte imbalance[68,69,79] (Na^+, K^+, HCO_3^-, Mg^{++})	Delirium	Multiple etiologies; check serum electrolytes
Dehydration[68,69]	Delirium	Poor skin turgor, orthostatic hypotension, *other* physical stigmata; check serum electrolytes, urea nitrogen
Water intoxication, syndrome of inappropriate ADH secretion[68,69,79]	Delirium	Check serum electrolytes, blood and urine osmolarities
Acute intermittent porphyria[67,80,81]	Chronic "emotional lability," delirium	Abdominal colic; peripheral and cranial neuropathy, increased urinary δ-aminolevulinic acid
Wilson's disease[71,82,83]	Schizophrenia-like, manialike syndrome	Kayser-Fleischer ring, stigmata of liver disease; Involuntary movement disorder; low serum copper, ceruloplasmin

3. Infectious
   Central nervous system

meningoencephalitis[68,70,84—86]	Delirium, paranoia, grandiosity (tertiary syphilis)	Viral, bacterial, fungal, protozoan organisms; cultures, serologies, especially for *Treponema pallidum*
"Slow virus" infection[87,88] (Jakob-Creutzfeldt disease; ?causative of other diseases as well	Hallucinations, rapidly developing dementia	Myoclonus; EEG may confirm
Systemic infection[70]	Delirium	Fever, signs of focal infection; check WBC, cultures
Infectious mononucleosis[89,90]	Schizophrenialike syndrome	Check peripheral blood smear, heterophile titer

continued

Table 3-2
continued

Disease	Symptoms	Comment
4. Collagen-vascular disease[68,71]		
Systemic lupus erythematosus	Paranoia, schizophrenialike syndrome, delirium	Psychotic symptoms may predate systemic symptoms; check ESR; LE cell preparation
Temporal arteritis[68,69]	Hallucinations, dementia	Temporal artery tenderness, high ESR
5. Cardiovascular/cerebro-vascular disease		
Myocardial infarction[68,69,71,92]	Delirium	Associated with emboli to brain, decreased cerebral perfusion (pump failure)
Congestive heart failure[68,71]	Delirium	Decreased cerebral perfusion
Tachy-(or brady-) dysrhythmias[68,71]	Delirium	Decreased cerebral perfusion, syncope common; check pulse, ECG
Hypertensive encephalopathy[70]	Delirium, dementia	Marked elevation of BP, grade III-IV retinopathy, focal neurologic deficits
Stroke[71,93]	Delirium, dementia, focal neurologic deficits	Often associated with BP elevation (multi-infarct dementia), may play a part in up to 36% of dementia
Subarachnoid hemorrhage[70]	Delirium	Headache, stiff neck, rapidly evolving obtundation
Migraine[70,94]	Delirium	Symptoms as prodromata to headache
6. Brain tumor[95—98] (abscess, hematoma, granuloma, neoplasm, parasitic cyst)	Dementia, schizophrenialike syndrome	Headache, focal neurologic deficits depending upon location; check CT scan

7. Degenerative brain disease

multiple sclerosis, other demyelinating diseases[99—102]	Dementia	Increased CSF γ-globulin; delayed cortical evoked potentials
Alzheimer's disease[71,103]	Dementia	Postmortem diagnosis or diagnosis of exclusion
Huntington's disease[71,104]	Dementia, chorea	Autosomal dominant gene
Parkinson's disease[70,105,106]	Dementia	Signs of extrapyramidal system dysfunction
Pick's disease[71,107,108]	Dementia	Postmortem diagnosis

8. Temporal lobe epilepsy (complex partial seizures)[109] — Hallucinations (ictal) Schizophrenialike syndrome (interictal) — History of psychomotor seizures; EEG with nasopharyngeal leads

9. Vitamin deficiencies

Vitamin B_{12} [68,71]	Delusions, hallucinations, dementia	Signs of posterior column and cortico-spinal tract dysfunction; check serum vitamin B_{12} level
Thaimine[68,71]	Wernicke-Korsakoff syndrome (see text)	
Nicotinic acid[67,68,71]	Delusions, delirium, dementia	Skin rash, diarrhea

10. Miscellaneous

Normal Pressure hydrocephalus[71]	Dementia	Gait disturbance, incontinence, check CT scan
Thrombotic thrombo-cytopenic purpura[110]	Anemia, decreased platelet count, fever, renal failure	Highly variable, catatonia reported
Temperature dys-regulation[68] (hyper-, hypothermia)	Delirium	Check body temperature
Reactive psychosis	Delusions, hallucinations	May be caused by the stress of any significant medical illness (see text)

necessity in the differential diagnosis of psychosis and may be diagnostic of many of the disorders listed in Table 3-2. (Most of these disorders are discussed more fully in earlier chapters on anxiety and depression.)

In addition to the complete history and physical examination, certain laboratory data are advisable in evaluating the psychotic patient (see above). The availability of the multichannel autoanalyzer (SMA-12) allows the determination of blood sugar, serum calcium, and renal and hepatic function with but one sample of blood. In addition, a relatively inexpensive "organic screen" might include serum electrolytes, a complete blood count with peripheral blood smear (with the caveat that vitamin B_{12} deficiency may be detectable only by determining a serum B_{12} level), a serology for syphilis, and an ESR. (The ESR is, of course, very nonspecific but may serve as the only early evidence of a malignant, autoimmune, or inflammatory process.)

Other laboratory studies might be ordered as dictated by the history and physical examination, although some would argue that thyroid hormone levels and CT scanning should be routine parts of this evaluation. More specific (and generally more expensive) studies are noted in Table 3-2. Finally, Pro and Wells advocate the use of electroencephalography as a diagnostic tool, stating that EEG changes "virtually always accompany delirium."[111]

Surgical Complications

Preoperative anticipation may provoke a psychotic disorganization. Depending upon the patient's psychic make-up, the symbolic importance of "being put to sleep," cut upon, and perhaps in some way disfigured, may pose an enormous threat to psychological integrity. The enforced passivity of the surgical patient may add to this threat. One need not invoke "castration anxiety" as a unifying explanation for all preoperative anxiety. The more literal threats of pain, disfigurement, or death may be sufficient to produce a psychotic state.

The postoperative stress of learning a dreaded diagnosis may also overwhelm the patient and lead to psychotic decompensation. As with the preoperative syndrome described above, this would probably best be classified as a *brief reactive psychosis*.

Postoperative psychosis may be a product of psychological, environmental, and/or biological factors.[114,115] Kornfeld et al, observing patients who underwent heart surgery, remarked, for example, that patients with dominant, "controlling" personality traits seem more vulnerable to the submissive postoperative state.[115] While such generalizations may be useful, a knowledge of the patient's individual vulnerabilities and of the literal and symbolic impact of surgery upon him may be most helpful in understanding a postoperative psychotic reaction.

It is generally accepted that the postoperative environment may play a significant disorganizing role. Profound *sensory deprivation* has long been recognized as a factor that may cause psychosis even in normal volunteers.[116] The postoperative milieu may be one of sensory deprivation unless attempts are made at providing orienting stimuli. This fact has been incorporated into the practices of most intensive care units, where visitors, clocks, and other such stimuli are strongly encouraged.

Obviously, certain types of surgery portend more severe troubles with sensory deprivation. The "black patch psychosis" associated with eye surgery is such an example.[117] (Interestingly, hallucinations have also been reported in patients with blindness due to cataracts, in which case eye surgery has been *curative* of the psychotic symptom.) [118] Extensive orthopedic surgery with prolonged postoperative immobilization may also result in significant sensory deprivation and psychosis.

The biologic factors that may contribute to postoperative psychosis are at least as varied as the lists of drugs and medical illnesses that have been previously discussed. Drug toxicity (or drug withdrawal—beware the "social" alcoholic!) should be strongly considered in the differential diagnosis of postoperative psychosis. Similarly, intraoperative factors, such as hypotension, should be considered. The possible contribution of infection, electrolyte disturbance, or other postoperative factors should be ruled out as well.

Postpartum psychosis may take the form of a major depressive episode (see chapter 2) or a manic or schizophreniform illness. In fact, it has been argued that postpartum psychosis does not warrant a separate diagnosis and that it simply represents an expression of underlying schizophrenia or affective illness. Certainly the stresses of pregnancy, parturition, and "new parenthood" are considerable and may conspire with the patient's psychological vulnerabilities to produce a psychotic reaction. One of us saw, for example, a 25-year-old woman with needs to be a successful executive while being the consummate mother and marital partner. The demands of her newborn, of her husband, and of an unsympathetic employer ultimately resulted in her having a psychotic reaction.

In addition to the psychological stresses of childbirth, there are organic changes that may contribute to the onset of psychosis. The new mother undergoes great shifts in circulating hormones, most significant being a drop in progestin levels. The precise significance of such shifts, vis à vis mood and thought, is unclear. While the dramatic drop in gestational hormone levels cannot in itself account for psychosis (psychosis remains a relatively rare complication of parturition), it may play an enabling role.

Other possible organic contributors to postpartum psychosis are, again, as varied as the list of drugs and medical conditions that have previously been outlined. One drug bears special mention because of its former common use in obstetrical anesthesia. *Scopolamine* has, in fact, fallen out of favor because of its common association with postanesthesia delirium.

Trauma

Brain trauma appears to increase the risk for subsequent schizophreniform psychosis beyond that expected for the general population. In the most extensive review of this subject, Davidson and Bagley conclude that the psychotic disturbance occurs independent of any genetic vulnerability and that it is most closely associated with temporal lobe injury.[119] Nasrallah et al have reported a previously healthy 22-year-old man who developed paranoid delusions within hours of wakening from coma following a right frontal lobe contusion.[120] This patient went on to follow a downhill course difficult to distinguish from undifferentiated schizophrenia.

Psychosis has also been reported as a psychological reponse to mutilating trauma.[121] The sudden adjustment to disfiguring or disabling injury may overwhelm more mature and adapative ego defenses.

Psychiatric Illnesses

Table 3-3 lists the "functional" illnesses to be considered in the differential diagnosis of psychosis. Again, one should invoke the functional/organic dichotomy advisedly. As our understanding of these disorders increases, this distinction becomes increasingly flawed.

Early in the assessment of a psychotic symptom one should ask himself, "Does this, in fact, reflect a psychotic illness?" In rural or more primitive cultures, for instance, hallucinations may be a cultural norm. The same may be said for certain fundamentalist religions whose tenets may seem to the uninitiated to be delusional.

A danger in diagnosing psychosis ("the departure from reality") is that there are few "hard" clinical data on which to depend. Instead, the clinician commonly uses his own perception of reality as the standard against which

Table 3-3
**Psychiatric Illnesses with Psychotic Features
("Functional Psychoses")**

1. Schizophrenic disorders
2. Mania
3. Major depression
4. Paranoid disorders
5. Brief reactive psychosis
6. Borderline personality disorder
7. Histrionic personality disorder
8. Factitious psychosis
9. No psychiatric illness (normality)

others are judged. (I do not hear the accusing voices my patient hears and do not perceive an imminent threat from the mafia. Moreover, I cannot follow his train of thought. I conclude, therefore, that he is hallucinating, delusional, and that he has looseness of associations.) This standard may not only be flawed (the mafia may, indeed, be after my patient!), but may at its worst be abused. There is but a step between not sharing my patient's perception of reality and not sharing his political or religious beliefs. Sadly, psychiatric diagnosis and hospitalization may be used simply to suppress the dissident views of people without psychiatric illness.

Schizophrenia is an all too common illness (roughly 1% lifetime prevalence) with often devastating morbidity. As defined by the *Diagnostic and Statistical Manual of Mental Disorders* (DSM-III), it is a chronic illness characterized by progressive deterioration of social function.[122] The inevitability of this deterioration has recently been challenged in longitudinal studies of schizophrenic patients. To make the diagnosis one must obtain a history of symptoms lasting 6 months or more. This time period may include a prodromal phase, wherein there is deterioration of function without clear psychotic symptoms, and a residual phase, wherein psychotic symptoms are attenuated but functional impairment persists.

Schizophrenia is a disorder of adolescence and young adulthood. By DSM-III convention, symptoms must have their onset before age 45. For reasons that are unclear, onset of symptoms and first hospitalizations seem to occur earlier in men than in women.[123]

Among the most salient psychotic symptoms of schizophrenia are those associated with the patient's disordered thinking. Bizarre *delusions* are commonly seen. These may have paranoid, grandiose, somatic, or religious overtones, in which case they are not distinctive from delusions encountered in other psychotic disorders. More specific to schizophrenia are *delusions of passivity* . These include delusions of being controlled, of having thoughts inserted into one's head, or of having thoughts forcefully withdrawn or broadcast.

Hallucinations are another nonspecific psychotic symptom encountered in schizophrenia. Most suggestive of schizophrenia (as opposed to other psychoses) are auditory hallucinations involving running commentary about the patient or involving two voices in discourse with one another.

The thought processes of the schizophrenic are typically marked by illogic and incoherence. The interviewer, unable to follow a logical thread in the patient's discourse, should note this finding as *looseness of associations* .

Blunted, bizarre, or inappropriate affect is typical of the schizophrenic disorders. It may be argued that this is a defense against the abject terror felt by the patient at a barely unconscious level.

The behavior of the schizophrenic patient is apt to be markedly disorganized or, at the opposite extreme, catatonic. The catatonic patient may be mute and stuporous and show odd posturing and "waxy flexibility" of the limbs. Or rarely he may exhibit extreme excitement and agitation which may culminate in exhaustion and death if not treated urgently.

The schizophrenic disorders are divided into several descriptive subtypes. *Catatonic*c-type schizophrenia is characterized by symptoms described immediately above. *Paranoid*-type illness is dominated by delusions and/or hallucinations with jealous, persecutory, or grandiose content. The *disorganized* type is marked by frequent incoherence, lack of organized delusions, and affect that is blunted, silly, or inappropriate.

Schizophreniform disorder is distinguished from schizophrenia only by its duration, which is between 2 weeks and 6 months. The major reason for distinguishing this from the schizophrenic disorders is that patients whose psychosis runs a briefer course seem more likely to recover full social function. In addition, affected patients do not seem to carry the genetic vulnerability for schizophrenia seen in the latter illness.[122]

The major affective disorders (mania, major depression) have been discussed in chapters 1 and 2. These disorders may have prominent psychotic features which at times makes the distinction from schizophrenia quite difficult.

The hallmark of *mania* is "one or more distinct periods with a predominantly elevated, expansive or irritable mood."[122] At least three accessory symptoms must also be demonstrated.[122] These include: (1) increase in social, sexual, or work activity; (2) increase in prolixity ("pressured speech"); (3) tangential thought production, flight of ideas or "racing thoughts"; (4) grandiosity (may be delusional); (5) decreased need for sleep; (6) distractibility; (7) poor judgment with financial, social, and other indiscretions which may have adverse consequences.

It is not unusual for the manic patient to manifest delusions, hallucinations, and bizarre behavior. If these are mood congruent, ie, consistent with the expansive, grandiose state of the patient, the diagnosis of mania may still be fairly clear. If, however, there are persecutory delusions or delusions of passivity or other "mood-incongruent" psychotic features, schizophrenia will inevitably enter the differential diagnosis. In such cases definitive diagnosis may be extremely difficult. A family history of affective illness shifts the diagnostic bias toward mania, as does a clear past history of depression or mania. Often only a longitudinal view of the patient makes clear a pattern of recurrent bipolar mood swings. With the luxury of retrospection it is not unusual to revise a working diagnosis from schizophrenia to manic-depressive illness, a revision with important prognostic and treatment implications.

The patient with *major depression* (see chapter 2) and with delusions or hallucinations that reflect his guilt, despondency, or nihilism presents a relatively minor diagnostic problem. Again, however, the presence of mood-incongruent psychotic features (delusions of persecution, of passivity, etc) is apt to raise the question of schizophrenia. The profoundly withdrawn depressed patient with psychomotor retardation may look similar to the catatonic schizophrenic, further confusing the issue. A past history or family history of affective illness may again be helpful. Barring this and barring other symptoms that point the way toward either depression or schizophrenia, one may reach a diagnostic impasse. As yet there are no biologic markers sensitive and specific enough to be reliable. It is fortunate that electroshock therapy may be helpful both for the patient with acute catatonic schizophrenia and for those with major depression.

Several points *may* be useful in making the difficult distinction between schizophrenia and a major affective disorder. First, if the salient clinical feature is a disturbance in *mood* (be it depressed or elated), one should think more of manic-depressive illness. Conversely, if thought disorder dominates the mental status, then schizophrenia is more likely. Second, flight of ideas and tangential thought production are typical of mania. The interviewer can usually follow the tangential direction of the patient's logic. The thought disturbance is a *quantitative* one. In contrast, the schizophrenic showing typical looseness of associations has a *qualitative* disturbance of thought that renders it illogical and not possible to follow. Finally, the interviewer is more likely to feel a sense of emotional contact with the manic or depressed patient; whereas a sense of distance is more common in interviewing the schizophrenic. Alas, all too often none of these criteria (particularly the last) are clear enough to solve the diagnostic dilemma.

Paranoid disorders have as their central feature persistent delusions of persecution or delusional jealousy. Affected patients do not show the more pervasive psychotic disturbances (thought disorder, hallucinations, etc) seen in schizophrenia. They typically function quite well and seem normal outside the realm of their delusion. These disorders are discussed more fully in chapter 8.

Brief reactive psychosis is a disturbance occurring in response to major stress. The psychotic response to physical trauma or other disaster is an example of this. Affected patients may show delusions, hallucinations, looseness of associations, and bizarre behavior. What distinguishes the disorder from schizophrenia and schizophreniform psychosis is its brevity (from hours to a maximum of 2 weeks). There is also usually a history of good premorbid adjustment, and there should be eventual full return of function.

Transient psychotic disturbances may also occur in patients with *borderline or histrionic personality disorders* . It is beyond the scope of this chapter to discuss the personality disorders, but these might be considered in a patient with brief psychotic experiences and a long-standing history of nonpsychotic maladaption to work and to relationships.

Psychosis has also been described as a conversion symptom.[124] Conversion symptoms may be highly variable and may fluctuate according to the clinical setting. As with any conversion phenomenon, conversion psychosis may be seen as an *unconscious* attempt to contain anxiety. Usually the symptom(s) can be seen to afford the patient some secondary gain (eg, being cared for) as well. To make the diagnosis of conversion psychosis with certainty, however, it must be shown that the symptom can be removed by psychological means (psychotherapy, behavioral modification, etc).

Conversion psychosis does not represent a true factitious disorder in that the symptoms are not under voluntary control. Pope et al[125] reported a chart review of 219 consecutive inpatients admitted for psychosis. Nine of these were found to meet DSM-III criteria for *factitious psychosis* . These criteria include: The symptoms appear to be under the voluntary control of the patient. The symptoms cannot be accounted for by another psychiatric diagnosis. The patient's purpose in producing symptoms is to assume the sick role.[122] Pope et al found a strong association to underlying borderline or histrionic personality disorders. In addition, none of the nine patients had a family history positive for psychosis. Ironically, the long-term outcome for Pope's patients with factitious psychosis proved to be quite poor—similar to that for his schizophrenic patients.

Hay has added an additional twist to the confusing question of factitious psychosis.[126] He reports six patients initially diagnosed as feigning schizophrenia. Five of the six went on to become frankly schizophrenic. Hay's message is clear: the diagnosis of factitious psychosis should be made with extreme circumspection in the absence of obvious reasons for the patient to "fake it."

Malingering represents a variation on the theme of factitious psychosis. Here again the symptoms are under voluntary control. In addition, the patient can be seen to be consciously motivated by some goal other than assuming the sick role. Such motives might include release from jail or from military duty.

Finally, we have observed in bereaved patients a phenomenon that should be distinguished from psychosis. Such patients may report feeling the "presence" of their lost loved one (usually a spouse) and may talk to the one dead. Patients are apt to be reluctant to reveal this to the physician out of fear of being deemed "crazy." When seen in the absence of other symptoms suggesting organic or functional psychosis, this finding seems to have no pathologic significance. Instead, it seems to represent a normal attempt by the ego to find solace as restitution for its loss.

REFERENCES

1. Lipowski ZJ: Delirium updated. *Compr Psychiatry* 1980;21:190-196.
2. Frost R: "Desert Places," in *Complete Poems of Robert Frost*. New York Holt,Rinehart & Winston, 1969.
3. Shaffer P: *Equus*. New York, Avon, 1974.
4. Erickson E: *Childhood and Society*, ed 2. New York, WW Norton, 1963.
5. Tsuang MT, Fowler RC, Cadoret RJ, et al: Schizophrenia among first-degree relatives of paranoid and nonparanoid schizophrenics. *Compr Psychiatry* 1974;15:295-302.
6. Cancro R: The role of genetic factors in the etiology of the schizophrenic disorders, in Grinspoon L (ed): *Psychiatry 1982 Annual Review*. Washington, American Psychiatric Press, 1982, pp 92-97.

7. Rosenthal D, Kety SS: *The Transmission of Schizophrenia.* Oxford, PergamonPress, 1968.

8. Taylor MA, Redfield J, Abrams R: Neuropsychologic dysfunction in schizophrenia and affective disease. *Biol Psychiatry* 1981;16:467-478.

9. Flor-Henry P: On certain aspects of the localization of the cerebral systems regulating and determining emotion. *Biol Psychiatry* 1979;14:677-698.

10. Weinberger DR, Cannon-Spoor E, Potkin SG, et al: Poor premorbid adjustment and CT scan abnormalities in chronic schizophrenia. *Am J Psychiatry* 1980;137:1410-1413.

11. O'Kasha A, Madkour O: Cortical and central atrophy in chronic schizophrenia. *Acta Psychiatr Scand* 1982;65:29-34.

12. Reveley AM, Reveley MA, Clifford CA: Cerebral ventricular size in twins discordant for schizophrenia. *Lancet* 1982;1:540-541.

13. Golden CJ, Moses JA, Zelazowski R, et al: Cerebral ventricular size and neuropsychological impairment in young chronic schizophrenics. *Arch Gen Psychiatry* 1980;37:619-623.

14. Heath RG, Franklin DE, Shraberg D: Gross pathology of the cerebellum in patients diagnosed and treated as functional psychiatric disorders. *J Nerv Ment Dis* 1979;167:585-592.

15. Luchins DJ, Weinberger DR, Wyatt RJ: Schizophrenia and cerebral asymmetry detected by computed tomography. *Am J Psychiatry* 1982;139:753-757.

16. Buchsbaum MS, Ingvar DH, Kessler R, et al: Cerebral glucography with positron tomography: use in normal subjects and patients with schizophrenia. *Arch Gen Psychiatry* 1982;39:251-259.

17. Wolkin A, Jaeger J, Brodie JD, et al: Persistence of cerebral metabolic abnormalities in chronic schizophrenia as determined by position emission tomography. *Am J Psychiatry* 1985;142:564-571.

18. Spokes EGS: Biochemical abnormalities in schizophrenia: the dopamine hypothesis, in Gurzon E (ed): *Biochemistry of Psychiatric Disturbances.* New York, John Wiley & Sons, 1980, pp 53-71.

19. Crow TJ, Owen F, Cross AJ, et al: Letter to the editor. *Lancet* 1978;1:36, cited in Hales RE, Frances AJ (eds): *American Psychiatric Association Annual Review.* Washington, American Psychiatric Press, 1985, Vol 4, p 27.

20. Crow TJ: The biology of schizophrenia. *Experientia* 1982;38:1275-1282, cited in Hales RE, Frances AJ (eds): *American Psychiatric Association Annual Review.* Washington, American Psychiatric Press, 1985, Vol 4, p 27.

21. Zemlan FP, Hitzemann RJ, Hirschowitz J, et al: Down-regulation of central dopamine receptors in schizophrenia. *Am J Psychiatry* 1985;142:1334-1337.

22. Bonney WE, Goodwin FK, Murphy DL: The "switch process" in manic-depressive illness. *Arch Gen Psychiatry* 1972;27:304-309.

23. Schildkraut JJ: The catecholamine hypothesis of affective disorders: a review of supporting evidence. *Am J Psychiatry* 1965;22:507-522.

24. Terenius L, Wahlstrom A, Lindstrom L, et al: Increased levels of endorphins in chronic psychosis. *Neurosci Lett* 1976;3:157-162.

25. Gunne LM, Lindstrom L, Terenius L: Naloxone-induced reversal of schizophrenic hallucinations. *J Neurol Transmission* 1977;40:13-19.

26. Kline NS, Li CH, Lehman HE, et al: Beta endorphin induced changes in schizophrenic and depressed patients. *Arch Gen Psychiatry* 1977;34:1111-1113.

27. Widerlov E, Lindstrom LH, Besov G, et al: Subnormal CSF levels of neurotensin in a subgroup of schizophrenic patients: normalization after neuroleptic treament. *Am J Psychiatry* 1982;139:1122-1126.

28. Krieger DT, Martin JB: Brain peptides. *N Engl J Med* 1981;304:876-885,944-951.

29. Gowdy JM: Immunoglobulin levels in psychotic patients. *Psychosomatics* 1980;21:751-756.

30. Pandey RS, Gupta AK, Chaturvedi UC: Autoimmune model of schizophrenia with special reference to anti-brain antibodies. *Biol Psychiatry* 1981;16:1123-1136.

31. Jankovic BC: Delayed skin hypersensitivity reactions to human brain S-100 protein in psychiatric patients. *Biol Psychiatry* 1982;17:687-697.

32. Knight JG: Dopamine-receptor-stimulating autoantibodies: A possible cause of schizophrenia. *Lancet* 1982;2:1073-1076.

33. Lidz T, Fleck S, Cornelison, AR: *Schizophrenia and the Family*. New York, International Universities Press, 1965.

34. Arieti S: *Interpretation of schizophrenia*. New York, Brunner, 1955.

35. Haley J: Testing parental instructions of schizophrenic and normal children. *J Abnorm Psychol* 1968;73:559-565.

36. Brown GW, Birley JLT, Wing JK: Influence of family life on the course of schizophrenic disorders: a replication. *Br J Psychiatry* 1972;121:241-258.

37. Vaughn CE, Leff JP: The influence of family and social factors on the course of psychiatric illness. *Br J Psychiatry* 1976;129:125-137.

38. Lipton FR, Cohen CI, Fischer E, et al: Schizophrenia: a network crisis. *Schizophr Bull* 1981;7:144-151.

39. Faris REL, Dunham HW: *Mental Disorders in Urban Areas*. Chicago, University of Chicago Press, 1939.

40. Hollingshead AB, Redlich FC: *Social Class and Mental Illness: A Community Study*. New York, John Wiley & Sons, 1958.

41. Sabatini R: *Scaramouche*. New York, Grosset & Dunlap, 1921.

42. Goldhamer H, Marshall AW: *Psychosis and civilization: two studies in the frequency of mental disease*. New York, Free Press of Glencoe, 1953.

43. Ursano RJ, Boydstun JA, Wheatley RD: Psychiatric illness in US Air Force Vietnam prisoners of war, five year follow-up. *Am J Psychiatry* 1981;138:310-314.

44. Drugs that cause psychiatric symptoms. *Med Lett Drugs Ther* 1981;23:9-12.

45. Erman MK, Guggenheim FG: Psychiatric side effects of commonly used drugs. *Drug Ther Hosp* 1981:55-64.

160

46. Propping P: Genetic disorders presenting as "schizophrenia." *Hum Genet* 1985;65:1-10.
47. Gilbert GJ: Quinidine dementia, letter.*Am J Cardiol* 1978;41:791.
48. Hall RCW, Popkin MK, Stickney SK, et al: Presentation of the steroid psychoses. *J Nerv Ment Dis* 1979;167:229-236.
49. Baldessarini RJ: Drugs and the treatment of psychiatric disorders, in Gilman AG, Goodman LS, Rall TW, et al (eds): *The Pharmacological Basis of Therapeutics*, ed 7. New York, MacMillan Publishing Co, 1985, p 425.
50. Gordon C: Differential diagnosis of cimetidine-induced delirium.*Psychosomatics* 1981;22:251-252.
51. Post RM, Kopanda RT: Cocaine, kindling and psychosis. *Am J Psychiatry* 1976;133:627-634.
52. Lesko LM, Fischman MW, Javaid JI: Iatrogenous cocaine psychosis, letter. *N Engl J Med* 1982;307:1153.
53. Levin M: Bromide hallucinosis. *Arch Gen Psychiatry* 1960;2:429-433.
54. Brown CE: The alcohol withdrawal syndrome. *Ann Emerg Med* 1982;11:276-280.
55. Unde TW, Redmond DE, Kleber HD: Psychosis in the opioid addicted patient: assessment and treatment. *J Clin Psychiatry* 1982;43:240-247.
56. Chouinard G, Jones BD, Annable L: Neuroleptic induced supersensitivity psychosis. *Am J Psychiatry* 1978;135:1409-1410.
57. Witschy JK, Malone GL, Holden LD: Psychosis after neuroleptic withdrawal in a manic-depressive patient. *Am J Psychiatry* 1984;141:105-106.
58. Feinberg JF: The Wernicke-Korsakoff syndrome. *Am Fam Physician* 1980;22:129-133.
59. Patterson WM, Logar WE, Vandewalle MB: PCP psychosis in a general hospital. *Milit Med* 1982;147:311-312.
60. DiSclafani A, Hall RCW, Gardner ER: Drug-induced psychosis: emergency diagnosis and management. *Psychosomatics* 1981;22:845-850.
61. Craig DH, Rosen P: Abuse of anti-Parkinsonian drugs. *Ann Emerg Med* 1981;10:98-100.
62. Shaul P, Farrell MK, Maloney MJ: Caffeine toxicity as a cause of acute psychosis in anorexia nervosa. *J Pediatr* 1984;105:493-495.
63. Louria DB: Trace metal poisoning, in Wyngaarden JB, Smith LH (eds): *Cecil Textbook of Medicine*, ed 17. Philadelphia, WB Saunders Co, 1985, p 2308.
64. Peterson GC: Organic mental disorders induced by drugs or poisons, in Kaplan HI, Freedman AM, Sadock BJ (eds): *Comprehensive Textbook of Psychiatry*, ed 3. Baltimore, Williams & Wilkins Co, 1980, p 1450.
65. Josephson AM, MacKenzie TB: Thyroid-induced mania in hypothyroid patients. *Br J Psychiatry* 1980;137:222-228.
66. Walker JI, Brodie HKH: Paranoid disorders, in Kaplan HI, Sadock

BJ:*Comprehensive Textbook of Psychiatry,* ed 4. Baltimore, Williams & Wilkins Co, 1985, pp 753-754.

67. Koranyi EK: Undiagnosed physical illness in psychiatric patients. *Ann Rev Med* 1982;33:309-316.

68. Liston EH: Delirium in the aged. *Psychiatr Clin North Am* 1982;5(1):49-66.

69. Steel K, Feldman RG: Diagnosing dementia and its treatable causes. *Geriatrics* 1979;34:79-88.

70. Lipowski ZJ: Organic mental disorders: introduction and review of syndromes, in Kaplan HI, Freedman AM, Sadock BJ (eds): *Comprehensive Textbook of Psychiatry,* ed 4. Baltimore, Williams & Wilkins Co, 1985.

71. Gershon S, Herman SP: The differential diagnosis of dementia. *J Am Geriatr Soc* 1982;30 (suppl):558-566.

72. Granet RB, Kalman TP: Hypothyroidism and psychosis: a case illustration of the diagnostic dilemma in psychiatry. *J Clin Psychiatry* 1978:39;206-263.

73. Portnoi VA: Thyrotoxicosis as a mimic of dementia and/or stroke-like syndrome. *Postgrad Med* 1979;66:219-221.

74. Reed K, Watkins M, Dobson H: Mania in Cushing's syndrome: case report. *J Clin Psychiatry* 1983;44:460-462.

75. Williams EY, Weeks LR: Premenstrual tension associated with psychotic episodes. *J Nerv Ment Dis* 1952;116:321-329.

76. Benson RC: Gynecology of obstretics, in Krupp MA, Chatton MJ (eds): *Current Medical Diagnosis and Treatment.* Los Altos, Calif, Lange Medical Pub, 1981, pp 428-483.

77. Endo M, Daiguji M, Asano Y, et al: Periodic psychosis recurring in association with menstrual cycle. *J Clin Psychiatry* 1978;39:456-466.

78. Yik KY, Sullivan SN, Troster M: Neuropsychiatric disturbance due to occult occlusion of the portal vein. *Can Med Assoc J* 1982;126:50-52.

79. Santy PA, Schwartz MB: Hyponatremia disguised as an acute manic episode. *Hosp Community Psychiatry* 1983;34:1156-1157.

80. Massey EW: Neuropsychiatric manifestations of porphyria. *J Clin Psychiatry* 1980;41:208-213.

81. Pepplinkhuizen L, Bruinrels J, Blom W, et al: Schizophrenia-like psychosis caused by a metabolic disorder. *Lancet* 1980;1:454-456.

82. Cartwright GE: Diagnosis of treatable Wilson's disease. *N Engl J Med* 1978;298:1347-1350.

83. Scheinberg IH: Wilson's disease, in Isselbacher KJ, Adams RD, Braunwald E, et al (eds): *Harrison's Principles of Internal Medicine,* ed 9. New York, McGraw-Hill Book Co, 1980, pp 491-494.

84. Binder RL, Dickman WA: Psychiatric manifestation of neurosyphilis in middle-aged patients. *Am J Psychiatry* 1980;137:741-742.

85. Ommen KJ, Johnson PC, Ray CG: Herpes simplex type 2 virus encephalitis presenting as psychosis. *Am J Med* 1982;73:445-448.

162

86. Wilson LG: Viral encephalopathy mimicking functional psychosis. *Am J Psychiatry* 1976;133:165-170.
87. Behan PO: Creutzfeldt-Jakob disease. *Br J Med* 1982;284:1658-1659.
88. Gilden DH: Slow virus diseases of the CNS. *Postgrad Med* 1983;73:113-118.
89. Bleich A, Munitz H, Wijsenbeck H: Schizophreniform episode with infectious mononucleosis. *Psychosomatics* 1982;23:1067-1068.
90. Rubin RC: Adolescent infectious mononucleosis with psychosis. *J Clin Psychiatry* 1978;39:63-65.
91. Shenberger KN, Meharg JG, Lane CD: Temporal arteritis presenting as ataxia and dementia. *Postgrad Med* 1981;69:246-249.
92. Hontela S, Schwartz G: Myocardial infarction in the differential diagnosis of dementias in the elderly. *J Am Geriatr Soc* 1979;27:104-106.
93. Wells CE: Role of stroke in dementia. *Stroke* 1978;9:1-3.
94. Feely MP, O'Hare J, Veale D, et al: Episodes of acute confusion or psychosis in hemiplegic migrane.*Acta Neurol Scand* 1982;65:369-375.
95. Cordingley G, Navarro C, Brust JCM, et al: Sarcoidosis presenting as senile dementia. *Neurology* 1981;31:1148-1151.
96. Kuhnley EJ, White DH, Granoff AC: Psychiatric presentation of an arachnoid cyst. *J Clin Psychiatry* 1981;42(2):167-168.
97. Binder RL: Neurologically silent brain tumors in psychiatric hospital admissions: three cases and a review. *J Clin Psychiatry* 1983;44:94-97.
98. Hamilton NG, Frick RB, Takahashi T, et al: Psychiatric symptoms and cerebellar pathology. *Am J Psychiatry* 1983;140:1322-1326.
99. Ramani SV: Psychosis associated with frontal lobe lesions in Schilder's cerebral sclerosis: a case report with CT scan evidence. *J Clin Psychiatry* 1981;42:250-252.
100. Case records of the Massachusetts General Hospital. *N Engl J Med* 1982;306:286-293.
101. Awad AG: Schizophrenia and multiple sclerosis. *J Nerv Ment Dis* 1983;171:323-324.
102. Kellner CH, Davenport Y, Post RM, et al: Rapidly cycling bipolar disorder and multiple sclerosis. *Am J Psychiatry* 1984;141:112-113.
103. Schneck MK, Reisberg B, Ferris SH: An overview of current concepts of Alzheimer's disease. *Am J Psychiatry* 1982;139:165-173.
104. Caine ED, Shoulson I: Psychiatric syndromes in Huntington's disease. *Am J Psychiatry* 1983;140:728-733.
105. Wells C: Chronic brain disease: an update on alcoholism, Parkinson's disease, and dementia. *Hosp Community Psychiatry* 1982;32:111-116.
106. Mindham RHS, Ahmed S, Clough CC: A controlled study of dementia in Parkinson's disease. *J Neurol Neurosurg Psychiatry* 1982;45:969-974.
107. Iivanainen M, Bergstrom L, Nuutila A, et al: Psychosis-like absence status of elderly patients. *J Neurol Neurosurg Psychiatry* 1984;47:965-969.

108. McKenna PJ, Kane JM, Parrish K: Psychotic syndromes in epilepsy. *Am J Psychiatry* 1985;142:895-904.
109. Adebimpe VR: Complex partial seizures simulating schizophrenia. *JAMA* 1977;237:1339-1341.
110. Read SL: Catatonia in thrombotic thrombocytopenic purpura: a case report. *J Clin Psychiatry* 1983;44:343-344.
111. Pro JD, Wells CE: The use of the electroencephalogram in the diagnosis of delirium. *Dis Cent Nerv Syst* 1977;38:804-808.
112. Smith JS, Kiloh LG: The investigation of dementia: results in 200 consecutive admissions. *Lancet* 1981:824-827.
113. Dubin WR, Field AL, Gastfriend OR: Postcardiotomy delirium: a critical review. *J Thoracic Cardiovasc Surg* 1979;77:586-594.
114. Sadler PD: Incidence, degree and duration of post-cardiotomy delirium. *Heart & Lung* 1981;10:1084-1092.
115. Kornfeld DS, Heller SS, Frank KA, et al: Personality and psychological factors in post-cardiotomy delirium. *Arch Gen Psychiatry* 1974;31:249.
116. Bexton WH, Heron W, Scott TH: Effects of decreased variation in the sensory environment. *Can J Psychol* 1954;8:70.
117. Weisman HD, Hackett TP: Psychosis after eye surgery. *N Engl J Med* 1958;258:1284-1289.
118. Levine AM: Visual hallucinations and cataracts. *Opthalmic Surg* 1980;11:95-98.
119. Davidson K, Bagley CR: Schizophrenia-like psychosis associated with organic disorders of the central nervous system: a review of the literature, in Herrington RN (ed): *Current Problems in Neuropsychiatry. Br J Psychiatry* 1969;4:113-184.
120. Nasrallah HA, Fowler RC, Judd LL: Schizophrenia-like illness following head injury. *Psychosomatics* 1981;22:359-361.
121. Henker TO: Body-image conflict following trauma and surgery. *Psychosomatics* 1979;20:812-820.
122. American Psychiatric Association: *Diagnostic and Statistical Manual of Mental Disorders,* ed 3. Washington, American Psychiatric Association, 1980.
123. Lewine RRJ: Sex differences in age of symptom onset and first hospitalization in schizophrenia. *Am J Orthopsychiatry* 1980;50:316-322.
124. McEvoy JP, Wells CE: Case studies in neuropsychiatry II: conversion pseudodementia. *J Clin Psychiatry* 1979;40:447-449.
125. Pope HG, Jonas JM, Jones B: Factitious psychosis: phenomenology, family history, and long-term outcome of nine patients. *Am J Psychiatry* 1982;139:1480-1483.
126. Hay GG: Feigned psychosis — a review of the simulation of mental illness. *Br J Psychiatry* 1983;143:10.

4 Hallucinations

Stephen M. Soreff

HALLUCINATIONS   The perception of something actually not there: the believed sensation which is not real.[1] Hallucinations may be auditory, visual, olfactory, tactile, gustatory, somatic or kinesthetic.[2]

Case report   A 22-year-old man hears voices of people not in attendance, sees sights of animals not there, and smells odors of materials not present. He recoils with fear. He has been under recent stresses, had taken an unidentified "pill," and had not been feeling himself of late. The interviewer, after a moment of disbelief, commenced a thorough evaluation.

FEATURES

The vast, restless sea of mental activity: driven by conflicts, battered by drugs, whipped by substance abuses, hammered by disease, and fanned by the environment, creates its own believed perceptions and reality -- hallucinations.

Mood

Patients exhibit a wide variety of emotional responses to their hallucinations.

Some people react with terror. The voices or images may present in a threatening, attacking, and frightening manner. A 65-year-old male patient on the seventh floor of the hospital became paralyzed with fear as he heard and saw a freight train roar through his room.

Others find the hallucinations discomforting and unpleasant. The voices arguing and discussing in their heads bother them. The smell of

164

burning rubber is not pleasant. They feel disturbed, annoyed, and inconvenienced but not necessarily alarmed by the sensation.

Still others derive a feeling of enjoyment, well-being, fulfillment, and thrill from the hallucination. Indeed, some seek certain substances to obtain such an experience. Many students have used LSD in order to feel a sense of wonder, euphoria, and awe.

Yet some will appreciate their hallucination with apathy. They have experienced hallucinations before or for too long a time. They recognize them as their problem, their struggle, and their symptom. They greet the event with indifference.

Finally, certain individuals will approach the hallucination with a sense of curiosity. They want to know the meaning, the cause, and the course of the sensation. They are intrigued by their perception and want to understand it.

Thought

The disordered thought processes constitute the key feature of the hallucinatory experience. This fundamental alteration of the perceptual system and its integration to an internal logic sequence creates a false, yet believed, sensation. The thought content of an hallucination involves three components: the varied sensations, the qualities of that experience, and the underlying inner reality of the event.

Sensory perceptions   Hallucinations occur in a wide variety of sensations.

Auditory hallucinations take many forms and have a variety of qualities. They may occur as a voice or voices: a person talking, a group discussing, or a crowd yelling. They may be a sound or sounds: a buzz, a bell, a river, a wind, an orchestra, or a train. The voices may be providing a commentary, be condemning, be commanding, be accusing, be supportive. The sounds may appear to be near, in one's head, or from afar. They may be a whisper, soft, natural, or loud.

Visual hallucinations occur in a number of ways. Individuals see people: lovers, departed loved ones, or strangers, animals, places, lights, dashes, or geometric patterns. They view them as single images in slide-like projections, or in continuous action. The objects may be inviting, interesting, or threatening. The vision may be dull, subdued, gentle, bright, vivid.

The olfactory hallucination experience takes different forms. People smell familiar, pleasant odors: food cooking, flowers, or the ocean. People sense unfamiliar, unpleasant smells: burning rubber or foul eggs.

Tactile hallucinations occur in many ways. Individuals feel objects: wood, stone, metal. They perceive insects or snakes crawling on their skin (*formication*), or they sense people not actually present.

Gustatory hallucinations cover a number of taste sensations. People may sense fine food. The experience might register as bitter and repulsive sensations. Or they may have metallic, unfamiliar tastes in the mouth.

Somatic hallucinations involve internal bodily sensations and include a variety of events. There is the perceptions of pain, for example. Or the sense of internal organs disarranged or in disarray. Alternately, patients may feel bizarre sensations, such as animals eating their insides or snakes wandering about their abdomen.

Kinesthetic hallucinations represent the perception of the body's orientation in space, is derived from sensations in muscles, joints, and semicircular canals, and takes the form of feeling physically disoriented. People may feel they are losing their balance, or they may perceive themselves as upside down.

When the hallucination occurs is important in both description and understanding of the experience. Most hallucinations happen when the person is awake. However, during the periods preceding and following sleep, people frequently have these perceptual experiences.

Hypnagogic hallucinations take place during the twilight between wake and full sleep.[3]

Hypnopompic hallucinations occur in the time between sleeping and being awake. Both hypnagogic and hypnopompic hallucinations are common experiences and are often not evidence of psychopathology.

Quality The hallucinatory experience has several qualities. First, it often is persistent and sustained.[4]

It continues and is not interruptable. Second, it remains unavoidable and undeniable. Third, it stands as an immediate and compelling event.

Reality The final and most important feature of the hallucination remains its reality. To the beholder, the hallucination is *real*. It stands as an actual, believed, perceived, and true experience. In contrast, with *pseudohallucination* the experiencer recognizes that the perception is not real; it comes from internal distortion of the event.

Along with hallucinatory experience, the patients may exhibit other mental status abnormalities and findings. These include delusions, obsessions, illusions, and disorientation. Where relevant, the discussion of the particular cause and situation will mention these features.

Behavior

Hallucinations lead to a wide range of behaviors. Hallucinations trigger these responses not only as a reaction to the perceptions themselves but also in direct relation to the accompanying affective context of the experience. The combination produces the following behaviors: withdrawal, flight, violence, and commanded activity.

Many people may respond to their hallucinations by *withdrawal*. They move into their own world, thoughts, visions, and creations. They may prefer an inner reality to the external experience. They dwell upon the images and mental adventures. They may derive pleasure and enjoyment from hallucinations. Or they may find such pain, turmoil, and ugliness from the perceptions that they may select withdrawal and isolation to protect themselves and others from the experience.

Others may take *flight* because of the hallucinations. They flee from the accusing voices, the condemning crowd, the threatening image, the offensive odors. A man ran to the emergency department to escape the warring voices in his head which both commented upon and bitterly judged him. A woman dashed from her hospital bed as she perceived a sailing vessel coming toward her.

Violence may erupt in response to a hallucinatory experience. People may assault others perceived to be attacking them. Or they may fight an imagined group of enemies.

Finally, one of the most dreaded results of these perceptions remains *command hallucinations*. Here, the patient responds directly to the message and direction of the hallucination. A voice commands a man to kill his brother, hurt himself, or amputate part of his body.[5] A woman reacts to voices ordering her to sacrifice her child. These patients respond to inner reality and directions which order destruction, devastation, and disaster.

Physical examination   Although no one physical finding is typical of the hallucinatory experience, there are a variety of responses to both the accompanying affect and resultant behavior and to specific causes. Anxiety, flight, and violence may be reflected in an elevated pulse and blood pressure. Alcohol withdrawal may produce tachycardia and a rise in temperature. Delirium may present with a number of neurologic signs and findings. Or marijuana may lead to infected conjunctiva, decreased temperature, and lowered blood pressure.

Laboratory Findings

Although no one test is appropriate to cover all hallucinatory experiences, certain studies are indicated by specific perceptual events. Olfactory hallucinations suggest EEG and CT scans with special emphasis upon the frontal and temporal regions. Similarly, visual hallucinations point toward a neurologic work-up, including EEGs and CT scans. Yellow vision occurring in people taking digitalis calls for obtaining blood level of that drug.

As the various diagnostic possibilities develop, particular physical findings and specific studies with their results will be advanced.

Interviewer's Reaction

Interviewers find themselves with two principal responses to the patients and their hallucinations: incredulity and fascination.

Many clinicians express feelings of incredulity in the face of the hallucinatory experience. They simply cannot believe that the patient actually believes the hallucination. They have trouble accepting the patient's acceptance of the perceptual reality. They wonder if the patient describing animals walking around the examining room "is for real."

The other major response remains a total sense of awe and fascination. For centuries hallucinations have intrigued theologians, philosophers, students, and physicians. They are thought to have power, prediction, and potential. Clinicians find themselves interested, curious, and enthusiastic toward eliciting the experience and discovering its origins.

PATHOGENESIS

Individual—their struggles, their hopes, their losses, their stresses, their pasts, and their convictions, create hallucinations. Hallucinations represent dramatic reflections of inner turmoil, conflicts, and pressures. They can be understood, like a host of other psychiatric symptoms, on the basis of psychodynamic formulations, unconscious strivings, and personality factors. Indeed, it is against the background, backdrop, and bedrock of the person that all subsequent biologic and environmental factors are discussed.

Psychodynamic Explanation

Wish fulfillment creates and propels the hallucinatory experience. Freud made reference to the wish-derived quality and function of the false perception.[6] The hallucination represents an unconscious wish, striving, or hope, and is a dramatic manifestation of the primary process desires.[7] For example, in the situation of condemning, vilifying voices, the individual may be seeking punishment for secret thoughts, feelings, or sins, eg, masturbation or a homosexual encounter. The auditory hallucinations provide the pain unconsciously wanted.[8] Hallucinations—their latent and manifest content—offer an important avenue to understanding the patient's wishes and underlying personality. Hallucinations can be appreciated and comprehended as dreams can.[9] They reveal the patient's unconscious universe.

Hallucinations result from mental excitement. Stresses—both inner and external—acting upon the individuals create these experiences. They represent the final common pathway, mechanism, and release from conflicts, strivings, turmoil, anguish, hope, apprehension, and pain.

Hallucinations provide a method to momentarily restore a loss. The experiencer retains in life and in attendance those who have died or are far away. After a couple lost their 6-year-old son to leukemia, they frequently heard his voice calling them. Occasionally the mother saw him standing in the stairway. The voice and image kept him alive and still part of them.

Hallucinations occur as a consequence of age function failure.[10] In essence, the experience happens because the critical determining ego judgment and assessment factors are either suspended or absent. The individual accepts the reality of perception; it is not mentally challenged or questioned.

Hallucinations are driven by and created from memories.[11] They represent expressions of past events, activities, and undertakings. Their occurrence provides dramatic intrusions of the past into the present. An old veteran was in his hospital bed. He was dying. Yet he dwelled on the "big one": the Battle of the Bulge. He talked to the troops; he saw the enemy. He lived then as he slipped away from now. Memory traces provide the substratum for hallucinations.

Intense convictions create their own hallucinatory manifestations. Be the conviction religious, political, scientific, or utopian, the beholders, if they wish hard enough, dwell long enough, and obsess long enough, may

Table 4-1
Pathogenesis of Hallucinations

	Auditory	Visual	Olfactory	Tactile	Other
Psychodynamic Explanation					
I. Wish fulfillment	X	X	X	X	X
II. Reaction to excitement	X	X	X	X	X
III. Restitution of loss	X	X			
IV. Ego Dysfunction	X	X	X	X	X
V. Pressure of memories	X	X			
VI. Intense conviction	X	X	X	X	X
VII. A mechanism	X	X	X	X	X
Environment					
Cultural Determinants					
Influence	X	X		X	
Reactions	X	X			X
(Hypnagogic/hypnopompic)					
Sensory deprivation					
Experimental	X	X			
Naturally occurring	X	X			
Medical	X	X	X	X	X

Intensity

Nonpsychotroic Drugs

Cardiac glycosides	X	X			
Bromides	X	X	X		X
Levodopa		X	X		
Amatadine hydrochloride		X			
Amphetamine	X	X	X		
Cimetidine	X	X			
Propranolol hydrochloride	X	X	X	X	
Narcotic antagonists		X			
Anticholinergic drugs	X	X		X	

Psychotropic Drugs

Anticholinergic Effects
    Regular dose
    Overdose
    Additive
	X	X		X	

Impramine hydrochloride		X		X (Hypnopompic)	
Disulfiram	X	X			

Alcohol

Hallucinosis	XX	X	X		X (Tinnitus)
Withdrawal Delerium (delirium tremens)	X	XX	X	X	

continued

Table 4-1
continued

	Auditory	Visual	Olfactory	Tactile	Other
Other Abused Substances					
Amphetamine	X	X	X		
Barbiturates	X	X		X	
Cocaine	X	X	X	X	X (Gustatory)
Hallucinogens LSD Dimethyltryptamine (DMT) Mescaline Peyote, psilocybin	X	XX		X	
Marijuana		X			
Phencyclidine (PCB)	XX	X		X	
Medical Illnesses					
Neurologic Narcolepsy	X	X			X (Hypnagogic/hypnopompic)
Tumors	X	X	X		X (Gustatory)
Migraine attacks		X			
Temporal lobe Epilepsy	X	X	X		X
Developing blindness		X			
Ear pathology	X				X (Tinnitus)
Severe conditions Pain Fever Starvation Delirium	X	XX	X	X	

Surgical Complications

Anesthesia					
Ketamine hydrochloride		X			
Eye Patch	X	X			
Phantom limb					X (Kinesthetic)
Cortex stimulation	X	X	X	X	X
Physical Trauma					
Head		X	X		
Frontal lobe					
Psychiatric Diagnosis					
Organic disorder	X	X	X	X	
Schizophrenia	X	X	X	X	X (Gustatory)
Major affective disorders					
Manic Episode	X	X			
Major depressive episode					
Conversion reaction	X	X			

produce their own perceptions. A man believed completely in extra-terrestrial life. He dedicated his existence to proving its presence. Ultimately, he told his friends how he communicated with extraterrestrial creatures.

Finally, a mental mechanism produces the false perception.[12] A two-step process occurs. First, the persons exercise denial. Their denial may be a feeling, a thought, a hope, or a fear. Second, the desired object is projected. A man lost his beloved father. He then heard his father calling him. He had at that moment denied the death and projected the voices onto a new reality.

Hallucinations represent the final common pathway of a series of psychodynamic processes.[13]

Biologic Explanation

An extensive array of *biochemical agents* have been implicated in the hallucinatory phenomenon. Their very range and diversity suggest the complexity of the situation. Mescaline and amphetamines as phenyl-alkylamine derivatives have compositions similar to dopamine, norepinephrine, and epinephrine. In contrast, LSD and psilocybin as tryptamine derivatives have structures similar to serotonin.[14] Additionally, such varied drugs and substances as digitalis, phencyclidine hydrochloride, cocaine, and alcohol withdrawal account for hallucinations. An endogenous route of generating hallucinations is through a transmethylation mechanism.[15] A methyl group is placed upon a compound producing a hallucinogen. Based upon these examples, one can reach two conclusions. First, a number of biochemical agents, medications, and abused substances trigger hallucinatory experiences. Second, as of yet, no one chemical substance has been demonstrated responsible for all hallucinations.

Stimulation, lesions, or trauma to *specific cortex* regions often result in particular hallucinatory experiences. Tumor of the temporal lobe will produce formed images. These may or may not be accompanied by auditory hallucinations. Lesions to the temporal lobes will also generate both olfactory and gustatory hallucinations. Lesions to occipital lobes will account for unformed images such as light flashes.[16]

The optical stimulation state, explored more fully in the environment section, suggests a bridge from the biochemical to the experiential.[17] Hallucinations occur when the individual is either under- or overstimulated. Monotony, sameness, and lack of input is one extreme. On the other, too much input, changes, and stimulation also will generate these perceptual experiences. Drugs such as mescaline, LSD, or amphetamines cause excessive CNS excitement, and thus hallucinations.

Genetics

The genetic contribution to an understanding of hallucinations remains less apparent than the other factors. However, a fascinating study by Rosenthal and Quinn of monozygotic quadruplets, concordant for schizophrenia, suggests an interesting hereditary role.[18] Of these identical four girls, three exhibited hallucinations. One's first hallucination was auditory; the other two had visual experiences. The authors conclude there is a basic genotype predisposing toward hallucinations, yet the actual expression of it remains plastic and variable.

Environment

Cultural determinants play key roles in the hallucinatory experience. First, they influence the perceptual event itself: its type, quality, and nature. Second, such cultural determinants help to govern the individual's reactions to his experiences. Currie and Currie report a dramatically significantly higher incidence of emergence deliriums, often accompanied by hallucinations, in literate patients compared with illiterate patients receiving the anesthetic ketamine hydrochloride.[19] As a result, the patients either view the hallucinations as evidence of pathology or as signs of normality. Taken collectively, the cultural factors point out the importance of clinicians seeing moods, thoughts, and behaviors within the context of the individuals' backgrounds, communities, traditions, religions, and social systems.[20]

One's cultural background influences the type of hallucinatory experience. Individuals with strong religious histories and traditions may find themselves experiencing hallucinations with a profound godly presence and commandment. A deeply involved young Baptist, as he began his manic episode, heard voices commanding him to go to the airport and receive Christ arriving on a jet plane. Ishmael in *Moby Dick* perceived the hypnagogic hallucination of being held by supernatural powers as syntonic with his belief system.[21] In another sphere, Vitols et al reported the interesting finding that black schizophrenic patients experienced a significantly greater number of hallucinations than did white schizophrenics on first admission to the same facility.[22]

Cultural factors also determine the individuals' reactions to hallucinatory experiences. On one hand, the individuals' community backgrounds may cause them to see a benign event as evidence of severe pathology. For example, an African student in the United States had a hypnopompic experience of both hearing voices and feelings of being struck on each arm. In this country such perceptual events are considered normal and of little consequence. Yet, the psychiatric reassurance failed, because in his country these experiences were proof of severe illness, the result of spiritual possession, and meant one was "being held by the spider."[23] On the other hand, many hallucinations experienced within religious contexts are held in their communities as natural and divine occurrences. A number of the Middle Age visions now judged as signs of mental illnesses were then culturally supported events.[24]

Sensory deprivation results in a wide and wild array of hallucinations. The acute and chronic dramatic diminution of sensory input propels the mind into a fascinating display of perceptual experiences. Experimental procedures, natural occurrences, and medical treatment may cause sensory deprivation.

In the 1950s a number of investigators conducted a series of studies allowing individuals to experience acute, often total sensory deprivation.[25] The participants had many perceptual distortions of both a significant magnitude and of a terrifying nature. Lilly suspended persons wearing only a blackened head mask in water at $34.5^{\circ}C$. They developed a rich, individualized fantasy experience and visual imagery.[26] Bexton et al placed college students in a soundproof room with their hands and feet in cardboard cuttings.[27] They wore translucent glasses which allowed only light without images to pass through. Most students could not tolerate the experiment for more than 72 hours. Those who persisted beyond 72 hours developed hallucinations.

A vast number of everyday and exceptional natural occurrences promote the development of hallucinations through sensory deprivation mechanisms.[28] Daily events include driving long distances for many hours on interstate highways, "turnpike trances," long solo flights, or continuously watching a monitor, eg, sonar or radar. Exceptional experiences involve being alone in the Antarctic, such as Admiral Byrd experienced, or adrift in a lifeboat, lost in the mountains, or as prisoner of war. A man alone in the mountains buried by a blizzard heard skiers and perceived people about him. Another man adrift for weeks ultimately saw the faces of his comrades on the rocks of an island on which he had landed. All these experiences had a common thread: isolation, monotony, stress, protracted time involvement, and limited stimuli.

Finally, medical or surgical treatments may produce immobility, limited stimulations, monotony, and isolation. The classic example was the use of tank-type respirators for patients with poliomyelitis. These patients had auditory, visual, olfactory, tactile, gustatory, and kinesthetic hallucinations.[29] Other incidents might include the room at the end of the corridor without visitors, staff, or windows, "isolation," a "burn" room, or a full body cast.

An extremely intense environment leads to hallucinations. For example, severe cold may induce a hallucinatory experience, as may thirst, hunger, and fever.[30] An array of "beyond" experiences, eg, crossing the river, being beckoned by departed relatives, and bright lights, have been reported by resuscitated patients.[31] Additionally, an overstimulating environment may precipitate hallucinations, eg, loud continual noises or bright, changing lights.

DIFFERENTIAL DIAGNOSIS

Nonpsychotropic Drugs

A wide range of medications produce hallucinatory experiences. These represent dramatic, often intense, events which prove disruptive to the patient, the family, and the staff. Generally, the hallucinations diminish and disappear with the drug's discontinuance. The visual hallucinations emerge as the most commonly encountered, although many other types occur. The hallucinations may appear in patients with clear sensorium or represent a part of a delirium.

Cardiac glycosides (the digitalis preparations) create a number of perceptual distortions. These include auditory hallucinations and visual disturbances. Often these events occur when the patient is digoxin-toxic. Efficacy is at 0.8 ng/mL; toxicity at 2.0 ng/mL and above.[32] Auditory hallucinations are frequent in the elderly. One woman reported accusing and quarreling voices with a digoxin level of 5.0 ng/mL.[33] These disappeared with digoxin discontinuance. Others experience seeing objects with yellow-green tints or edges (chromatopsia) when they are digitalis-toxic.[34]

Bromides, although less used in recent years, cause hallucinations. They come in the form of bromide salts, eg, bromisovalum. Signs of toxicity occur above serum bromide levels of 50 mg/100 mL.[34] The level usually builds over time with bromides having a long half-life. Auditory and visual hallucinations are common. Frequently, the hallucinations possess a self-referential quality.[35] One patient reported God warning her. Another common sensation of bromide intoxication involves the feeling of floating in air. Olfactory hallucinations also occur.

Antiparkinsonian drugs —*Levodopa, amantadine hydrochloride, and bromocriptine*—produce hallucinations. All act by increasing the available amount of CNS dopamine. Levodopa serves as a precursor of dopamine; amantadine causes enhanced release of dopamine; and bromocriptine functions as a specific dopamine receptor agonist.[36] Dopamine has emerged as the major biochemical etiologic agent of schizophrenia.[14] Levodopa results in visual hallucinations usually, although olfactory hallucinations have also been reported.[37] Amantadine produces visual hallucinations which, in contrast to levodopa, develop insidiously and slowly over months of therapy.[38] Bromocriptine is also responsible for visual hallucinations.[39]

Amphetamines and a host of sympathomimetic drugs lead to hallucinations. Amphetamines are prescribed for narcolepsy, attention deficit disorders, and used to be commonly enlisted for weight control. Hallucinations include the auditory (frequently hearing accusatory voices), visual (distorted body and facial images), tactile (formication), and olfactory.[34,40] A whole spectrum of sympathomimetic drugs, which include common "cold" preparations, decongestants, nose drops, and bronchodilators, produce hallucinatory experiences similar to amphetamines.[41,42]

Cimetidine, a drug widely employed to diminish gastric acid secretion, produces both auditory and visual hallucinations. Cimetidine acts competitively as a histamine H_2 receptor antagonist.[43] It produces perceptual disturbances rapidly and upon discontinuance results in prompt cessation of these symptoms.[44] Both auditory and visual hallucinations occur frequently in individuals on cimetidine who are in serious medical situations and in intensive care units (ICUs).[45]

Propranolol hydrochloride produces a variety of hallucinatory experiences: auditory, visual, olfactory, and tactile. This drug was the first β-adrenergic blocking agent used. Physicians prescribe it for treatment of hypertension, cardiac arrhythmias, and angina pectoris. Early on in its application, hallucinations had been noted.[46] In one study, 18% of patients treated for hypertension with propranolol had visual hallucinations, frequently quite vivid and often recurrent.[47] For example, one patient saw a dead body near his bed and spiders composing his pillow. Others describe auditory hallucinations as well as visual ones, with voices commenting about their behavior.[48] In one case, a patient reported smelling smoke while on propranolol.[49] Another had crawling sensations about the skin.[50]

The narcotic antagonists generate visual hallucinations.[51] These include naloxone hydrochloride (Narcan) and levallorphan tartrate (Lorfan), the latter ten times more potent than the former. These drugs are used for respiratory depression induced by narcotics.

Anticholinergic drugs represent a major pharmacologic cause of hallucinatory experiences. These drugs are prescribed for a variety of reasons: belladonna or atropine as an antispasmodic; benztropine mesylate (Cogentin) as an antiparkinsonian drug; scopolamine as a "sedative;" or cyclopentolate hydrochloride as a mydriatic. Visual, auditory, and tactile hallucinations have been reported.[52]

Psychotropic Drugs

Psychotropic drugs are responsible for a number of hallucinatory experiences. These events represent side effects which are often dose-related. They cause great patient discomfort, clouding a frequently difficult diagnostic and therapeutic picture.

Anticholinergic-induced hallucinations occur with psychotropic drugs in a variety of settings. These hallucinations encompass auditory, visual, or tactile perceptual distortions.[52]

First, a number of psychotropic drugs have significant and potent anticholinergic activity: antidepressants, eg, amitriptyline hydrochloride; antiparkinsonian drugs, eg, trihexyphenidyl hydrochloride; and antipsychotic medications, eg, thioridazine (Mellaril). In particularly sensitive individuals, at high dosages, or in the elderly, they may trigger an anticholinergic hallucinatory experience.[53] Decreasing or eliminating the drug usually ceases the side effect.

Second, the anticholinergic effect of any of these drugs may be accentuated by an overdose. Again, the result is the picture of anticholinergic psychosis. A student in a fit of anger took all of her boy friend's trihexyphenidyl. During the following 24 to 48 hours in the ICU, she heard loud voices, saw terrifying objects, and felt things crawling over her.

Third, the combination of a number of psychotropic drugs, each with anticholinergic properties, may produce the same hallucinatory experience.[54] Not infrequently, certain patients are taking an antipsychotic drug, an antiparkinsonian drug to prevent reactions to the first medication, and a tricyclic antidepressant. Or they may be receiving an antipsychotic drug and an antiparkinsonian drug.[55] The additive effect is anticholinergic hallucinations.

Imipramine hydrochloride, a tricyclic antidepressant, has been implicated in the production of visual hallucinations. The effect is different from the just cited anticholinergic reaction. Klein reports these image experiences were similar to those noted by persons on hallucinogens.[56] Visions included spider webs, snowfall, doses of light, yellow sparkles turning into bugs. In Klein's study of 209 inpatients started on imipramine, 12 (6%) had these experiences. Of the 12, nine were schizophrenic. None of the 12 had a delirium. Imipramine has also been advanced as the cause of hypnopompic hallucinations.[57] These represent perceptual distortion occurring in the zone between sleeping and waking. Again, the visual hallucinations predominate, but auditory and tactile forms have been reported. One woman on imipramine reported seeing a red glow and people in her room. These terrifying visions ceased when the drug was discontinued.

In both examples imipramine's production of hallucinations may be different, either through an anticholinergic effect or through triggering an underlying schizophrenic reaction.

Disulfiram (Antabuse) has also been reported to cause hallucinations.[58] As a dopamine β hydroxylase inhibitor, it increases the available dopamine. The hallucinations have most frequently been noted in patients also taking monoamine oxidase inhibitors (MAOIs).

Alcohol

Alcohol hallucinosis designates an important withdrawal syndrome. The hallucinations are predominantly auditory but occasionally visual or olfactory. It occurs in persons with clear sensoriums, and presents usually between 12 hours to two days after reduction or cessation of heavy alcohol consumption.[59] The voices are terrifying, threatening, and accusing, and frequently refer to the patient in the third person, eg, "Let's get him." The patients experiencing these hallucinations have long histories of alcohol abuse and, not uncommonly, seek flight or help to escape the voices. Quite often tinnitus in the form of a loud sound, clicking sensation, fluttering noise, or fading sound also accompanies the alcohol withdrawal. This represents heightened activity of the middle ear muscles.[60] Of critical diagnostic significance, these patients remain oriented to person, place, and time in this condition.

Alcohol withdrawal delirium (delirium tremens) represents a severe form of alcohol withdrawal marked by disorientation, hallucinations, fever, and, not infrequently, seizures. It occurs among heavy drinkers usually between two to five days following decrease or termination of their alcohol intake. The visual hallucinations dominate the picture. The patients see fearful, attacking, often fantastic animals which may appear in diminutive size.[60] Such experiences may be accompanied by auditory, olfactory, and tactile hallucinations. Patients not only report bugs on them, but they may also feel them crawling over them. The central effect of these hallucinations emerges as one of terror, massive anxiety, and overwhelming fear.

Other Abused Substances

Amphetamines are responsible for a variety of hallucinations. They often have a paranoid or persecutory quality to them. Amphetamines produce vivid auditory, visual, and olfactory hallucinations.[61] Commonly, these events occur during and following amphetamine ingestion or intravenous (IV) administration. However, they may also appear during amphetamine withdrawal.

Barbiturates cause auditory, visual, and tactile hallucinations.[62] These occur during barbiturate withdrawal and present clinically similarly to the perceptual distortions of delirium tremens. This delirium manifests itself usually within seven days after the termination of chronic excessive barbiturate consumption.

Cocaine, in both acute intoxication and chronic use, over 6 months, generates in addition to a wide range of hallucinations, a unique and fascinating array of tactile events: "cocaine bugs."[63] Cocaine acts as a strong CNS stimulus, producing cortical arousal, heightening the activity of the reticular activating system, and triggering temporal lobe electrical discharges. Protracted use leads to chronic mydriasis, reflecting increased norepinephrine effects. Hallucinations include the auditory (voices calling, or whispering); olfactory (smelling gasoline, urine, garbage, or feces); and gustatory (unpleasant tastes). The tactile events center about the so-called cocaine bugs. This paresthesia is also called Magnan's sign and refers to the sensation of bugs or insects moving either over or under the skin. The cocaine bugs occur early with chronic use; the visual hallucinatory experiences develop later.

Cocaine's visual experiences involve "snow lights," geometric patterns, dysmegalopsia, and dysmorphopsia. Snow lights are pseudohallucinations appearing as light reflected off snow and occurring in the peripheral visual fields. The geometric designs present in black and white as lines, curved or straight and as points which may vibrate or develop in complex constructs. Dysmegalopsia is a disturbance in which people and objects appear larger than they actually are. In dysmorphopsia the shapes of objects become distorted, eg, an ashtray becomes a chicken or frying pan.

The hallucinogens produce a remarkable display of visual hallucinatory experiences and, rarely, auditory and tactile perceptual disturbances.[64] The common hallucinogens are LSD, dimethyltrytamine (DMT), mescaline, peyote, and psilocybin. The hallucination commences usually within an hour after ingestion and disappears after four to 12 hours. The images often develop as a slide show or appear as a movie. Patients report kaleidoscopic visual hallucinations. The visual experiences are intense, dramatic, and frequently either intriguing and fascinating "pleasant journeys," or alarming and terrifying "bad trips." Typical hallucinogen-induced images include religious symbols, small animals, and people.[64] The hallucinogens' principle biochemical action involves CNS norepinephrine release. Additionally, flashbacks, a repeat of the original hallucination, may occur.

Marijuana causes both visual hallucinations and flashbacks of these. Observers report seeing vivid slide shows or movies after tetrahydrocannabinal (THC) inhalation.[65] They note dramatic geometric patterns, with bright colors: violet, black, green, red, and orange. The shapes include symmetrical snowflakes, pinwheels, tunnels, circles, and fingerprint whorls. Frequently the pattern moves.

Phencyclidine (PCP) causes auditory, visual, and tactile hallucinations.[66] The auditory type is the most common. The hallucinations may have a religious quality. They may be accompanied by neurologic symptoms and signs, eg, nystagmus, ataxia, and altered sense of pain at touch. One potential mechanism of PCP, as well as its hallucinogen action, involves its induction of cerebral artery spasm.[67]

Medical Illnesses

Hallucinations, in several ways, may serve as a dramatic vivid signal of medical illness. They may herald the onset of a complex disease process. They may present as the sole manifestation of an underlying disease. Or they may occur in a cluster of compelling other symptoms.

Narcolepsy not only principally presents as sudden irrestible sleep episodes, but also with significant hallucinatory experiences.[68] The disease consists of four major symptoms: sleep attacks, cataplexy, hallucinations, and sleep paralysis. The hallmark of the condition involves sleep attacks occurring suddenly, often during activity and lasting usually for 15 minutes. Its onset is usually in the second decade. The hallucinations are hypnagogic and hypnopompic and are either auditory or visual. Patients report them as dreamlike states and find them frequently frightening. The disease mechanism is thought to involve patients going directly into REM sleep from the waking state and not passing through the intervening sleep stages (see chapter 7). This explanation accounts for these two types of hallucinations, as well as the cataplexy and sleep paralysis representative of REM sleep.

Brain tumors, depending on their location, will manifest themselves as different types of hallucinations.[16] Temporal lobe tumors reveal themselves in several ways: olfactory, gustatory, auditory, or visual hallucinations. The olfactory and gustatory (uncinate fits) hallucinations may be the principle presentation of the lesion or may precede seizures of the jacksonian type. The visual events are formed and may be accompanied by auditory experiences. In contrast, the occipital lobe tumors reveal themselves as unformed pictures, eg, light flashes.

Migraine attacks frequently include spectacular visual hallucinations as well as other visual distortions and events. Patients report visual hallucinations, such as seeing themselves across a railroad track, and perceptual alterations, such as people and objects appearing smaller than they actually are, and colors changing.[69] Richards has described some of these visual displays as resembling pre-twentieth century fortifications as seen from the air.[70] They consist of a series of lines or bars. The pattern also seems to expand outward during the attack. In the classic migraine, the prodromal phase (lasting 10 to 20 minutes) involves ipsilateral vasoconstriction of CNS-supplying arteries and contralateral neurologic signs, eg, hemianopsia, hemiparesis, aphasia, and/or headaches (hemicranium) lasting for hours. The visual events occur during the vasoconstriction period.

A temporal lobe epilepsy episode often commences with a hallucinatory event.[71] It may take the form of an ill-defined yet definite odor or taste, olfactory or gustatory hallucinations, called uncinate fits. Or it may involve auditory or visual hallucinations. The visual experience is often panoramic in quality.[72] Other common initiating symptoms include deja-vu or jamais-vu phenomena, dreamy states, flashbacks, or moments of fear. The fit consists of automatic movements of the mouth (eg, lip smacking), autonomic changes, (eg, usually pupil dilation and pallor), stereotype repetitive movements, amnesia, and postictal confusion and disorganization. Electroencephalography demonstrates spikes and other dysrhythmias in the temporal lobes. These are often better revealed during sleep tracing or using nasopharyngeal leads.

Failing vision leads to visual hallucinations. Generally eye disease results in unformed images, eg, light flashes of zigzag lines. However, White reports a number of patients with eye pathology, eg, macular degeneration, choroideraemia, and cataracts, who reported complex visual hallucinations.[73] They noted the abrupt onset of brightly colored pictures of children, animals, and in one case a circus troupe. Light appeared to trigger these vivid images. As sight deteriorated and blindness ensued, the hallucinations diminished. Aging and eye pathology correlate with the occurrence of visual hallucinations.[74]

Ear pathology produces noises in the ears, tinnitus. Tinnitus encompasses a wide range of sounds: buzzing, hissing, roaring, and whistling. Diseases of the middle ear and the eustachian tube often present with low-frequency vibratory sensations, such as roaring, pops, or clicks. In contrast, cochlea and light nerve lesions cause high-pitched tones which are nonvibratory. Some individuals in response to their growing deafness may develop auditory hallucinations.

A number of severe, critical, stressful medical conditions lead to hallucinations. Severe, prolonged, unrelenting pain may produce an hallucinatory experience. High *fever* has been associated with hallucinations. An extremely febrile woman with a pneumococcal empyema manifested a silly, inappropriate affect and auditory hallucinations. *Starvation*, hunger and thirst may cause hallucinations as the mind struggles to find a food and drink solution. *Pellagra*, a deficiency of niacin, results in dermatitis, diarrhea, and dementia with hallucinations.

Delirium, regardless of the cause, presents with clouded consciousness, hallucinations, illusions, speech often incoherent, psychomotor disturbances, disorientation, disordered sleep, and memory loss.[75] Hallucinations may play a prominent role in the clinical condition.

Surgical Complications

Ketamine, a general anesthetic, produces hallucinations, usually visual.[76] It has been classified as a dissociative anesthesia because it causes an intense sensation of dissociation between the patients and their environment. It is administered either IV or intramuscularly (IM) and causes visual perceptual disturbances, delirium, or excitement in about half the adult patients receiving it. It also accounts for flashbacks occurring for weeks following its use. These experiences result from emergence excitement.[77] Ketamine acts directly on the cortex and limbic system.

Eye surgery and its resultant application of *patch* results in auditory and visual hallucinations.[78] These experiences occur within the constellations of symptoms of disorientation and delirium called "cataract delirium" and "black-patch delirium." Its onset is usually in the second postoperative day, although it may commence immediately following surgery or may develop a week after surgery. It emerges at night when auditory cues are diminished. The hallucinations represent the patient's response to severe stress and sensory deprivation.[79]

The phantom limb experience follows immediately after amputation. This has been described as a kinesthetic hallucination in which the patient perceives changes, sensations, activity, movement, and positions in the absent limb. Patients most appreciate experiences in the distal portion of the extremity, particularly the hand and its digits, especially the thumb and the index finger. They describe the extremity's shape as diverse and over time note that the digits move toward the stump. The process of digit retreat to and into the stump is called telescoping. The hallucinatory experiences reflect the limb and its distal section representation in the thalamus and cortex. The entire phantom limb phenomenon is normal and natural.

Phantom pain involves the appreciation of pain where the limb would have been. It does not occur in all cases of amputation. It happens frequently when the limb has been the cause of protracted pain and rarely is found in cases of nondiseased limb amputations, eg, wartime situations.[80] A history of family members who have sustained phantom pain correlates to patients developing phantom pain. A 24-year-old-man sustained severe burns, especially to the left leg, as a result of a motorcycle accident. In the ensuing year and a half his leg had extensive surgery in attempts to save it. During that time he experienced intense leg pain. Following amputation, he continued to have severe "leg" pain which persisted despite nerve blocks and stump revisions.

Cortex electrical stimulation during neurosurgical procedures yields a fascinating array of hallucinations. Penfield and Perot, through an extensive number of direct stimulations of the cortex, not only reproduced the patient's seizure experience in order to remove the focus, but also vastly and dramatically enhanced our understanding and knowledge of the brain.[81] Electrostimulation of the lateral surface of the nondominant temporal lobe produced visual hallucinations. Integrated images involving both visual and auditory hallucinations were derived from activation of the first temporal convolution bilaterally. Stimulation of Brodmann's areas 41 and 42 led to simple noises, but electrical triggering of the lateral surface, first temporal convolution bilaterally, resulted in orchestrated voices. Similarly, activation of Brodmann's areas 17, 18, and 19 gave rise to seeing lights, and zigzag lines of geometric patterns, whereas stimulation of the posterior temporal convolution produced complete pictures and scenes. Stimulation of the parietal cortex produced body image distortions, the phantom limb experience, and paresthesias. Meanwhile, electrostimulation of the temporal lobe also caused olfactory and gustatory hallucinations. Stimulation deep at the sylvian fissure at the transverse gyri led particularly to taste sensations.

Physical Trauma

Head trauma may result in hallucinations as part of the organic presentation.[82] It arises along with disorientation, lability of affect, and fluctuating levels of consciousness. Specifically, trauma to the frontal lobe yields either visual or olfactory hallucinations.[83] These may represent damage to the optic and the olfactory nerves.

Psychiatric Diagnosis

Here we will emphasize hallucinations within the context of organic mental disorders, schizophrenia, major affective disorders, and conversion reactions.[84] They also compose part of the picture in other psychiatric disorders.

In the organic brain syndromes, hallucinations have often a prominent role. They may serve as the major focus, the initiator of the evaluation, or one of a range of distressing signs and syndromes. Delirium, a global cognitive disturbance of rapid onset, features hallucinations, usually visual, within the constellation of attention difficulty, illusions, misperceptions, incoherence, altered sleep cycle, and dramatic changes in psychomotor activity.

In organic hallucinosis, the hallucination provides the dominant event, where there is no cloud consciousness like delirium, intact intellectual functioning, no major affective quality nor delusional quality, and there is a specific organic etiology.

Substance-induced organic mental disorders have been discussed above.

The *schizophrenic* hallucinatory experiences are marked by a number of features. Schizophrenic patients experience a wide range of hallucinations. These include auditory, visual, olfactory, tactile, and gustatory. Robert et al found through careful interviewing of schizophrenic inpatients that 83% had olfactory hallucinations.[85] The majority perceived the odors as unpleasant. Additionally, some patients report bizarre internal feelings and sensations, eg, turning organs or transmitting from their spinal cord. In late paraphrenia, occurring in elderly patients, they may hallucinate phantom boarders.[86]

The nature of the hallucinations may change during the course of the disease.[87] During the acute schizophrenic episode, the auditory hallucinations often have an accusatory, demanding, and commanding quality to them. The patients feel helpless and the victim of them. However, while the illness is in remission, the hallucinations may not disappear, but rather adopt a more supportive, positive, alternative-suggestive feature. The patients may find they have more control over them in this stage.

The auditory hallucinations have a number of qualities. They may appear as thoughts or ideas arguing about, discussing, or commenting upon the patient. They often occur in the second or third person.[88] The patients perceive them as separate from themselves and initially beyond their control. The major hallucinatory message generally remains accusatory, persecutory, and derogatory.

External factors can influence the hallucinatory process. Specifically, actively hallucinating schizophrenic patients, when given a job to perform, will experience a decrease in the perceptual disorder during the task.[89] Conversely, the same patients involved in passive behavior will note an increase in such perceptions. Cultural issues affect this process. Non-Western settings commonly have a higher incidence of hallucinations, especially visual, than do Western., Further, Ndetei and Vadher, looking at an English hospital schizophrenic patient population from Africa, West India, and Asia, found greater frequencies of hallucinations in those groups than in the English.[90]

Finally, a reminder that psychodynamic mechanisms contribute to the schizophrenic's hallucination formation. Modell comments on the object quality and relationship of the hallucination.[91] The patients may develop such experiences in part to replace an earlier loss. They have a relationship with hallucinations.

A **manic episode**, within the context of manic-depressive illness, not infrequently includes hallucinations within its symptoms of heightened activity, pressured speech, grandiosity, distractibility, flight of ideas, and decreased sleep. Most commonly, these patients experience auditory hallucinations. Many times mania is initially thought to be an acute schizophrenic episode.[92] The DSM-III views these hallucinations as evidence of the psychotic level of the disease and these perceptual disorders may either be congruent with mania or incongruent. A woman during a manic attack began buying new cars because voices she heard over the switched-off television ordered her to do so.

Similarly, a *major depression* may also present with hallucinations. Again, the DSM-III sees these perceptual events as signs of a psychotic level and the hallucinations may either be mood-congruent or incongruent. The clinician must not only pay attention to the perceptual disturbance but also focus on the history, the family history, and the other parts of the mental status. (See chapter 2 for a complete discussion of major affective disorders.)

Conversion reactions may take the form of a hallucination. Here, the patient does experience a hallucination. The perceptual event does provide an avenue to solve an unconscious conflict, to handle a prohibited drive while avoiding guilt, to escape from a stressful situation, and to offer a "sick role."[93] A 35-year-old married woman came to the emergency department to report seeing scenes of her brother's funeral. He had committed suicide 2 years before. She described them in detail with an air of indifference; had a clear sensorium; and felt deep anguish in her marriage. She was admitted to the psychiatric unit. She neither had a schizophrenic disorder nor a major affective one. Qualities of the hallucinatory conversion reaction include complex, complicated vivid detail, naive presentation, and la belle indifference.[94] These symptoms often provide unconsciously sought secondary gain.

Hallucinations may also occur in other psychiatric disorders. In children, hallucinations usually reflect late-onset psychoses but also present within the realm of nonpsychotic conduct and emotional disorders.[95] Here auditory experiences predominate followed by visual and olfactory. Patients with a factitious psychosis may present with hallucinations.[96] The report is under voluntary control with the goal of gaining the patient status.

The tapestry of an hallucination has been woven from the fibers of the person, the personality, the biology, the culture, and the ecology. Its appearance is varied. Its presentation is compelling, fascinating, and inviting of investigation.

REFERENCES

1. American Psychiatric Association: *A Psychiatric Glossary,* ed 5. Washington, American Psychiatric Association, 1980.
2. Drever J: *A Dictionary of Psychology.* Baltimore, Penguin Books, 1960.
3. McDonald C: A clinical study of hypnogogic hallucinations. *Br J Psychiatry* 1971;118:543-547.
4. Hoch PH: *Differential Diagnosis in Clinical Psychiatry.* New York, Science House, 1972.
5. Hall DC, Lawson BZ, Wilson LG: Command hallucinations and self-amputation of the penis and hand during a first psychotic break. *J Clin Psychiatry* 1981;42:322-324.
6. Freud S: Wish fulfillment in *Standard Edition of the Complete Psychological Works of Sigmund Freud,* Strachey J (trans), London, Hogarth Press, 1953, Vol 5, pp 550-572.
7. Fenichel O: *The Psychoanalytic Theory of Neurosis.* New York, WW Norton, 1945.
8. Linn EL: Verbal auditory hallucinations: mind, self, and society. *J Nerv Ment Dis* 1977;164;8-17.
9. Kolb LC, Brodie HK: *Modern Clinical Psychiatry,* ed 10 Philadelphia, WB Saunders Co, 1982.
10. Rabkin R: Ego functions and hallucinations. *Am J Psychiatry* 1966;123:481-484.
11. West LJ: A clinical and theoretical overview of hallucinatory phenomenon, in Siegel RK, West LJ (eds): *Hallucinations: Behavior, Experience, and Theory.* New York, John Wiley & Sons, 1975, pp 287-311.
12. LaBarre W: Anthropological perspectives on hallucination and hallucinogens, in Siegel RK, West LJ (eds): *Hallucinations: Behavior, Experience, and Theory.* New York, John Wiley & Sons, 1975, pp 9-52.
13. Horowitz MJ: A cognitive model of hallucinations. *Am J Psychiatry* 1975;132:789-795.
14. Spokes EGS: Biochemical abnormalities in schizophrenia: the dopamine hypothesis, in Curzon G (ed): *The Biochemistry of Psychiatric Disturbances.* New York, John Wiley & Sons, 1980, pp 53-71.
15. Wyatt RJ, Cutler NR, DeLisi LE, et al: Biochemical and morphological factors in the etiology of the schizophrenic disorders, in American

Psychiatric Association: *Psychiatry Annual Review*. Washington, American Psychiatric Press, 1982, pp 112-153.

16. Merritt HH: *A Textbook of Neurology*, ed 6. Philadelphia, Lea & Febiger, 1979.

17. Hartmann E: Dreams and other hallucinations: an approach to the underlying mechanism, in Siegel RK, West LJ (eds): *Hallucinations: Behavior, Experience, and Theory*. New York, John Wiley & Sons, 1975, pp 71-79.

18. Rosenthal D, Quinn OW: Quadruplet hallucinations. *Arch Gen Psychiatry* 1977;34:817.

19. Currie MA, Currie AC: Ketamine: effect of literacy on emergence phenomena. *Ann R Coll Surg Engl* 1984;66:424-425.

20. Farazza AR, Oman M: Overview: foundations of cultural psychiatry. *Am J Psychiatry* 1978;135:293-303.

21. Schneck JM: Hypnagogic hallucinations in Herman Melville's *Moby Dick*. *NY State J Med* 1977;77:2145-2147.

22. Vitols MM, Waters HG, Keeler MH: Hallucinations and delusions in white and negro schizophrenics. *Am J Psychiatry* 1963;120:472-476.

23. Williams MA, Abernathy V: Being held by the spider. *Am J Psychiatry* 1978;135:232-233.

24. Kroll J, Buckrach B: Visions and psychopathology in the middle ages.*J Nerv Ment Dis* 1982;170:41-49.

25. Zisking E: An explanation of mental symptoms found in acute sensory deprivation: researches 1958-1963. *Am J Psychiatry* 1965;121:939-946.

26. Lilly JC: Mental effects of reduction of ordinary levels of physical stimuli on intact healthy persons. *Psychiatr Res Rep Am Psychiatr Assoc* 1956;5:1-9.

27. Bexton WH, Heron W, Scott TH: Effects of decreased variation in the sensory environment. *Can J Psychol* 1954;8:70-76.

28. Solomon P, Lieberman PH, Mendelson J, et al: Sensory deprivation. *Am J Psychiatry* 1957;114:357-363.

29. Mendelson J, Solomon P, Lindemann E: Hallucination of poliomyelitis patients during treatment in a respirator. *J Nerv Ment Dis* 1958;126:421-428.

30. Siegel RK: Introduction, in Siegel Rk, West LJ (eds): *Hallucinations: Behavior, Experience, and Theory*. New York, John Wiley & Sons, 1975, pp 1-7.

31. Negorsky VA: A neurophysiological analysis of "hallucinations" experienced by post resuscitation patients. *Resuscitation* 1984;11:1-8.

32. Oates JA: Wilkinson GR: Principles of drug therapy, in Isselbacher KJ, Adams RD, Braunwald E, et al (eds): *Harrison's Principles of Internal Medicine*, ed 10. New York, McGraw-Hill Book Co, 1983, pp 392-402.

33. Gorelick DA, Kussin SZ, Kahn I: Paranoid delusions and auditory

hallucinations associated with digoxin intoxication. *J Nerv Ment Dis* 1978;166:817-819.

34. Slaby AE, Lieb J, Tancredi LR: *Handbook of Psychiatric Emergencies,* ed 2. Garden City, NY, Medical Examination Publishing Co, 1981.

35. Levin M: Bromide hallucinosis. *Arch Gen Psychiatry* 1960;2:429-433.

36. Vance ML, Evans WS, Thorner MO: Bromocriptine. *Ann Intern Med* 1984;100:78-91.

37. Goodwin FK: Psychiatric side effects of levodopa in man. *JAMA* 1971;218:1915-1920.

38. Hausner RS: Amantadine: associated recurrence of psychosis. *Am J Psychiatry* 1980;137:240-242.

39. Abramowicz M (ed): Drugs that cause psychiatric symptoms. *Med Lett DrugsTher* 1984;26:75-78.

40. Griffith JD, Cavanaugh J, Held J, et al: Dextroamphetamine. *Arch Gen Psychiatry* 1972;26:97-100.

41. Escobar JF, Karno M: Chronic hallucinations from nasal drops. *JAMA* 1982;247:1859-1860.

42. Sankey RJ, Nunn AJ, Sills AJ: Visual hallucinations in children receiving decongestants. *Br Med J* 1984;288:1369.

43. Jefferson JW: Central nervous system toxicity of cimetidine: a case of depression. *Am J Psychiatry* 1979;136:346.

44. Bowden CL, Barnhart CC: Toxic psychosis with cimetidine. *Am J Psychiatry* 1979;136:725-726.

45. Arneson GA: More on toxic psychosis with cimetidine. *Am J Psychiatry* 1979;136:1348-1349.

46. Greenblatt DJ, Koch-Weser J: Adverse reactions to propranolol in hospitalized medical patients: a report from the Boston Collaborative Drug Surveillance Program. *Am Heart J* 1973;86:478-484.

47. Fleminger R: Visual hallucinations and illusions with propranolol. *Br Med J* 1978;1:1182.

48. Gershon E, Goldstein RE, Moss AJ, et al: Psychosis with ordinary doses of propranolol. *Ann Intern Med* 1979;90:938-939.

49. Renick RA, O'Kane J, Sparling JG: A case report of toxic psychosis with low-dose propranolol therapy. *Am J Psychiatry* 1981;138:850-851.

50. Kurland ML: Organic brain syndrome with propranolol. *N Engl J Med* 1979;300:366.

51. Hall, RCW: *Psychiatric Presentations of Mental Illness.* New York, SP Medical & Scientific Books, 1980.

52. Dysken MW, Merry W, David JM: Anticholinergic psychosis. *Psychiatric Annals* 1978;8:452-456.

53. Perl M, Hall RCW, Gardner ER: Behavioral toxicity of psychiatric drugs, in Hall RCW (ed): *Psychiatric Presentations of Medical Illness.* New York, SP Medical & Scientific Books, 1980, pp 311-336.

54. Heiser JF, Gillin JC: The reversal of anticholinergic drug-induced

delirium and coma with physostigmine. *Am J Psychiatry*
1971;127:1050-1054.

55. El-Yousee MK, Janowsky DS, Davis JM, et al: Reversal of
antiparkinsonian drug toxicity by physostigmine: a controlled study.
Am J Psychiatry 1973;130:141-145.

56. Klein DF: Visual hallucinations with imipramine. *Am J Psychiatry*
1965;121:1965-1968.

57. Schlauch R: Hypnopompic hallucinations and treatment with
imipramine. *Am J Psychiatry* 1979;136:219-220.

58. Hartmann E: Dreams and other hallucinations: an approach to the
underlying mechanism, in Siegel RK, West LJ (eds): *Hallucinations:
An Approach to the Underlying Mechanism.* New York, John Wiley &
Sons, 1975, pp 71-79.

59. Victor M, Hope JM: The phenomenon of auditory hallucinations in
chronic alcoholism. *J Nerv Ment Dis* 1958;126:451-481.

60. Sararay SM, Pardes H: Auditory elementary hallucinations in alcohol
withdrawal psychosis. *Arch Gen Psychiatry* 1967;16:652-658.

61. Deiker T, Chambers HE: Structure and content of hallucinations in
alcohol withdrawal and functional psychosis. *J Stud Alcohol*
1978;39:1831-1840.

62. Wilford BB: *Drug Abuse.* Chicago, American Medical Association,
1981.

63. Siegel RK: Cocaine hallucinations. *Am J Psychiatry* 1978;135:309-
314.

64. Siegel RK: Hallucinations. *Scientific Am* 1977;237:132-140.

65. Siegel RK, Jarvik ME: Drug-induced hallucinations in animals and
man, in Siegel RK, West LJ (eds): *Hallucinations: Behavior,
Experience, and Theory.* New York, John Wiley & Sons, 1975, pp 81-
161.

66. Allen RM, Young SJ: Phencyclidine-induced psychosis. *Am J
Psychiatry* 1978;135:1081-1084.

67. Altura BT, Altura BM: Phencyclidine, lysergic acid diethylamide, and
mescaline: cerebral artery spasms and hallucinogenic activity. *Science*
1981;212:1051-1052.

68. Wells CE, Duncan GW: *Neurology for Psychiatrists.* Philadelphia, FA
Davis, 1980.

69. Hachinski VC, Porchawka J, Steele JC: Visual symptoms in the
migraine syndrome. *Neurology* 1973;23:570-579.

70. Richards W: The fortification illusions of migraines. *Sci Am*
1971;225:88-96.

71. Blumer D: Temporal lobe epilepsy and its psychiatric significance, in
Benson DF, Blumer D (eds): *Psychiatric Aspects of Neurologic
Disease.* New York, Grune & Stratton, Inc, 1975, pp 171-198.

72. Taylor MA, Sierles F, Abrams R: The neuropsychiatric evaluation, in
Hales RE, Frances AJ (eds): *American Psychiatric Association Annual
Review.* Washington, American Psychiatric Press, 1985, Vol 4, pp
109-141.

193

73. White HJ: Complex visual hallucinations in partial blindness due to eye disease. *Br J Psychiatry* 1980;136:284-286.
74. Berrios GE, Brook P: Visual hallucinations and sensory delusions in the elderly. *Br J Psychiatry* 1984;144:662-664.
75. Lipowsky ZI: Transient cognitive disorders (delirium, acute confusional states) in elderly. *Am J Psychiatry* 1983;140:1426-1436.
76. Marshall RE, Wollman H: General anesthetics, in Gilman AG, Goodman LS, Gilman H (eds): *Goodman and Gilman's The Pharmacological Basis of Therapeutics,* ed 8. New York, MacMillan Publishing Co, 1980, pp 276-299.
77. Dundee JW, Knox JWD, Black GW, et al: Ketamine as an induction agent in anaesthetics. *Lancet* 1970;1:1370-1371.
78. Weisman AD, Hackett TP: Psychosis after eye surgery. *N Engl J Med* 1958;258:1284-1289.
79. Ziskind E, Jones H, Filante W, et al: Observations on mental symptoms in eye patched patients. *Am J Psychiatry* 1960;116:893-900.
80. Siegfried S, Zimmerman M (eds): *Phantom and Stump Pain.* New York, Springer-Verlag, 1981.
81. Penfield W, Perot P: The brain's record of auditory and visual experience. *Brain* 1963;86:595-696.
82. Weisz GM: Psychiatry and the management of an accident service, in Howells JG (ed): *Modern Perspectives in the Psychiatric Aspects of Surgery.* New York, Brunner/Mazel, 1976, pp 534-548.
83. Hecaen H, Albert ML: Disorders of mental functioning related to frontal lobe pathology, in Benson DF, Blumer D (eds): *Psychiatric Aspects of Neurologic Disease.* New York, Grune & Stratton Inc, 1975, pp 137-149.
84. American Psychiatric Association: *Diagnostic and Statistical Manual of Mental Disorders,* ed 3. Washington, American Psychiatric Association, 1980.
85. Robert SL, Hollender MH, Mehrhof EG: Olfactory hallucinations. *Arch Gen Psychiatry* 1961;5:121-126.
86. Rowan EL: Phantom boarders as a symptom of late paraphrenia. *Am J Psychiatry* 1984;141:580-581.
87. Larkin AR: The form and content of schizophrenic hallucinations. *Am J Psychiatry* 1979;136:940-943.
88. Linn EL: Verbal auditory hallucinations: mind, self, and society. *J Nerv Ment Dis* 1977;164:8-17.
89. Margo A, Hemsley DR, Slade PD: The effects of varying auditory input on schizophrenic hallucinations. *Br J Psychiatry* 1981;139:122-127.
90. Ndetei DM, Vadher A: A comparative cross-cultural study of the frequencies of hallucination in schizophrenia. *Acta Psychiatr Scand* 1984;70:545-549.
91. Modell AH: An approach to the nature of auditory hallucinations in schizophrenia. *Arch Gen Psychiatry* 1960;3:259-266.
92. Taylor MA, Gaztanaga P, Abrams R: Manic-depressive illness and

acute schizophrenia: a clinical, family history, and treatment-response study. *Am J Psychiatry* 1974;131:678-682.

93. Modai I, Sirota P, Cygielman G, et al: Conversive hallucinations. *J Nerv Ment Dis* 1980;168:564-565.

94. Fitzgerald BA, Wells CE: Hallucinations as a conversion reaction. *Dis Nerv Syst* 1977;38:381-383.

95. Garralda ME: Hallucinations in children with conduct and emotional disorders: I. The clinical phenomena. *Psychol Med* 1984;14:589-596.

96. Pope HG, Jonas JM, Hudson JI, et al: An empirical study of psychosis in borderline personality disorder. *Am J Psychiatry* 1985;142:1285-1290.

5 Somatization

Charles V. Ford

The differential diagnosis of the patient who exhibits abnormal illness behavior (somatization) is an essential component of the practice of medicine. Surveys have shown that a significant proportion of the patients who present themselves in physicians' offices (a) have no disease, (b) have complaints which are substantially in excess of the objective evidence of the pathology, or (c) their illness is associated with considerable "psychological overlay."[1]

SOMATIZATION covers a wide range of illness behavior and is the process by which a patient uses the body to express psychological feelings or ideas for some personal gain.[2]

From this definition it can be seen that somatization may accompany genuine physical illness, or be a process which stimulates a disease. In its most extreme form, abnormal illness behavior includes the repetitive simulation of diseases with dramatic presentations to medical facilities in order to obtain hospitalization—the Munchausen syndrome.[2]

The following discussion of the differential diagnosis of the somatizing patient will not take into account all of the various possibilities of somatizing behavior but instead focus upon the four specific syndromes that have been identified as the "somatoform disorders": hypochondriasis, conversion disorder, psychogenic pain disorder, and somatization disorder. The physician must keep in mind, however, that somatization is a very broad concept and is not limited to the four disorders under consideration.

HYPOCHONDRIASIS

Definition

"Hypochondriasis is defined as a concern with health or disease in oneself which is present for the major part of the time. The preoccupation must be justified by the amount of organic pathology and must not respond more than temporarily to clear reassurance given after a thorough examination of the patient."[3] This definition is basically the same as the diagnostic criteria specified in the American Psychiatric Association's *Diagnostic and Statistical Manual of Mental Disorders,* third edition[4] now known colloquially as DSM-III. However, DSM-III further specifies the exclusionary criteria of a concurrent diagnosis of other mental illnesses which cause the symptoms.

There is a clinical pragmatism to Pilowsky's suggestion that hypo-condriasis be divided into two major categories, primary (see above) and secondary forms (hypochondriasis due to other coexisting mental illness).[4] The clinician must first identify the presence of hypochondriacal behavior and then proceed to evaluate the patient to determine the presence or absence of an underlying etiology.

Case report A 58-year-old married mother of three adult children presented herself repetitively at the office of her primary care physician. Although she had been a frequent user of medical care facilities throughout her life, her physical symptoms had accelerated over the preceding 3 years. Her complaints focused upon several organ systems. She claimed that she was nauseated every morning upon awakening and that this sensation would not remit for several hours. She also expressed worry about her heart. She frequently monitored her pulse and had noted some premature ventricular contractions. She was also preoccupied with her blood pressure even though her very mild essential hypertension was well controlled by use of diuretics. Repeated examinations by the primary care physician failed to disclose any significant organic pathology. Electrocardiography and other tests of cardiac function were within normal limits with the exception of an occasional premature ventricular contraction (PVC). Blood pressure, as mentioned, was within normal limits and repeated examination of the patient's gastrointestinal (GI) system and gall-bladder function failed to yield any abnormality. In view of her complaints, which had resulted in an increasing frequency of office visits, her physician investigated her psychosocial history.

It was discovered that the patient was worried and concerned about a husband whose job had transferred him to another city and who was having to maintain a separate residence. The patient could not accompany her husband because her grown daughter, a very anxious and phobic individual, required the patient's continuing psychological support in her home city. In addition, the patient was worried about another grown son who had been married four times and who was unable to maintain steady employment. The wife of yet another son had died recently and the patient found herself thinking about death and worrying about the care of her two grandchildren from that marriage. Exploration of the patient's psychological symptoms indicated that there had been changes in behavior over the past several years which had occurred in an insidious fashion. The patient had stopped her usual regular attendance at church and reported that her previous perfectionistic housekeeping had deteriorated and that she was no longer proud of the way her home looked. She also indicated that her appetite was poor, which she associated with the nausea, and that she had lost between 10 and 12 lbs over the preceding 3 years. In addition, she stated that her worries kept her up at night and that she slept poorly.

The patient appeared mildly depressed but when questioned about this she denied any particular mood disturbance other than her worries about her children and her husband. However, she did report that her mother had suffered from periodic episodes of depression and had once been hospitalized and received electroconvulsive therapy (ECT). She described both parents as being rigid perfectionists, as were her sisters, one of whom had also been treated for depression in the past.

The patient's past psychosocial history with the exception of that mentioned was unremarkable. She described her husband as a "good man and a good provider." She expressed some confusion and dismay over the problems that the children had experienced and said, "My husband and I worked so hard to give them everything."

Features

Mood The mood of the hypochondriacal patient is often best described as constricted with an undercurrent of depression which, at times, is associated with mild anger or resentment. The patient often appears tense and anxious. When questioned about a mood disturbance the patient almost inevitably relates his feelings to his concern about his physical complaints. It is not infrequent for the patient to be unable to describe his feelings at all. Many patients fit the description by Sifneos of *alexithymia,* (literally: no words for feelings").[5] Persons with alexithymia are unable to give verbal expression to their emotions but rather focus minutely upon details such as symptoms. They tend to be not psychologically minded, have impoverished fantasy lives, and, interestingly, do not recall their dreams.

Because of the hypochondriac's difficulty in expressing his mood states, it is important for the interviewer to pay close attention to observing the patient's mood rather than merely questioning the patient about it. Often the diagnosis of underlying depression must be made on the basis of behavioral observations, or reports of vegetative symptoms, rather than the patient's own recognition of being depressed. The patient described above had a major unipolar depression which underlay her hypochondriacal complaints. Both the somatic complaints and the patient's mood and behavior improved significantly with the institution of antidepressant medication.

Patients with the purer form of hypochondriasis, primary hypochondriasis, do not fit the diagnostic criteria for major depression but they do have a constricted mood and demonstrate obsessiveness. Patients whose underlying diagnosis is that of one of the monosymptomatic hypochondriacal states, which are closely related to schizophrenia and/or paranoia, are often shy, introverted, and retiring in manner. Patients who exhibit transient hypochondriasis due to physical illness or because of environmental stresses frequently demonstrate anxiety as the primary mood disturbance. Occasionally schizophrenic patients will present with hypochondriacal concerns or somatic delusions. Inappropriate or flat affect is characteristic of schizophrenia.

Thought   By definition, the thought content of the hypochondriac is preoccupied with somatic symptoms. Efforts to engage these patients in conversation or to question aspects of their personal lives almost inevitably result in a return, sooner or later, to their preoccupation with physical symptoms. Life events are typically evaluated in regard to these physical symptoms and problems. Instead of being seen as causal for illness, such events are regarded as having been caused by illness. As mentioned above, many of the patients are alexithymic and one often finds the patient to be preoccupied with minute and often irrelevant details. It is not unusual for the hypochondriacal patient to give an extremely detailed medical history. They tend to remember the dates of their illnesses and their hospitalizations with precision as well as all of their diagnoses and attempted treatments in the past, including side reactions. For example, a hypochondriac might report such details as the frequency, color, and consistency of bowel movements on a day-to-day basis.

Patients who exhibit hypochondriasis secondary to depression are often morbidly preoccupied with the possible implications of their reported physical symptoms. For example, they may be fearful that the symptoms referable to the heart may be indications of rapidly decreasing function and perhaps even death. These patients therefore may have a hopelessness associated with their physical symptoms. Patients who have one of the monohypochrondriacal syndromes often are preoccupied with their symptoms to a delusional extent. Efforts to dissuade them from talking about such a symptom are often useless because the patient attributes essentially all life events to the symptom. For example, a young man with delusions of bromosis (a condition in which patients believe they emit an offensive odor) may claim that all of his social and occupational difficulties are due to his symptom.[6]

Behavior Patients not only make frequent office visits to see physicians but also use the telephone to an excessive extent as they seek continual reassurance for their symptoms and/or report new symptoms and their worries about them. If the patient feels unsatisfied with one physician and his responses, which is not at all unusual, he moves on to another physician to seek further opinions and medical care. This behavior has been described as "doctor shopping" as the patients move from doctor to doctor and sometimes from medical center to medical center in their efforts to find an explanation for their medical symptoms.

When the physician inquires closely, other abnormal behavior will also be found in these patients. For the patient with primary hypochondriasis, it is not unusual to find that they live rather constricted lives, both socially and in terms of their recreational pursuits. Some of these patients are engaged, self-sacrificingly, in the care of other persons such as a sick family member or friend.

A patient with secondary hypochondriasis due to underlying depression often exhibits a pervasive disability which is in excess of the degree of physical disability that a person with organic disease might exhibit.[7] Similarly, the patient with one of the monohypochondriacal syndromes may be markedly socially constricted and demonstrate significant alterations in behavior which are all explained by the delusional symptom. Patients with monosymptomatic hypochondriasis are often the most intense of the doctor shoppers and the patient with a perceived physical defect (dysmorphophobia) may go from plastic surgeon to plastic surgeon until he finds one who will operate upon the imagined defect.[8]

Physical examination and laboratory findings The physical examination and laboratory findings for the hypochondriacal patient are frequently completely within normal limits. Despite this, the patient continues to be fearful and frequently requests further investigation of his complaints. However, it is not unusual to find abnormalities in the physical examination or an occasional mildly abnormal laboratory result. Some degree of concurrent physical disease does not rule out hypochondriasis. In fact, many persons over the age of 40 years will have one or more chronic diseases, often mild in symptomatic expression, which most individuals would not feel to be physically disabling. It is important for the physician to differentiate between the possible coincidence of mild physical abnormalities, which are of little significance physiologically, and the disabling complaints of which the patient obsessively complains.

Interviewer's reaction One of the most important diagnostic clues in diagnosing the hypochondriac is that of the emotional reactions that they elicit in physicians.[9] The hostile-dependency and intentions of these patients frequently elicits irritation and at times overt anger. It has been said that a "crock" cannot be diagnosed as such until the physician fails to find anything that might be of potential interest to the patient. Such patients are frequently described as unattractive and boring.[10] It is not unusual for the physician to want to stifle their complaints and get them out of the office as quickly as possible. Telephone calls are often received with a high degree of irritation by the physician.

All of these adverse emotional reactions are concretely demonstrated by the wide variety of pejorative terms by which these patients are labeled by physicians. In addition to crock, other names for such patients are "gourds," "problem patients," "thick-chart patients," and "PPP" ("piss-poor protoplasm"). Patients who elicit negative responses in the physician should trigger internal questions as to the differential diagnosis of one of the somatizing disorders.[9] The above responses from interviewers occur in all interviews of the various forms of hypochondriasis but the monosymptomatic hypochondriacal patient may elicit the most irritation. The intensity of complaints and the reluctance of the patient to accept even transiently any type of explanation or reassurance make them even more frustrating to manage than the typical crock.

Pathogenesis

Psychodynamic explanation Several psychodynamic explanations have been offered to explain hypochondriasis. Among these explanations are that the hypochondriacal symptoms serve as an ego defense mechanism. The individual both fears disease and the consequences of disease but also unconsciously desires to be sick in order to achieve the benefits of the sick role. Although the patient may secretly fear the effects of physical disease, the illness serves to explain deficits in the self, such as problems in sexual or social functioning and occupational achievement, that the patient may experience.[11]

Hypochondriasis can also be seen as determined by the patient's need to suffer. Many of these patients have life histories that are consistent with a masochistic lifestyle.[12] They may be fearful that they do not deserve help and therefore the sick state serves to defend against any guilt that they might experience by being more successful in life. Yet another psychodynamic explanation is that the hypochondriacal symptoms may represent an identification with someone of importance in the patient's life who had similar physical symptoms.

Biologic explanations Although hypochondriasis is generally seen as a psychiatric syndrome and, by definition, there is no underlying physical illness to account for the symptoms, there may be some biological contributions. For example, these patients may, by virtue of constitutional factors, have a decreased sensitivity to pain or in some other way be particularly prone to awareness of their physiologic status.[11]

Genetics Concerns of a possible genetic input to hypochondriasis consist largely of the noted familial incidence; a significant proportion of these patients have a parent who was hypochondriacal. However, an increased familial incidence may also reflect environmental factors. Another confounding variable relates to the fact that many of these patients have an underlying affective disorder. Recent research has suggested that susceptibility to the affective disorders has a significant genetic component.

Environment Environment can contribute to hypochondriasis in a number of ways. Perhaps the most important is the cultural component. Persons who come from cultures that do not stress psychological explanations for human distress are much more likely to produce persons who somatize their distress.[13,14] As noted above, many of these patients come from families in which there was a model for the hypochondriacal complaints. Similarly, many hypochondriacs have had experience with someone in their background who was ill and this individual may have experienced benefits from the sick role. Thus, the hypochondriacal patient may have learned that illness has certain benefits and thus their somatizing symptoms can be interpreted as "learned behavior." Another environmental factor in the pathogenesis of hypochondriasis is the role of psychosocial stress. It has been shown that when a person feels stressed there is a concurrent sense of increased vulnerability and as a consequence bodily symptoms may be overinterpreted in their possible relationship to disease.[15]

Differential Diagnosis

Nonpsychotropic drugs Medications can result in hypochondriacal preoccupations on two different bases. The first is that many drugs have a wide variety of physiologic effects other than that of their intended indication. Adverse drug reactions may result in complaints that appear hypochondriacal in nature. The physician must be alert to all of the known side reactions to drugs and when in doubt review them in the *Physician's Desk Reference* .[16] A second cause of hypochondriasis due to the prescription of nonpsychotropic drugs is the fact that many drugs have the capability to induce depression. The *organic affective disorders* may be associated with a wide variety of physical symptoms. Among the drugs that can cause depression are cimetidine, digitalis, and many of the antihypertensive agents.[17]

Psychotropic drugs The differential diagnosis of hypochondriasis resulting from the effects of drugs prescribed for psychotropic indications is usually not difficult. If the patient is receiving psychotropic drugs then the physician has already considered the possibility that the patient's symptoms may have psychological input. However, many psychotropic drugs have side reactions as mentioned above and when a patient sees several physicians concurrently it is entirely possible that the result is polypharmacy with all of its attendant capabilities for drug cross-reactions as well as side reactions.

Alcohol The length of time required to diagnose alcoholism in the medical patient is often remarkable. The physician may see a patient who chronically abuses alcohol for an extended period of time before the underlying cause of the patient's multiple symptoms become apparent. The physician may be inclined to interpret the patient's complaints as due to hypochondriasis because the patient has led the physician astray by not reporting the abuse of alcohol. In addition, alcoholism and depression are often closely associated and alcohol has an effect upon many physiologic systems of the body. As a general rule, alcoholism must always be considered as a part of the differential diagnosis in patients who frequently use medical services and/or have multiple somatic complaints.

Other abused substances The major problem in the differential diagnosis of patients with hypochondriasis and substance abuse is the possibility of iatrogenic habituation. Patients with hypochondriasis rarely use street drugs but in their repetitive visits to physicians they may be prescribed a variety of pain medications and/or minor tranquilizers, such as diazepam, which have a high capacity for abuse.

Medical illness Medical diseases have traditionally been the major alternative explanation for the various hypochondriacal conditions. As a general rule, physicians initially accept a patient's physical complaint at face value and assume that they reflect some type of underlying physiologic diagnosis. For example, a complaint such as nausea (as illustrated in the patient described above) may be interpreted as possibly reflecting a peptic ulcer and the patient is evaluated for such a disorder.

The diagnosis of hypochondriasis may be made in error. When a physician fails to find, after an extensive workup, a physical disease to account for multiple symptoms, the physician then may make a diagnosis of hypochondriasis by default. The patient may subsequently have the emergence of new symptoms. Cushing's syndrome is an example of such a disease process. All new symptoms which a hypochondriac develops must be carefully re-evaluated before being attributed to hypochondriasis. Hypochondriasis does not confer immunity from disease.

Surgical complications Patients with hypochondriasis often undergo an excessive number of surgical interventions as physicians search to find the cause of the patient's multiple somatic complaints. As a consequence of these surgical interventions, the patient may develop complications of an iatrogenic nature (eg intra-abdominal adhesions) which may lead to future symptoms upon which the patient focuses attention. At times it may be difficult to determine whether symptoms result from the patient's hypochondriacal preoccupations or represent pathophysiologic change which has occurred as a result of these surgical interventions.

Physical trauma The major concern in the differential diagnosis of hypochondriasis in regard to physical trauma relates to the psychological after effects of physical trauma. It is quite normal following a surgical operation or severe illness for a patient to experience what is known as the posttraumatic syndrome. In this syndrome the patient frequently exhibits symptoms of anxiety, grief, and preoccupation with concern about vulnerability of the body.[18] The posttraumatic syndrome should be considered a normal response to a life-threatening situation and is not *per se* a pathologic state. At times a patient who is predisposed to hypochondriacal behavior or who is already a confirmed hypochondriac may seize upon a traumatic event and incorporate it into his hypochondriacal repertoire. The management of such patients with posttraumatic syndrome must take into account an assessment of the extent of symptoms with regard to the degree of trauma.

The "humpty dumpty syndrome" is a hypochondriacal disorder associated with disability which occasionally follows trauma, particularly industrial injuries.[19] Patients exhibiting this syndrome typically have characteristics consisting of long working hours prior to the accident, premature and excessive responsibility, and minimal occupational flexibility. It has been suggested that the injury allowed a collapse of the ego mechanism of reaction formation and the patients then give in to their previously unmet dependency wishes.

Psychiatric diagnosis   As mentioned above, hypochondriasis is generally considered as consisting of either primary hypochondriasis, or secondary hypochondriasis which is then assumed to be due to an underlying psychiatric diagnosis.

Among the most common of the underlying psychiatric diagnoses are those related to depression. Patients with depression frequently demonstrate multiple physical symptoms including pain.[20] There is the potential to confuse these symptoms either with the possibility of underlying physical disease and/or with the diagnosis of primary hypochondriasis. The diagnosis of primary hypochondriasis is based on the features of a pervasive long-standing life style that has emphasized preoccupation with health and illness. With a somatizing depression there should be a time of onset, even if it extends back 2 or 3 years (see case report above). In addition, the patient with depression will have experienced changes in behavior associated with the onset of somatic preoccupation, eg, a decrease in participation in previously enjoyed activities.

Hypochondriasis must also be distinguished from schizophrenia. Schizophrenics may focus upon their bodies as a way of explaining other pervasive deficits in their lives. However, this somatic preoccupation frequently has a somewhat bizarre and unusual quality reflecting delusional thought rather than just obsessive preoccupation. Schizophrenics and other prepsychotic individuals are more likely to present with one of the monosymptomatic hypochondrial states.

Patients with anxiety disorders may at times also be confused with hypochondriacs. Anxious patients frequently experience a number of physiologic symptoms such as increased muscle tension, increased heart rate, diaphoresis, and hyperventilation syndrome.[21] Differentiation from hypochondriasis can be made on the fact that the hypochondriac demonstrates obsessional thinking about the body but has minimal physiologic changes whereas the anxious patient will generally manifest the physiologic concomitants of anxiety.

It may be difficult to distinguish the patient with an obsessional disorder from the hypochondriacal states because primary hypochondriasis may in itself represent one form of obsession.

In reference to the other somatoform disorders, one must keep in mind that hypochondriasis is a general term which can also encompass some of the psychogenic pain disorders. (These will be discussed below.) The differentiation of hypochondriasis from somatization disorder (Briquet's syndrome) is based largely on the fact that hypochondriacs worry about symptoms but rarely have the pseudoneurologic symptoms characteristic of somatization disorder. Somatization disorder will also be discussed below in detail.

CONVERSION DISORDERS

Conversion disorders are a medical entity known since antiquity. The terminology has changed through the years; previously they were called hysterical conversion neuroses or conversion reactions. The current diagnostic criteria, as specified by the DSM-III[4] are (1) that the diagnosis is based upon a physical symptom that cannot be explained by a known disease process, (2) is determined by unconscious mental processes, and (3) has either a precipitating psychosocial stress and/or secondary gains to help explain its psychogenesis. The diagnosis of conversion disorder cannot be made if the symptom is primarily pain or sexual dysfunction. Other exclusionary criteria are a concurrent diagnosis of either somatization disorder (see below) or schizophrenia.

Conversion disorder most usually involves the voluntary motor system or sensation. These are often called "pseudoneurologic" symptoms. Examples of conversion-type symptoms include hemiparalysis or hemianesthesia, tunnel vision, and globus hystericus. Conversion disorders are diagnosed more frequently in women but are by no means exclusive to them.[22,23] Similarly, they are found more frequently, but not exclusively, in unsophisticated persons.[22,23]

Case report   A 36-year-old thrice divorced black practical nurse was referred with symptoms of left hemiparesis and partial left hemianesthesia. These symptoms waxed and waned and were inconsistent with normal physiologic function. All laboratory tests were negative with the exception of some atypical lymphocytes seen on a peripheral blood smear and not believed to be of significance.

The patient's symptoms began acutely while she was at work at her job in a hospital located in a rural southern town. Of note was the fact that the patient was supporting in her home a 21-year-old abusive and nonworking boy friend, an 11- year-old daughter, and a 15-year-old daughter who had just given birth to an illegitimate child. Also of importance was the fact that 5 months previously an aunt, who had raised the patient, had died of a cerebral vascular accident at the same hospital where the patient worked. Her father, an uncle and a grandmother had also all died of strokes.

Mental status examination revealed an obese black woman who appeared to be her stated age and was unremarkable except for her initial hostility at being seen by a psychiatrist. Her intelligence was judged to be normal but she was psychologically unsophisticated.

During hospitalization the patient's symptoms showed progressive resolution and on discharge she accepted a recommendation of a referral to her local mental health clinic to talk about issues related to stress in her home situation.

Features

Mood   The moods that patients with conversion disorder exhibit can be quite variable. Traditionally, these patients were thought to be characterized by that which we called *la belle indifference* . This term refers to an inappropriate indifference to one's symptoms rather than worry and concern about them. However, systematic clinical research has demonstrated that la belle indifference occurs infrequently in patients with conversion disorder and may present in patients who have genuine organic disease.[24]

The patient described above initially displayed symptoms of anger and hostility at the insinuation that her symptoms might be of psychic etiology. Such a mood is not uncommmon in patients with conversion disorder, but other patients may demonstrate symptoms of pervasive anxiety or depression.

Thought   As with the variation of mood in patients with conversion disorder, these patients' thought processes and content are also quite variable. Some patients appear to be preoccupied with their physical symptoms; others seem to ignore the symptoms. Most of these patients are currently involved in a psychosocial crisis and similarly the patients may either ignore these or, to the contrary, be preoccupied with them.

Behavior There is no specific behavioral pattern characteristic of patients with conversion disorder. However, many of these patients are quite histrionic and are quite comfortable at playing the sick role ("a la Camille"). Much more typical is the behavior of relatives and other persons with whom the patient has a close relationship. These people are often quite concerned about the patient's symptoms and frequently demonstrate increased involvement with the patient as compared with their behavior prior to the onset of the conversion disorder.

Physical examination and laboratory findings By definition, the physical examination and laboratory findings cannot account for the symptoms which the patient is exhibiting. Often sophisticated tests will demonstrate that indeed there is a normal neurophysiologic function. Commonly the patient's symptoms will be incompatible with anatomy and physiologic function, eg, aphonia in the presence of a normal cough.[25]

At times a patient will have a concurrent physical and/or abnormal laboratory finding which is coincidental but does not explain the symptom. The patient described above had an incidental abnormal blood smear, probably reflecting a recent viral infection. Physicians must be cautious to not seize upon coincidental findings to explain the patient's symptoms. However, one phenomenon frequently seen is that the patient does indeed have a mild degree of organic pathology but that it has been exaggerated. It is as if the patient were fearful that the physician might not detect it without a little bit of assistance. The physician may be led astray and identify the exaggeration but miss the underlying neurologic abnormality. A careful physical and neurologic examination of patients with conversion disorder is mandatory because, in some, a neurologic disease will emerge later to explain the original symptom.[26]

Interviewer's reaction Physicians are rarely indifferent to patients with conversion disorders. Instead of the objective attitude that usually accompanies medical care of a patient with organic disease, physicians treating patients with conversion disorder tend to have one of two reactions. One is amusement and curiosity. Conversion is sufficiently rare to pique the physician's interest and perhaps elicit pride in being able to make the diagnosis. A second reaction, which physicians may experience on occasion, is anger. There may be resentment that the patient is engaged in manipulation or a belief that the behavior is fraudulent. This anger may be expressed in ways such as the performance of brusque physical examinations including testing for anesthesia with pinpricks sufficiently deep to draw blood! Another unnecessarily abusive technique is to allow a "paralyzed" hand to fall on the patient's face.

Pathogenesis

Psychodynamic explanation Conversion disorder has been traditionally explained by psychodynamic concepts. Symptoms may be interpreted as symbolically communicating a feeling or idea that is otherwise blocked from consciousness. The symptom may be viewed as a compromise between a strong instinctual drive (eg, anger) and the superego prohibition of the expression of such a drive. For example, the symptom of a paralyzed right arm may be interpreted as the patient's wish to strike out in anger, but the paralysis prohibits the action. Other psychodynamic explanations for conversion involve identification with another person, often someone close to the patient who has experienced a similar symptom or who has died. From the case history described above it could be speculated that the patient's paralysis represented a feeling that she could no longer continue to carry her burden of responsibility, and/or the symptoms represented identification with one or more of her multiple relatives who had died from complications of stroke.

Biologic explanations Recent neuropsychological research has been, tentatively, confirmatory of neurophysiologic theories of the etiology of conversion disorders. Such theories date back to the clinical observations and speculations of the French neurologists Briquet and Charcot. Many of these patients differ from normals in their vigilance and their increased field dependency.[27] In addition, neuropsychological testing has demonstrated that patients with repetitive conversion disorders have cerebral dysfunction of both hemispheres with the dominant hemisphere (involved in verbal expression) more impaired than that of the nondominant hemisphere.[28] Many patients with conversion have concurrent neurologic disease and one investigator observed that many patients with conversion had a history of recent head trauma.[29] It can be hypothesized that concurrent CNS disease may, in some poorly understood way, influence the function of the brain in a manner which facilitates expression of conversion symptoms.

Genetics Patients with somatization disorder (Briquet's syndrome), as discussed below, have a high familial incidence of the disorder and/or sociopathy in male relatives. Because the diagnosis of Briquet's syndrome is made largely upon a history of repetitive conversion symptoms it is possible that the familial incidence reflects genetic input. These data must be interpreted with the utmost caution because an increased familial incidence may be explained equally well as being reflective of environmental factors.

Environment Environmental factors are considered to be very important in the pathogenesis of conversion disorders. In the overwhelming majority of these patients, an acute psychosocial stressor in the patient's environment will antedate the symptom.[24] For example, in the case described above, the responsibility upon the patient was suddenly increased by the addition of an illegitimate child to the family. Other important environmental factors in the pathogenesis of conversion are the changes which may occur in the environment as a result of the patient's syndrome. These changes are commonly called the secondary gains. At times, the secondary gains can be quite remarkable and the conversion disorder may be seen as a manipulation which changes the behavior of those persons close to the patient or in some way changes the degree of responsibility and demands upon the patient.[30] Other environmental factors which are important in the pathogenesis of conversion include those which are related to the culture. If there are cultural prohibitions of certain types of behavior, eg, the expression of anger by a woman, then conversion symptoms may serve as a means for her to communicate in a more socially acceptable manner the feelings which she is experiencing. Conversion disorders appear to be more common among rural, unsophisticated persons.[31] The patient mentioned in the case above came from a rural southern background, was uneducated, and had never traveled beyond her community.

Differential Diagnosis

Nonpsychotropic drugs Many prescribed, and over-the-counter drugs have multiple idiosyncratic side effects. At times a physician, unaware of a rare side effect, may attribute a symptom to a conversion symptom when in actuality it is due to the drug. An example is "yellow vision" accompanying digitalis toxicity.[32]

Psychotropic drugs As with nonpsychotropic drugs, the psychotropic drugs have a wide variety of side effects. Among the more striking of these, and which may be mistakenly interpreted as a conversion symptom by an unaware observer, are those related to the extrapyramidal nervous system. For example, some patients may develop acute muscular spasms such as opisthotonos or oculogyric crisis in response to phenothiazines. Such reactions have at times been mistakenly interpreted as conversion disorders; eg, when prochlorperazine (Compazine) has been described for nausea.

Alcohol   Alcohol is a CNS depressant and in low dosages may serve to reduce inhibitions. As such, the patient may engage in a variety of behaviors and/or verbal utterances that are different from the unintoxicated state. However, these are rarely confused with conversion disorders. One complication of alcoholism which may be confused with conversion is the Wernicke-Korsakoff syndrome. Patients who, as a result of their alcoholism, become thiamine-depleted may present with acute symptoms of confusion, ataxia, and extraocular muscle palsies.[33] This is an acute medical emergency which must be treated with thiamine, but a poorly informed observer might confuse the symptoms as being of psychogenic origin.

Other abused substances   There are a wide variety of behavioral and psychiatric states which may be induced by abuse of such substances as cocaine, mescaline, or Jimson weed. However, these substances rarely produce symptoms of the voluntary motor system that might be confused with conversion. Theoretically, a state of altered consciousness might facilitate the development of conversion.

Medical illnesses   A variety of medical illnesses may be confused with conversion disorder and present difficult diagnostic problems. Those diseases in which conversion is most likely to be falsely diagnosed and later proved to have an organic etiology are those which reflect some type of degenerative process of the connective tissue or the nervous system.[34] Other neurologic diseases which frequently present difficulty in differential diagnosis with conversion disorder are multiple sclerosis and seizure disorder. The complicating factor for both of these diseases is that conversion may coexist with the organic disease.[35,36] The patient may, because of experience with genuine symptoms of the disease, learn how to "model" conversion symptoms. Differentiation between organic or psychogenic causes may be, for all practical purposes, impossible. Factors pointing toward a psychogenic etiology are evidence of recent psychological stress and/or changes in the environment as a result of the symptom. It must be emphasized, however, that such events may also occur with genuine organic disease.

Surgical complications   Patients who have a proclivity for somatization have more surgical procedures than do normal persons. Surgery is a physical stress; once an operation has been performed there is obviously a physical disorder (severed and healing tissue) which must be taken into account. In addition, general anesthesia raises the possibility of CNS dysfunction secondary to cerebral anoxia or a cerebral vascular accident. Surgery also represents a psychological stress; there may be changes in body image or implications of further disease, pain, or disability.

Despite the fact that the situation would appear ripe for the development of conversion symptoms, they appear to be uncommon, or at least not frequently diagnosed, in the postoperative period. Perhaps this is because the patient's dependency needs are being met by the assumption of the sick role. However, rare conversion disorders do occur postoperatively. One patient reported in the literature could not swallow his food following successful reconstruction of his esophagus. This symptom persisted despite demonstration of normal physiologic function as demonstrated by barium swallow. The patient proved to have a confused concept of his internal body image; he did not believe his esophagus was connected to his stomach. In addition, his symptoms provided massive secondary gains as his family attempted to get him to eat.[37]

Physical trauma Conversion disorder following physical trauma is not unusual. In the series of patients reported by Whitlock, over half the patients had recently suffered an episode of head injury.[29] Physical trauma is not only damaging to the soma but also is an anxiety-producing experience which requires some reorganization of the ego. As such, it may be defended against in a variety of means. One such mechanism is conversion. Patients with apparent conversion phenomena following physical trauma should also be carefully evaluated for possible CNS abnormalities. It is entirely possible that the conversion symptom has been facilitated by cerebral injury. It is not uncommon for a patient's symptom and disability to continue after apparent physical recovery from an injury. This appears to be more frequently seen when the accident is compensable in some manner; this syndrome has been called "accident neurosis" or "compensation neurosis." At times an accident serves to resolve certain problems in the victim's life and therefore the disability is maintained because of the secondary gains. Accident neurosis following industrial injuries has been called a modern form of male hysteria.[38]

Psychiatric diagnosis Conversion disorders may be either a component of, or confused with, many other psychiatric diagnoses. The most difficult and most common problem in the differential diagnosis of conversion disorder is that of malingering. The determination of malingering carries with it the implied motivation that the person is seeking to deliberately obtain some type of secondary gain, usually relief from duties such as in the military service, or financial gain such as obtaining financial rewards and litigation for presumed injuries. Therefore it has been stated that to diagnose malingering is actually to make an accusation rather than a diagnosis.[39] The difference between malingering and conversion rests upon whether or not the patient has conscious awareness that he or she is producing the symptom. From a practical standpoint an examiner cannot read minds, and therefore cannot clearly make this determination. Thus, ultimately, the diagnosis of malingering depends upon the patient's confession of such behavior or careful detective work demonstrating that the symptom is not present when the patient believes himself to be unobserved. It is probable that malingering and conversion actually lie on a continuum, the difference being conscious recognition. To some degree patients with conversion disorder recognize that the symptom is not of organic etiology yet on the other hand most malingerers probably have some "hysterical" traits.[40]

One group of symptoms that may be mistakenly attributed to conversion disorder are those which constitute the catatonia syndrome. They include muscular rigidity, mutism, stereotypic behavior, and posturing. The diagnosis of catatonia is suggested by the presence of more than one symptom in this group and the concurrence of a thought disorder. Catatonia does not have a single etiology and may be caused by bipolar affective disorder, schizophrenia, drug overdose, viral encephalitis, and other disorders.[41,42]

Conversion disorder can serve as a defense against other psychiatric illness. For example, conversion may serve to defend against the awareness of depression. An elderly person who has experienced a loss, such as the death of a spouse, may develop a conversion disorder and become preoccupied with the physical symptom, thereby defending against feelings of grief and depression.[43]

Conversion disorder can also be seen as a coping mechanism reflecting a situational adjustment reaction as a way of handling acute environmental stresses and situations. For example, conversion has been reported as a normal and useful coping mechanism in servicemen incarcerated in prisoner of war camps.[44] Conversion phenomena are also occasionally seen as a part of the picture of the symptomatic presentation of acute schizophrenia. In such a situation the conversion symptoms may be evidence of severe ego disruption.

Repetitive conversion disorders form the basis for the diagnosis of somatization disorder. Some persons appear prone to use the conversion phenomenon as a coping mechanism and repeatedly call upon it as a way of handling life events. Somatization disorder will be discussed below as a separate diagnostic entity.

PSYCHOGENIC PAIN

Psychogenic pain is a new psychiatric diagnosis established in DSM-III.[4] Previously this disorder was largely subsumed under the category of conversion disorder. Many patients with psychogenic pain share characteristics similar to conversion disorder but the creation of a separate diagnosis of psychogenic pain does allow for a broader concept of the disorder.

Prolonged and severe pain is the predominant disturbance in psychogenic pain disorder. Because pain can present as a symptom of physical and organic illness, psychogenic pain must be further qualified as being inconsistent with the anatomical distribution of the nervous system, or when no organic cause can be found to account for the pain, or when the pain is clearly in excess of that which would be anticipated with the demonstrated physical pathology. Further diagnostic criteria for the diagnosis of psychogenic pain require evidence that the pain has a relationship to an environmental stress, which is apparently related to a psychological need or conflict, and/or that the presence of the pain enables the patient to obtain a secondary gain not otherwise forthcoming from the environment. An exclusionary criterion for the diagnosis of psychogenic pain disorder is that the pain not be a symptom of another mental disorder.

Case report   A 56-year-old widow from Appalachia was referred to a medical center for evaluation of long-standing facial pain. The pain had been treated multiple times by her local physicians and dentists; in fact, five different sets of dentures had been constructed in an effort to relieve her pain.

Of note, the patient's right facial pain began shortly after two important environmental stressors. The first was the suicide of her husband, who had been chronically disabled with arthritis for years, and the second was that her elder son had left home to enter the armed forces. The patient used exactly the same gesture with her hand to describe the location of the pain in her face that she used to describe the path of the bullet which had killed her husband! Prior to the onset of her pain, which she considered to be disabling, the patient had been a hard worker, supplementing the meager income of the family tobacco farm with her work as a seamstress in a local shirt factory. With the onset of the patient's pain, and her perceived disability, a younger son had remained at home to care for her. His life had completely revolved around her complaints since that time and he had felt too guilty to marry or leave home for any other reason.

Concurrent symptoms, in addition to the pain, indicated that the patient had insomnia of both the terminal and middle type, and had a decreased appetite with a weight loss of 22 lbs. There was a positive family history of affective disorder in a sister and mother.

Past history indicated that the patient grew up on a small farm marked by severe economic deprivation. The patient's mother died when the patient was 11 years old and it was necessary for the patient to leave school at that time.

Features

Mood The mood of patients who complain of chronic pain is almost always that of depression. A controversy continues as to whether or not pain is a symptom primarily of depressionn or whether depression is secondary to the experience of chronic pain.[45] Other mood states seen frequently in patients with chronic pain are those of anxiety and anger.[46] Many of the patients appear tense, anxious, and are constantly worried. Other patients present a picture of irritability and resentment—the resentment often being expressed toward previous medical caretakers who had failed to relieve their symptoms of pain.

Thought Patients with psychogenic pain are focused upon the symptom to a remarkable degree. Their conversation indicates preoccupation with the symptom and all problems and disabilities in their life are frequently related to the pain. Complaints such as, "If it weren't for the pain, I could...," are frequently heard. The patients frequently use words that reflect pain as a manner of communication. For example, "I get sore when...," or, "My daughter's behavior hurts me." Another common theme is the feeling of deprivation, resentment, and of having been exploited in life. Often, the patients come from backgrounds which were deprived, and a history of an abusive parent is not uncommon. Frequently they are self-sacrificing, hard-working persons who feel that they have not been given their fair share in life. Concurrent with this past history is information suggesting that they are being used or exploited by other persons in their lives, usually family members. All in all there is an undercurrent theme of a masochistic life style which pervades the histories and the thought content of these "pained" patients.[47,48]

Behavior When seen in an interview setting the pain patient's behavior is not particularly striking. At times there may be wincing and histrionic behavior suggestive of pain, but it is remarkable how frequently this behavior disappears when the patient becomes engaged in conversation. Their histories reveal a perceived sense of disability and activities are reported as highly restricted despite the apparent mobility demonstrated in interview situations. Typically they have given up many of their usual activities such as employment, church activities, social activities, and often, sexual activity. All of these difficulties are attributed to the pain. Other family members have usually responded to the patient's symptom of pain by assuming the patient's basic responsibilities (see case report above).

Another characteristic behavior of pain patients, and one of importance to physicians, is the fact that these patients often "doctor-shop." They seek consultation with physician after physician, often with the angry demand that something be done to find the cause of their pain. Implicit in many of these consultations is the charge that previous physicians were inadequate or incompetent and therefore unable to find the underlying reason for the pain. Some of these patients travel from medical center to medical center receiving repetitive diagnostic evaluations, all of which prove to be either negative or to yield only inconsequential findings.

Physical examination and laboratory findings By definition, patients with psychogenic pain must have physical findings that do not explain the intensity of the patient's perception of pain, but often in the course of the examination the physician will find that the patient appears to be unusually sensitive to pain in general. There are no consistent laboratory findings. It is not unusual, however, for there to be some evidence of an organic physical problem and one is often left with the impression that although the patient may have a minor physical abnormality the patient's perception, experience and communication is far in excess of that which would be anticipated.

Interviewer's reaction A physician's initial reaction to a pain patient may be a feeling of superiority or pride that the patient has at least sought out a more intelligent physician for medical care. The patients initially are flattering and make statements to the effect that, "At last I have found a competent physician." However, such feelings are usually short-lived and the interviewer begins to develop feelings of irritation as the patient's hostile-dependent behavior becomes more obvious and manifest. The patient's undercurrent anger, irritability, and feelings of entitlement strain the relationship. Requests for addicting medications, demands for the relief of the pain, and frequent after-hours office calls all contribute to negative reactions toward these patients. It has been suggested that the emergence of such negative feelings are themselves diagnostic clues to the underlying nature of the problem.[9]

Pathogenesis

Psychodynamic explanation Psychodynamic issues are considered to be major factors in the etiology of psychogenic pain syndromes. Pain is an important part of the developmental process of the personality. It is the crying of the infant in pain from hunger, a dirty diaper, or other discomfort, which brings the mother back to the child. Therefore the sensation of pain may be associated with the reunion and gratification of dependency needs. The infliction of pain is frequently used as punishment of children. Thus pain becomes closely associated with guilt and penitence. A third issue is related to child abuse. It has been noted that a number of patients with pain syndromes were physically abused by parents during their childhood. It is hypothesized that many of these children were otherwise emotionally deprived and/or ignored. Frequently, following such periods of abuse, the parents made efforts at restitution and increased concern. Thus pain may be associated, perversely, with love and attention.

The pain-prone patient has been described by Blumer and Heilbronn [47] and by Engel.[48] Engel described these patients as depressive, pessimistic individuals who unconsciously did not believe that they deserved success or happiness and felt that they must pay a price for it. Their life histories often included episodes that could have been avoided, in which they had been hurt, defeated, or humiliated. Pain-prone individuals often seem to develop pain at times when things are going well in their lives and perhaps unconsciously they feel that they do not deserve such happiness. Blumer and Heilbronn[47] described pain-prone patients as often alexithymic and denying anger and depression. However, themes of guilt, dependency, and masochism are prominent and combined with a preoccupation with bodily suffering. Other authors have noted that patients with pain syndromes are actually a very heterogeneous group. The pain-prone personalities described above are but one segment of a very diverse and varied population.[49]

Biologic explanations Many patients with pain syndromes actually have a physical disorder. As noted above most persons would not interpret their sensation of pain as do patients with psychogenic pain. There are wide individual differences in the capacity to tolerate pain and many patients amplify their symptoms.[11] Such differences may result from different biologic substrates for the sensitivity of pain. Other very important individual factors include concurrent anxiety and/or depression; any of these affects may have a biologic origin.

Genetics Pain behavior often seems to run in families. Certainly the histories of patients with pain disorders often are replete with stories of family members who have suffered from a variety of physical ailments, often with pain being a prominent symptom. It is difficult to determine whether such a familial incidence of painful syndromes represents a genetic or biologic vulnerability or merely represents psychodynamic factors such as identification. It has also been noted that various ethnic groups vary considerably in their expression of pain, and apparently in their perception of pain. For example, the Irish are noted to be stoical and to tend to deny the perception of pain.[50] Although it might be tempting to interpret such findings as reflecting genetic factors inherent in different ethnic groups, it is more probable that pain is used as a culturally determined method of relating to other persons. Pain may also have meanings to the individual that are culturally determined.[51] In one study of pain responses of subjects of different ethnic and racial backgrounds who had been acculturated over several generations in the United States, ethnic differences no longer were prominent.[52]

Environment Environmental factors are considered to be very important in the perpetuation of painful syndromes. For example, it is noted that pain very frequently follows an industrial or other compensable type of injury. The continuation of disability payments and relief from other responsibilities is frequently a powerful disincentive to the patient's recovery.[53] The symptom of pain represents one method by which the disability is continued. Disability payments are not the only reinforcers of pain behavior. Often the symptom of pain elicits different responses from intimate persons in the patient's environment such as a spouse, and not infrequently there is encouragement from others in the environment for the patient to maintain the pain syndrome. For example, a disabled spouse may meet the needs of the healthy spouse who may wish to take control of the family finances.[54] From this perspective pain frequently needs to be interpreted within a systems theory context: the pain allows for continuation of a steady state within the environment.[2]

Differential Diagnoses

Nonpsychotropic drugs Medications as a rule are not associated with inducing pain syndromes. However, any drug which may increase anxiety and/or depression may thereby increase the patient's perception of pain. Drugs which may increase anxiety include caffeine or pseudoephedrine. Drugs which may be associated with inducing depression include the antihypertensive agents, digitalis, cimetidine, and others.

Psychotropic drugs Psychotropic drugs are not as a rule associated with the etiology of psychogenic pain syndromes. However, many patients who present with psychogenic pain have previously seen a number of physicians. It is not unusual that one or more of these physicians has prescribed a variety of psychotropic drugs. Among these are habituating drugs such as the benzodiazepines, barbiturates, or meprobamate. Rarely have these categories of drugs been effective in helping a patient in relief of pain and it is not unusual that the patient has become habituated to one of them. It has been reported that meprobamate and barbiturates may actually have some antianalgesic effect.[55] Medications such as the neuroleptics and tricyclic antidepressants are usually associated with some relief of pain. This may be through the relief of anxiety, the treatment of underlying depression, or via a direct analgesic effect.[56]

Alcohol The abuse of alcohol is not generally associated with psychogenic pain syndromes. A possible complication of long standing alcohol abuse which might become confused with a psychogenic pain syndrome is that of peripheral neuritis. The patient may complain of burning of the soles of the feet or the palms of the hands and other poorly defined pains.

Other abused substances The addiction to narcotic agents, particularly agents such as meperidine hydrochloride or codeine, must be an important part of the differential diagnosis of a psychogenic pain disorder. Many patients with severe pain claim that it can be relieved only by a narcotic agent and seek prescriptions from physicians. What is actually underlying the complaint of pain is addiction to a narcotic. Through the pain complaint the drug is obtained in a socially approved manner. A suspicion of narcotic addiction should be raised any time the patient demands a specific agent. Frequently the patient will complain to be "allergic" to all other agents than that which is requested, or state that other side effects make it impossible for him to use other drugs. These patients frequently reject alternative treatment techniques and also make many visits to emergency rooms or make telephone calls with overt or latent requests for renewal of their analgesic agents. Their medical histories tend to be vague and it frequently proves to be difficult to obtain their medical records.

Medical illnesses A complete discussion of the medical illnesses which have pain associated with them, and therefore must be considered a part of the differential diagnosis of psychogenic pain, would fill medical textbooks. It is sufficient to say that pain is a symptom of almost any disease and the patient's complaints must be considered in the context of all diseases affecting the organ system associated with the complaint of pain. Psychogenic pain disorder should be given prominence in the differential diagnosis of complaints of pain when the description of pain is unusual. Often the complaints of pain (as noted above) have a particular dramatic or vivid quality to them, for example, "It feels like someone stuck a knife into my back and then turned it," or, "Someone has driven a spike between my ears."

Many medical illnesses such as rheumatoid arthritis are associated with varying degrees of chronic pain. The degree of disability and perception of pain that a patient will experience with such a disease appears highly variable and dependent upon individual personality factors, rather than upon the extent or duration of the disease process.[57] It should be noted that it is the degree of amplification of the symptom and the use of the symptom in regard to environmental events that is important rather than the absolute presence or absence of a disease with the capacity to cause pain.

It is important that psychogenic pain disorder be differentiated from other physical illnesses which may have psychological etiologies but have symptoms reflective of pain. For example, muscle tension headache may have significant psychogenic components but because there is a demonstrable organic findings (increased muscle contractions), psychogenic pain disorder is not an appropriate diagnosis.

Surgical complications Most patients recover from surgical interventions at a relatively rapid rate and use narcotics for relief of pain for only two to three days following the operation. However, some patients continue to complain of severe pain extending far beyond the usual time of recovery. These patients present difficult differential diagnostic problems because the question is always raised as to whether the patient is healing properly or whether there was an unexpected complication of surgery. Included in the differential diagnosis must be the question of addiction to narcotics prior to the operation and if the complaint of pain represents a means of continuing the habituation. Another consideration is that of phantom pain. Phantom pain is determined by many factors but has some physiologic basis. Syndromes of phantom pain are likely to be more severe when the personality of the patient is rigid or compulsively self-reliant or if there had been a period of long-standing pain in the extremity prior to amputation.[58] At times phantom pain represents an unresolved grief over the lost body part. Phantom pain is not limited merely to loss of a limb. It has been reported in such situations as phantom ulcer pain and phantom breast pain following mastectomy. In regard to mastectomy, patients who are more likely to experience phantom breast pain are those who did not receive much emotional support from their surgeons, who were younger, and who had a poorer relationship with husbands.[59]

Physical trauma   Complaints of pain following trauma tend to be more prominent when the trauma, as noted above, represents a compensable injury. Persistent pain following athletic injuries is noted less frequently than pain following industrial accidents. However, one must not be too quick to attribute complaints of persistent pain following trauma to motivation in obtaining secondary gains. The perception of pain may be closely related to the posttraumatic syndrome. In this syndrome patients often exhibit symptoms of depression and severe anxiety, disorders known to be associated with and to facilitate the perception of pain. The perception of pain may also be more intense if circumstances surrounding the episode of physical trauma had a particular psychologic significance. For example, the continuation of severe pain may be the unconscious representation of feelings of guilt and a need to suffer because of feelings of responsibility over causing an accident injuring themselves and possibly others, as with an automobile accident.

Psychiatric disease   The most important diagnosis to consider in regard to complaints of persistent and chronic pain of apparent psychogenic etiology is depression. Depression is closely associated with chronic pain and, in fact, some authors feel that it is essentially an inevitable consequence of experiencing pain. Thus the depression may be a secondary feature to a chronic pain syndrome rather than primary. However, it has also been noted that patients who seek treatment for depression frequently have concurrent complaints of pain. In one series of depressed private practice patients, 57% had recurring pain.[60] In another series a high frequency of pain syndromes were noted in patients with depression. For example, 77% had headaches and 37% complained of chest pain.[20] Complaints of facial pain have a very high correlation with underlying major depression.[61] An effort should be made to determine whether or not depression preceded the onset of pain or whether the depression appeared as the consequence of pain. However, for practical purposes, all patients who have concurrent symptoms of depression and pain should be treated for their depression.

Complaints of pain may be part of the symptomatic picture of schizophrenia. These complaints frequently have a delusional quality and are somewhat bizarre. Differentiation from other forms of psychogenic pain disorder should be made on the basis of demonstration of a schizophrenic thought disorder.

Recurrent complaints of pain frequently are associated with somatization disorder (see below). Chronic pelvic pain is a specific syndrome more frequently associated with somatization disorder. A large proportion of these patients will have histories consistent with hysterical personality disorder, antisocial personality, or somatization disorder.[62]

Complaints of persistent pain may be associated with narcotic addiction (see above) and/or malingering. With malingering the patient consciously and deliberately makes a complaint of pain without experiencing the pain. By definition, malingering is the effort by a person to obtain a concrete secondary gain, such as financial compensation, via simulated symptoms.

SOMATIZATION DISORDER

Somatization disorder is a new diagnostic entity created for the latest edition of the DSM-III.[4] The disorder is based on the earlier concept of "hysteria," subsequently relabeled with the eponym "Briquet's syndrome." Hysteria is a disorder which has been described over several thousands of years of medical history. The term has been used indiscriminately and has lost any specific diagnostic meaning. The term Briquet's syndrome was introduced in the late 1960s in an effort to rigorously define a specific and stable syndrome which encompassed the prior concept of hysteria.[63] Because reliability and validity data have yet to be accumulated for somatization disorder the following discussion will of necessity be based on work reported in regard to Briquet's syndrome with which there is a fairly high diagnostic concordance.[64]

One diagnostic criterion for somatization disorder is that a patient must report a history of physical symptoms of several years duration with the onset of symptoms before the age of 30. From a list of 37 possible symptoms the diagnosis requires complaints of at least 14 medically unexplained symptoms for women and 12 medically unexplained symptoms for men. In order to count as a symptom the patient must have taken some action in regard to the symptom such as having seen a physician or having taken a medication other than aspirin. The interviewer need not be certain that the symptom had actually been present; merely the report of the symptom is sufficient. Among the symptoms contained in the list are such items as the patient's stating that she believed herself to be sickly a good part of her life; conversion or pseudoneurologic symptoms; vague GI symptoms; a variety of gynecologic and/or psychosexual symptoms;

symptoms reflecting unexplained pain; and cardiovascular symptoms such as palpitations or dizziness. The overwhelming majority of patients reporting somatization disorder have been women, although there have been a few isolated reports of the disorder in men.[65]

Case report   A 43-year-old married female was admitted to the hospital for the tenth time in 9 years. Her hospital admission was precipitated by the patient's complaint of abdominal pain described as, "It feels like a cup of fire poured inside my belly." Medical work-ups failed to disclose any cause of the patient's pain, which gradually resolved during her hospitalization. It was noted that she received exceptional reinforcement for the sick role from her husband and children. The children did all of her housework and her husband drove 90 miles each way daily in order to see her while she was in the hospital. A review of the patient's past medical history indicated that the patient responded positively to 31 of the 37 items on the somatization check list. In addition, the patient had a history of at least one brief psychiatric hospitalization precipitated by a disabling conversion symptom. The type of symptoms that the patient complained of included primary urinary retention, severe dyspareunia, diplopia, diffuse skin pain, and poor memory.

Mental status examination revealed a cheerful, apparently non-distressed woman who stated her somatic complaints in a graphic and florid fashion. She specifically denied any psychological component to her pain and was cognitively intact without evidence of a thought disorder. The patient's past history was related dramatically with many inconsistencies as to date and symptoms.

Included in the medical history were a large number of minor surgical procedures such as biopsies and, in addition, the patient had undergone three gynecologic surgical procedures.

The patient's childhood history was notable in that her younger sister had suffered from poliomyelitis with residual paraplegia. The patient reported that "I carried my sister 3 miles to school every day in my arms." The patient had been married twice. She worked intermittently until age 28, at which time a diagnosis of "scleroderma" was made by a physician. From that time, despite the fact that the diagnosis was never confirmed in any of her subsequent medical evaluations, she considered herself disabled and never returned to work.

Features

Mood   The mood of the patient with somatization disorder is highly varied. Traditionally the patient displays an indifference to the symptoms (la belle indifference) and when hospitalized appears to be remarkably comfortable with the situation. The degree of illness suggested by the symptoms, eg, paraplegia, is not accompanied by the degree of worry and concern that the symptoms might suggest. Rather, the patient may be dressed in a provocative nightgown, primping herself while lying back in a hospital bed with fluffed-up pillows. However, this degree of bland indifference tends to exist only so long as the patient's needs are being met by the symptoms. If the symptoms fail to successfully defend against the ideas or affect which initiated the symptoms, then the patient may exhibit anxiety or depression. Similarly, if the symptoms fail to engender support from medical caregivers, husband, boy friend, or family, then the patient may also respond with anxiety, depression, or anger.

Thought   The thought content of patients with somatization disorder, as evidenced by their speech, indicates a preoccupation with their various illnesses, present and past, which are often recounted with a dramatic flair. Past illnesses are not recalled as minor episodes but often are remembered as life-threatening, eg, being saved by a surgeon just before the rupture of an inflamed and swollen appendix. Similarly, other life events are remembered dramatically and often with a degree of exaggeration. For example, in the patient described above, she "carried" her sister 3 miles to school daily. Patients tend to think and to relate their histories in a dramatic and global fashion rather than with precise detail. Dates and circumstances frequently change from interviewer to interviewer because the patients demonstrate a quality known as "affective truth." In other words, the patient's history is more determined by how the patient feels from moment to moment rather than by strict attention to detail.

Behavior   Consistent with her speech, the behavior of the patient with somatization disorder tends to be histrionic and dramatic. When the patient's needs are being gratified she may be very cooperative but problems may result in angry outbursts, temper tantrums, and other forms of impulsive behavior. The patient's past behavior is often characterized by impulsiveness including sexual promiscuity and suicidal gestures or manipulations. Many of these patients have abused addicting substances such as minor tranquilizers, pain medications, and/or alcohol.[66]

Physical examination and laboratory findings   The physical examination and laboratory studies in these patients are usually within normal limits. Abnormal findings are usually inconsequential and do not explain the patient's symptoms. They may be regarded as coincidental findings of no particular significance. At times the patients do have chronic illnesses that become incorporated into their somatization behavior. Symptoms are then exaggerated and the disease is often used, when convenient, to manipulate other people.

Interviewer's reaction The medical caregivers of these patients are often initially positively inclined toward patients with somatization disorder. The patients often display an engaging manner and the dramatic presentation of their symptoms frequently creates a sense of urgency that something must be done for the patient which stimulates feelings of wanting to help. However, with the passage of time physicians begin to find themselves increasingly angry and irritated because of the patient's dependency, frequent telephone calls, and manipulative attempts to obtain various medications. After the experience of evaluating multiple symptoms which did not prove to have an organic etiology it is not unusual for physicians to become quite angry and rejecting of the patients who come to be regarded as frauds or fakes.

Pathogenesis

Psychodynamic explanation Modern explorations of Briquet's syndrome (hysteria, somatization disorder) have focused upon the phenomenology and have been less concerned with the pathogenesis of the disorder. Traditional views of hysteria have emphasized the sexual aspects of the disorder. It is hypothesized that conflicts regarding sexuality are repressed from consciousness and then expressed through somatic symptoms. The sexual view of hysteria predates Freud and was reflected in the writings of both the ancient Egyptians and Greeks.[67] It is important to note that current diagnostic criteria continue to place a heavy emphasis upon symptoms such as dyspareunia. From a phenomenologic standpoint, it is of interest that many of these patients have conflicts concerning their feminine identity, may have engaged in sexual acting out, and have received a number of surgical interventions in the pelvic area of the body.[68] Thus the issue of underlying sexual conflicts continue to be considered as part of the syndrome whether or not they are viewed within traditional psychoanalytic theories.

Biologic explanations Ancient explanations of hysteria revolved around the theory of the wandering uterus. These theories were more or less laid to rest in the nineteenth century by the French neurologists

Briquet and Charcot who emphasized the CNS origins of the symptoms. They regarded hysterics as having a brain predisposed, perhaps by heredity, to developing conversion symptoms.[69,70] These theories were subsequently supplanted by psychodynamic explanations. However, recent work by neurologists have indeed suggested that the brains of patients who exhibit multiple conversion disorders do differ from normal controls in neuropsychologic functioning.[71] One recent report suggests that patients with multiple conversion symptoms (Briquet's syndrome) have dysfunction of both the dominant and nondominant hemispheres of the brain with relatively greater dysfunction of the dominant hemisphere. The consequence of this impairment is difficulty with verbal expression of emotional states.[28]

Genetics There is a definite increased familial incidence of both Briquet's syndrome and sociopathy in patients with these disorders. In addition to a higher incidence of Briquet's syndrome in the relatives of patients than in normal controls, there is also a higher incidence of alcoholism and sociopathy in their male relatives than would be expected by chance.[72] It has been suggested that Briquet's syndrome and sociopathy are basically the same disorder with the difference in symptomatic expression being determined by gender.[73,74] It should be noted, however, that increased familial incidence is not the same as a genetic disorder and that environmental factors could similarly affect the incidence in families. Because most patients come from lower socioeconomic backgrounds, the increased prevalence of alcoholism and greater social stress may be common factors. However, one recent finding, yet to be confirmed, indicates that patients with Briquet's syndrome have a significantly higher incidence of type A blood than would be expected by chance.[75] This type of evidence is consistent with a genetic component.

Environment The environment is considered to be an important aspect of the pathogenesis and the perpetuation of the symptoms of the patient with somatization disorder. These patients have frequently had a chaotic childhood.[72,73] The home was frequently marked by marital strife. Physical abuse and violence were not uncommon. In addition, one or the other of the parents may have been involved with an addictive drug, particularly alcohol. Lower socioeconomic status for many of these patients added the burden of economic deprivation. Patients frequently made premature excursions into sexual behavior, often had pregnancies at an early age and/or married to leave the home environment. As a consequence, the developmental tasks of later adolescence were frequently uncompleted at the expense of premature responsibility for children. The men that these patients marry often have a similar background, and problems with sociopathy, irresponsibility, and alcoholism are not uncommon.[76]

Illness behavior may have been learned during childhood as a way to obtain special favors or to manipulate for advantage. In the case listed above, the patient's younger sister had polio and was accorded special privileges within the large family.

As adults these patients have learned to utilize illness as a coping mechanism. It serves as an adequate excuse both to others and to the patient herself as a rationale for not fulfilling adult responsibilities. Illness and acute symptoms can also be used at times of acute stress. For example, a woman may use an acute physical symptom in an effort to return a philandering husband to the home or to obtain rest in a hospital when exhausted from caring for children.

Differential Diagnosis

Patients with somatization disorder provide a wide variety of differential diagnostic problems. Symptoms not only can be easily confused with physical illness but underlying the physical symptoms there may be a number of psychiatric and/or characterologic problems.

Nonpsychotropic drugs The somatizing patient is frequently under the medical care of several physicians simultaneously. These patients may be treated symptomatically and have prescriptions for a wide variety of medications. Often the various physicians treating the patient are unaware of the medications being prescribed by others and the patients may have a small pharmacy in the medicine cabinet at home. Because of this polypharmacy there is the possibility of a variety of side reactions, adverse reactions, or drug cross-reactions. Patients may present with a wide variety of physical symptoms that are drug-related. Another problem and potential complication, is that because of the patient's proclivity to impulsive suicidal gestures they may grab the first medication available in the medicine chest and thereby overdose on a wide variety of unusual substances, leading to uncommon problems in the medical management of the overdosage.

Psychotropic drugs The somatizing patient (Briquet's syndrome) is frequently prescribed a variety of psychotropic medications. The most common of these are the benzodiazepines prescribed in an effort to reduce the patient's anxiety. However, the patient frequently does not use the medication as prescribed and may present herself to her physician with a variety of different problems related directly to the drug itself. For example, problems of confusion or somnolence may be due to excessive use of the medications. Episodes of psychosis, seizures, and other neurologic symptoms may result from abrupt withdrawal of benzodiazepines if they have been taken in sufficiently high doses. Other psychotropic drugs frequently prescribed for these patients because of their episodes of "depression" include the tricyclic antidepressants. Side reactions from these medications include a wide variety of cardiovascular and anticholinergic effects. Concomitant with the patient's propensity to somatize, patients may also present with symptoms such as acute urinary retention or episodes of palpitations or tachycardia.

Alcohol The patient with somatization disorder frequently comes from a home in which alcohol was abused. The patient herself may also be an alcohol abuser, sometimes secretively. Because of the propensity to substance abuse, latent alcoholism must be a serious consideration in the differential diagnosis and a potential cause of the patient's various physical complaints. Symptoms include the toxic effects of alcohol such as alcoholic gastritis, hepatic toxicity with elevated liver enzymes, and peripheral or CNS neuropathy secondary to vitamin deficiencies. In addition, these patients may present acutely with vitamin deficiencies, or with withdrawal syndromes, including tremulousness, autonomic nervous system hyperactivity, and frank delirium tremens with seizures.

Other abused substances Pain is a frequent symptom of the somatizing patients. As a consequence they frequently obtain prescriptions for a wide variety of analgesics, some of which are habituating. It is not unusual for these patients to be demanding of medications with a potential for abuse including analgesic compounds which contain barbiturates (Fiorinal) or drug compounds which contain codeine (Emperincodeine). Other drugs of abuse are codeine, meperidine, pentazocine, and propoxyphene. The patient's somatic complaints may be used as a means of obtaining further medications when the underlying disorder is addiction. Many of the physical complaints may be the direct result of the addiction itself and/or a consequence of withdrawal. Episodes of hyperactivity of the autonomic nervous system, seizures, and confusion may not represent new organic symptoms reflecting underlying CNS disease, but rather symptoms of narcotic withdrawal.

Medical illnesses The symptoms of somatization disorder may simulate any known medical illness. As is the case with pain patients, a textbook of medicine would be required to explore the complete differential diagnosis of these patients' symptoms with regard to possible medical illnesses. The medical illnesses that are most likely to be confused with somatization disorder are those with insidious onset and vague and nonspecific multisystem manifestations. These include the collagen disorders (see the case above) and the endocrinopathies.

Examples of diseases that may be confused with somatization disorder include systemic lupus erythematosus (SLE) and systemic mastocytosis. SLE may present with multiple vague physical complaints, such as joint pain, and nonspecific psychiatric symptoms.[77] Systemic mastocytosis may similarly be manifested by numerous poorly defined symptoms of the cutaneous, GI, cardiovascular, and respiratory systems. Vague neuropsychiatric symptoms are also common.[78]

Patients may have a medical diagnosis established by a physician, often on inadequate grounds, which is carried through future hospitalizations and episodes requiring medical care (see the case above). The diagnosis may be ruled out only after many years when the disease has failed to progress as would have been expected.

As with all forms of somatization, these patients are by no means immune from disease and thus any new complaint must be carefully evaluated. However, the general rule to be observed is that no invasive diagnostic or therapeutic procedure should be undertaken without objective evidence of a pathophysiologic process.

Surgical complications   The somatizing patient has had an excessive number of surgical interventions. Studies suggest that these patients have surgical operations two to three times more frequently than do normal controls.[79] Because of this amount of surgery there are increased opportunities for complications, either acutely or chronically. The most common problems are those following abdominal surgery, often for symptoms which prove to have little objective evidence of disease. Episodes of abdominal pain may be considered as potentially due to partial bowel obstruction from adhesions. Somatizing patients also have a large number of operations for pelvic complaints. It is not unusual for future complaints to be considered as secondary to complications of prior surgery. For example, a hysterectomy may be followed by a variety of procedures to suspend the bladder or to attempt to correct other urinary tract complaints.

Surgery provides increased opportunity for complaints referable to the part of the body operated upon. Physicians may feel guilt or responsibility and be progressively engaged by the patient's manipulative behavior.

Physical trauma   The usual somatic complaints are those referable to disease rather than to trauma. However, one cautionary note is in order: a high degree of clinical suspicion should be entertained when the patient has unexplained trauma. As noted before, women with Briquet's syndrome not only come from chaotic family backgrounds in which physical abuse was common, but they frequently marry alcoholic men.[76] Physical abuse is by no means rare in these marriages and the woman who presents with trauma of a poorly explained origin may be a victim of wife abuse.

Psychiatric diagnosis   The diagnosis of Briquet's syndrome is usually not confused with other psychiatric syndromes when sufficient clinical time is invested into obtaining a complete history of repetitive somatizing behavior and a complete mental status examination is performed. However, at times, particularly with acute presentations or with inadequate evaluations, these patients may be confused with several other psychiatric disorders.

Depression is a frequent consideration in the differential diagnosis. On close examination, the depression of which the patients complain is usually situational in its etiology and takes the form of dysphoric unhappy feelings rather than major depression. Although the patient may complain dramatically of severe depression and even voice suicidal ideation, it is remarkable how often these dysphoric feelings remit when circumstances in the patient's environment change for the better. More prolonged episodes of dysphoria may represent atypical depression. The disorder "hysteroid dysphoria" is considered by some clinicians to be a form of atypical major depression.[80] Phenelzine sulfate (Nardil) has been suggested as a specific therapy for this particular disorder.[81] A note of caution must be raised. Phenelzine is a monoamine oxidase inhibitor and requires careful adherence to diet and the contraindication of many drugs including the narcotics. As a consequence it may be difficult to prescribe the drug safely for these impulse-driven patients.

The patient with Briquet's syndrome may also appear in a state of acute agitation, markedly anxious, tense, and agitated. This particular affective state may be mistaken for panic disorder or other forms of anxiety disorder. Again, as with depression, the patient's affect tends to be highly situationally related and the patient's anxiety and agitation abate quickly when there is relief from the distressing factors. In other words, the anxiety appears to be generated more from external environmental events than from internal conflicts of a neurotic nature. Conversely, patients who have panic disorder may focus on somatic complaints and sometimes resemble patients with somatization disorder.[82]

The most common disorder that may be indicated as a false-positive on the Briquet's checklist is schizophrenia.[83] Schizophrenics frequently have had a wide variety of unusual body and psychological experiences and therefore may respond to a large number of items in regard to past medical history. Differentiation of somatization disorder from schizophrenia depends upon the demonstration of the typical schizophrenic thought process disorder—the sine qua non of schizophrenia. Although patients with Briquet's syndrome may appear to be transiently psychotic when under severe psychic distress, the disorder is not considered one of the psychoses. Presence of delusions or hallucinations of other than the most transitory type should suggest a psychotic disorder rather than a somatization disorder.

Drug addiction must be differentiated from somatization disorder. Many addicts repetitively seek consultation from physicians complaining particularly of pain syndromes as well as other physical complaints in an effort to obtain prescriptions of narcotics. Although drug addiction and somatization disorder may coexist, the continual search for addictive substances is not the predominant feature of somatization disorder. A careful history will demonstrate that the somatization disorder frequently preceded addiction and has existed somewhat independently of the addictive state.

Somatization disorder (Briquet's syndrome) is at times confused with hypochondriasis. Because the diagnosis of Briquet's syndrome is a phenomenologic diagnosis there is the potential of overlap in the diagnostic criteria between the two disorders. However, as a general rule, the patient with hypochondriasis, while fearful of disease and complaining of many symptoms, does not exhibit the characteristic loss of function typical of conversion disorders. Patients with hypochondriasis tend to be obsessional and the disorder has a much closer relationship with major depression than does Briquet's syndrome. Patients with Briquet's syndrome typically demonstrate a hysterical cognitive style as opposed to the obsessional style characteristic of the hypochondriac.[2] This differentiation is of more than academic interest. The hypochondriac frequently benefits from the administration of antidepressant medication, while as a general rule the patient with somatization disorder does not. The prescription of antidepressant medications for a patient with somatization disorder may merely increase the likelihood of drug interactions and potential overdose.

SUMMARY

A review of the various somatization disorders suggests that there are no clear-cut differences between them nor is there a clear-cut differentiation between physical disease and the process of somatization. Somatization may be used as a coping mechanism by a patient, whether or not organic disease is present. Similarly, in many different psychiatric diseases somatization may be a part of the clinical picture either because of physical symptoms which accompany the disorder (eg, tachycardia with anxiety disorder, constipation with depression) or the need to express thoughts and feelings through bodily symptoms and nonverbal means of communication.

As a general statement, both conversion disorders and psychogenic pain syndromes should be considered as symptoms rather than as specific diagnoses. Underlying each may be a wide variety of psychiatric diagnoses. For example, conversion disorders may be coping mechanisms in response to acute stressful situations or they may be psychological defenses against underlying severe depression. As a repetitive coping mechanism, they take on a characterological style which is termed somatization disorder. Similarly, psychogenic pain disorders may be the symptomatic expression of hypochondriasis or somatization disorder. Very frequently psychogenic pain disorders are the primary symptom of underlying major depression. The division of conversion disorder and psychogenic pain disorder is somewhat arbitrary. In the past pain syndromes were regarded to be a form of conversion disorder.

Each patient who presents with somatization disorder requires careful evaluation of the physical symptoms to rule out organic disease. When somatization is strongly suspected, invasive diagnostic and therapeutic procedures are not indicated unless there is objective evidence of a pathophysiologic process. Further delineation of the specific form of somatization requires careful mental status examination and past medical and psychiatric history. Although such a procedure is frequently time-consuming, it proves to be highly cost-efficient because these patients' physical symptoms return them again and again to medical care.

REFERENCES

1. Culpan R, Davies B: Psychiatric Illness at a medical and surgical outpatient clinic. *Compr Psychiatry* 1960;1:228-235.

232

2. Ford CV: *The Somatizing Disorders: Illness as a way of life.* New York Elsevier, 1983.

3. *Diagnostic and Statistical Manual of Mental Disorders,* ed 3. Washington, American Psychiatric Association, 1980.

4. Pilowsky I: Primary and secondary hypochondriasis. *Acta Psychiatr Scand* 1970;46:273-285.

5. Sifneos PE: *Short-term Psychotherapy and Emotional Crisis.* Cambridge, Mass, Harvard University Press, 1972.

6. Bishop ER: An olfactory reference syndrome—Monosymptomatic hypochondriasis. *Clin Psychiatry* 1980;41:57-59.

7. Lesse S: Marked depression—a diagnostic and therapeutic problem. *Dis Nerv Syst* 1968;29:169-173.

8. Andreasen NC, Bardach J: Dysmorphophobia: Symptom or disease? *Am J Psychiatry* 1977;134:673-676.

9. Nesheim R: Caring for patients who are not easy to like. *Postgrad Med* 1982;72:255-266.

10. Cohen A: The physician and the "crock," in Usdin GL (ed): *Practical Lectures in Psychiatry for the Medical Practitioner.* Springfield, Ill, Charles C Thomas Publisher, 1966, pp 22-30.

11. Barsky AJ, Klerman GL: Overview: Hypochondriasis, body complaints, and somatic styles. *Am J Psychiatry* 1983;140:273-283.

12. Lipsitt DR: Medical and psychological characteristics of "crocks." *Psychiatr Med* 1970;1:15-25.

13. Katon W, Kleinman A, Rosen G: Depression and comatization: A review, pt I. *Am J Med* 1982;72:127-135.

14. Katon W, Kleinman A, Rosen G: Depression and somatization: A review, pt II. *Am J Med* 1982;72:241-247.

15. Mechanic D: Social psychologic factors affecting the presentation of bodily complaints. *N Engl J Med* 1972;286:1133-1139.

16. *Physicians' Desk Reference,* ed 37 Oradell, NJ, Medical Economics, 1983.

17. Hall RCW, Stickney SK, Gardner ER: Behavioral toxicity of nonpsychiatric drugs, in Hall RCW (ed): *Psychiatric Presentations of Medical Illness: Somatopsychic disorders.* New York, Spectrum Publications, Inc, 1980, pp 337-406.

18. Horowitz MJ, Wilner N, Kaltreider N, et al: Signs and symptoms of post traumatic stress disorder. *Arch Gen Psychiatry* 1980;37:85-92.

19. Ford CV: A type of disability neurosis: The "Humpty Dumpty syndrome."*Int J Psychiatry Med* 1978;8:285-294.

20. Mathew RJ, Wienman ML, Mirabi M: Physical symptoms of depression. *Br J Psychiatr* 1981;139:293-296.

21. Katon W: Panic disorder and somatization. *Am J Med* 1984;77:101-106.

22. Folks DG, Ford CV, Regan W: Conversion symptoms in a general hospital. *Psychosomatics* 1984;25:285-295.

23. Ford CV, Folks DG: Conversion disorders. An overview. *Psychosomatics* 1985;26:371-383.

24. Raskin M, Talbott JA, Meyerson AT: Diagnosis of conversion reactions: Predictive value of psychiatric criteria. *JAMA* 1966;197:102-106.
25. Weintraub MI: *Hysterical Conversion Reactions: A Clinical Guide to Diagnosis and Treatment* . New York, SP Medical & Scientific Books, 1983.
26. Slater E: Diagnosis of hysteria. *Br Med J* 1965;1:1395-1399.
27. Bendefeldt F, Miller LL, Ludwig AM: Cognitive performance in conversion hysteria. *Arch Gen Psychiatry* 1976;33:1250-1254.
28. Flor-Henry P, Fromm-Auch D, Tapper M, et al: A neuropsychological study of stable syndrome hysteria. *Biol Psychiatry* 1981;16:601-626.
29. Whitlock FA: The aetiology of hysteria. *Acta Psychiatr Scand* 1967;43:144-162.
30. Caplan LR, Nadelson T: The Oklahoma complex: A common form of conversion hysteria. *Arch Intern Med* 1980;140:185-186.
31. Folks DG, Ford CV, Regan W: Conversion symptoms in a general hospital. *Psychosomatics* 1984;25:285-295.
32. Anderson GJ: Clinical clues to digitalis toxicity. *Geriatrics* 1980;35:57-65.
33. Victor M, Adams RD, Collins GH: *The Wernicke-Korsakoff Syndrome.* Philadelphia, FA Davis Co, 1971.
34. Watson CG, Buranen C: The frequency and identification of false positive conversion reactions. *J Nerv Ment Dis* 1979;167:234-247.
35. Merskey H, Buhrich NA: Hysteria and organic brain disease. *Br J Med Psychol* 1975;48:359-366.
36. Caplan LR, Nadelson T: Multiple sclerosis and hysteria: Lessons learned from their association. *JAMA* 1980;243:2418-2421.
37. Nicassio P, Arnold E, Prager R: Behavioral treatment of hysterical dysphagia in a hospital setting. *Gen Hosp Psychiatry* 1981;3:513-517.
38. Allodi FA: Accident neurosis: whatever happened to male hysteria? *Can Psychiatr Assoc J* 1974;19:291-296.
39. Szasz TS: Malingering: "Diagnosis" or social condemnation? *Arch Neurol Psychiatry* 1956;76:432-443.
40. Cameron NA: *The Psychology of Behavior Disorders* . Boston, Houghton-Mifflin, 1947.
41. Gelenberg, AJ: The catatonic syndrome. *Lancet* 1976;1;1339-1341.
42. Stoudemire A: The differential diagnosis of catatonic states. *Psychosomatics* 1982;23:245-252.
43. Weddington WW: Conversion reaction in an 82 year old man. *J Nerv Ment Dis* 1979;167:368-369.
44. Wolf S, Ripley HS: Reactions among allied prisoners of war subjected to three years of imprisonment and torture by the Japanese. *Am J Psychiatry* 1947;104:180-193.
45. Reuler JB, Girard DE, Nardone DA: The chronic pain syndrome: Misconceptions and management. *Ann Intern Med* 1980;93:588-596.
46. Engel BT: Some physiological correlates of hunger and pain. *J Exp Psychol* 1959;57:389-396.

234

47. Blumer D, Heilbronn M: The pain-prone disorder: A clinical and psychological profile. *Psychosomatics* 1981;22:395-402.
48. Engel GL: "Psychogenic" pain and the pain-prone patient. *Am J Med* 1959;36:899-918.
49. Prokop CK, Bradley LA, Margolis R, et al: Multivariate analysis of the MMPI profiles of patients with multiple pain complaints. *J Pers Assess* 1980;44:246-252.
50. Zborowski M: Cultural components in responses to pain, in Jaco ED (ed): *Patients, Physicians and Illness.* Glencoe, Ill, Free Press, 1958, pp 256-268.
51. Zola IK: Pathways to the doctor—from person to patient. *Soc Sci Med* 1973;7:677-689.
52. Flannery RB, Sos J, McGovern P: Ethnicity as a factor in the expression of pain. *Psychosomatics* 1981;22:39-50.
53. Krusen EM, Ford DE: Compensation factor in low back injuries. *JAMA* 1958;166:1128-1133.
54. Bursten B, D'Esopo R: The obligation to remain sick. *Arch Gen Psychiatry* 1965;12:402-407.
55. Noyes R: Treatment of cancer pain. *Psychosom Med* 1981;43:57-70.
56. Moore DP: Treatment of chronic pain with tricyclic antidepressants. *South Med J* 1980;73:1585-1586.
57. Ford CV, Callahan LF, Brooks RH, et al: Psychological test results are not correlated with objective measures of function in rheumatoid arthritis. Proceedings of the 15th European Conference on Psychosomatic Research, in press.
58. Parkes CM: Factors determining the persistence of phantom pain in the amputee. *J Psychosom Res* 1973;17:97-108.
59. Jamison K, Wellisch DK, Katz RL, et al: Phantom breast syndrome. *Arch Surg* 1979;114:93-95.
60. Lindsay PG, Wyckoff M: The depression-pain syndrome and its response to antidepressantts. *Psychosomatics* 1981;22;571-577.
61. Lesse S: Atypical facial pain syndromes of psychogenic origin: complications of their misdiagnosis. *J Nerv Ment Dis* 1956;124:346-351.
62. Gross RJ, Doern H, Caldirola D, et al: Borderline syndrome and incest in chronic pelvic pain patients. *Int J Psychiatr Med* 1980;19:79-96.
63. Guze SB: The diagnosis of hysteria: What are we trying to do? *Am J Psychiatry* 1967;119:960-965.
64. De Souza C, Othmer E: Somatization disorder and Briquet's syndrome. *Arch Gen Psychiatry* 1984;41:335-336.
65. Smith GR, Monson RA, Livingston RL: Somatization disorder in men. *Gen Hosp Psychiatry* 1985;7:4-8.
66. Guze SB, Woodruff RH, Clayton PJ: Hysteria and antisocial behavior: Further evidence of an association. *Am J Psychiatry* 1971;127:957-960.
67. Veith I: *Hysteria, A History of a Disease* . Chicago, University of Chicago Press, 1965.

68. Bibb RC, Guze SB: Hysteria in a psychiatric hospital. *Am J Psychiatry* 1972;129:244-248.
69. Mai GM, Merskey H: Briquet's concept of hysteria: An historical perspective. *Can J Psychiatry* 1981;26:57-63.
70. Havens L: Charcot and hysteria. *J Nerv Ment Dis* 1966;141:505-516.
71. Miller L: Neuropsychologic concepts of somatoform disorders. *Int J Psychiatry* 1984;14:31-46.
72. Arkonac O, Guze SB: A family study of hysteria. *N Engl J Med* 1963;268:239-242.
73. Cloninger CR, Guze SB: Female criminals: Their personal, familial and social background. *Arch Gen Psychiatry* 1970;23:554-558.
74. Cloninger CR, Guze SB: Psychiatric illness and female criminality: The role of sociopathy and hysteria in the antisocial woman. *Am J Psychiatry* 1970;127:303-310.
75. Rinieris PM, Stefanis CN, Lykouras EP, et al: Hysteria and ABO blood types. *Am J Psychiatry* 1978;135:1106-1107.
76. Woerner PI, Guze SB: A family and marital study of hysteria. *Br J Psychiatry* 1968;114:161-168.
77. Hall, RCW, Stickney SK, Gardner ER: Psychiatric symptoms in patients with systemic lupus erythematosus. *Psychosomatics* 1981;22:15-24.
78. Lewis RA: Mastocytosis, in Wyngaarden JB, Smith LH (eds): *Cecil Textbook of Medicine*, ed 16. Philadelphia, WB Saunders Co, 1982 pp 1819-1820.
79. Cohen ME, Robins E, Purtell JJ, et al: Excessive surgery in hysteria. *JAMA* 1953;151:977-986.
80. Liebowitz MR, Klein DF: Hysteroid dysphoria. *Psychiatr Clin North Am* 1979;2:555-575.
81. Liebowitz MR, Quitkin FM, Steward JW, et al: Phenelzine and imipramine in atypical depression. *Psychopharmacol Bull* 1981;17:159-161.
82. Sheehan DV, Ballenger J, Jacobson G: Treatment of endogenous anxiety with phobic hysterical and hypochondriacal symptoms. *Arch Gen Psychiatry* 1980;37:51-59.
83. Woodruff RA, Clayton PJ, Guze SB: Hysteria: An evaluation of specific diagnostic criteria by the study of randomly selected psychiatric clinic patients. *Br J Psychiatry* 1969;115:1243-1248.

6 Eating Problems: Anorexia and Binge Eating

Stephen M. Soreff

Eating represents a major statement of an individual's state. Through food behavior patients reveal their basic condition and well-being. Through eating problems they signal disturbances within and among themselves. This chapter confronts the two principle eating problems: anorexia and binge eating. Anorexia conveys the message of something being wrong. Binge eating dramatically notes stress and problems.

ANOREXIA A single or constellation of reactions to food resulting in a diminished appetite, no interest in meals, or an aversion to eating and generally culminating in weight loss.

Case report A 20-year-old woman chemistry graduate student begins to lose weight massively following the use of diet pills and a "too" successful diet. She complains of headaches and tension, but disclaims any emotional stresses. Meanwhile, she both pursues thinness and maintains a vigorous schedule. Moving toward the appearance of "just skin and bones" she denies concerns, dismisses inquiry, and declines help. This interviewer finds her perplexing, intellectual, and amazing.

Features

Mood Anorexia involves two sets of affecive experiences. The first deals with patients' particular reactions toward food and eating. The second depicts the individual's underlying and overriding mood.

Specific reactions to food   Food and eating provoke a wide variety of feelings. These suggest the central position of food not only in daily survival, but also as part of family interactions, community rituals, and individual reactions. Eating is full of symbols, eg, the Jewish kosher traditions and the historic Catholic prohibition of meat on Fridays. It produces a host of personal responses.

Some react with revulsion and disdain toward food. They loath its presence; they avoid it. Meals enrage them; dining destroys them. Others respond to food with indifference. Eating is simply something they have to do. Still others experience anxiety. Eating will lead to obesity and away from thinness.

Some feel guilt, shame, and are ashamed by eating. Because of prior associated pain or because of feared weight gain, meals become an ordeal.

In certain patients, food triggers violent reactions: nausea and vomiting. For some, eating proves painful. Ingestion and digestion initiate physical discomfort and displeasure.

Global affects leading to anorexia   Depression represents the greatest cause of anorexia. In the context of melancholia, despair, feelings of hopelessness and worthlessness, and dejection, the appetite shrinks. Depressed patients lose interest in eating as they withdraw from and lose interest in life.

Anxiety so pervades the patients' lives that eating becomes irrelevant. The anxious, worried, and tense patients find themselves too overwhelmed to eat. They have no appetite.

Apathy provides the other general emotion which eclipses appetite. Because of dementia or brain lesions, the apathetic patients do nothing with interest or enthusiasm. Indifference to life also means indifference to eating.

Thought   The thought contents both initiate the anorexia and reflect attitudes toward food.

A number of obsessions may plague the anorectic patients. They endlessly pursue thinness. They dread any weight gain and completely fear obesity. They think about food all the time—its forms, its preparation, its qualities, and its texture.

Food may become a delusional focus. Some patients feel special power or danger in eating. They know their food has been poisoned. As one patient said, "They are controlling my thoughts through a potion added to my suppers!"

For other patients, distortion of body and self image preclude eating.[1] Although appearing remarkably like a skeleton, certain anorectic patients complain about their "fatness." They perceive obesity in the face of cachexia. Patients with a significant medical illness may deny they are losing weight in the face of their clothes being "too big or too loose."

Misconceptions may be behind weight loss. A childhood notion, often unexpressed, involves the idea of oral conception.[2] Such a view, if carried into adolescence, equates eating to becoming pregnant.

Finally patients may develop phobias and specific aversions toward foods. Eating certain things will make them sick.

Behavior The anorectic patients demonstrate a wide range of behaviors. Some patients show clear evidence of eating avoidance. They refuse to eat; they miss meals; they decline to come to dinner; or they deny any need for food.

Some are secretive and hoard food, yet they do not eat. They will store, stockpile, and hide large quantities of groceries. One anorectic patient used to secrete all her desserts in her hospital night table. They guard and treasure their often bizarre collection of foods.

Their level of activity proves to be extremely indicative of their problem. The anorectic demonstrates super hyperactivity in the face of weight loss, eg, excessive running and excesses in exercising. Yet, for other patients with decreased appetite, there emerges diminished activities. Less food means less energy. Patients have sleep disturbances, nocturia, fatigue, and loss of sexual interest.

Some patients engage in deliberate activities to lose weight. They vomit after meals secretly, abuse laxatives, use enemas, and take diuretics.

On the other hand, other patients struggle to eat to reverse the anorexia. They attempt small frequent feedings and they try high protein diets. They want to but cannot gain weight. In an extreme, some patients exhibit binge eating. They consume large quantities of food rapidly. This is often followed by vomiting or depression or both.

Compulsive behavior dominates the clinical picture for some anorectic patients. They engage in endless rituals, eg, hand washing.

Some patients engage in a variety of activities which take priority over eating. The alcoholic patients may drink to the exclusion of regular meals. The total anxious patients may have no time to eat. The "manic" patients have no time to eat; they are "too busy" to sit down for a meal.

Finally, often strikingly bizarre actions may occur in anorectic patients. Some patients will gaze at themselves in mirrors. Others despite their dramatic cachectic condition will love to prepare gourmet food for others.

Physical examination and laboratory findings These observations and results reflect two phenomena: the effects of starvation and the changes caused by deliberate weight reduction.

Physical examination Severe weight reduction produces a variety of profound physical effects. The patients appear cachectic and cadaverous. Their clothes fit badly; faces appear drawn; bones protrude. They exhibit a bradycardia and hypotension. Their cool skin reflects their hypothermia. They develop lanugo hair—silky, fine, lightly pigmented hair, especially about the face and ears. They have dependent edema. Odontologically, the carbohydrate binge eaters have extensive cavities, and the vomiters have decalcification and erosions.[3] Women have amenorrhea.[4] Not infrequently, anorectic patients have bilateral parotid enlargement.[5]

Laboratory findings A vast array of laboratory studies echo the starvation and the attempts toward thinness.[6] Blood work shows leukopenia and relative lymphocytosis. Bone marrow demonstrates hypocellularity and large amounts of gelatinous acid mucopolysaccharide.[7] Sedimentation rates are low as is the plasma fibrinogen level. Hypercarotenemia has been regularly noted in patients with anorexia nervosa.[8] These included specific evaluations of serum B-carotene, vitamin A, esters; vitamin A, alcohol; and vitamin A, acid.

Cholesterol levels may vary. In starvation, serum cholesterol is decreased.[9] Yet, there appears to be a hypercholesterolemia in anorexia nervosa patients along with decreased bile acid excretion. Indeed, this increase results specifically from an elevation of the low-density lipoprotein cholesterol.[10]

Endocrine studies show a number of facets to weight reduction, starvation, and anorexia nervosa.[11] Patients have thyroxine (T_4) in the low normal range with tri-odothyronine (T_3) levels decreased. They have incomplete suppression of cortisol to the dexamethasone challenge. The glucose tolerance test demonstrated an abnormal, diabeticlike pattern. Anorexia nervosa patients had both higher growth hormone levels and lower 17-ketosteroid levels than normal. Additionally, these anorectic patients showed a luteinizing hormone pattern similar to prepubertal and pubertal girls. Anorexia nervosa women have an increase in their catechol estrogens and men have a decrease in their testosterone level.

Electrolytes and plasma pH determination may suggest the use of diuretics or persistence of vomiting. Patients may have hyponatremia and hypokalemia. They may also have alkalosis.

Electrocardiographic (ECG), electroencephalographic (EEG) and computed tomographic (CT) scans provide useful information. Patients starving frequently have, on their ECG, flattened or inverted T waves, ST segment depression, and the QT interval lengthened. The EEG may reflect electrolyte disturbances or show CNS pathology. Anorexia nervosa patients on CT scan demonstrate significantly enlarged cortical sulci and interhemispheric fissures. [12]

Interviewer's Reaction

When one encounters a cachectic patient, one is seized by a series of reactions. First, there is the medical need and commitment to find the cause, to halt the weight loss, and to restore the patient to fullness. Second, one has a moment of appreciation—how did the patient lose weight when I cannot! Third, with the anorexia nervosa patient, there are particular responses: wonderment, amazement, disbelief, frustration, distance, and puzzlement.

PATHOGENESIS

Psychodynamics

Loss causes depression; depression leads to anorexia. This simple, ageless human equation accounts for many significant weight reductions. Death, disfigurement, devastation, disaster, divorce, and disease trigger sadness, despair, and desolation. [13] Meals cease to be meaningful, enjoyable, or even bearable. Appetite diminution emerges as one of the first casualties of a loss. A 65-year-old man's wife suddenly, unexpectedly died. He became anorectic, withdrawn, dejected, and sullen. He lost 35 lbs in a month.

Separation, an attenuated form of loss, similarly produces anorexia. A wife left by a husband on a long Navy patrol loses her appetite. A young man, an only child, goes to college leaving his widowed mother alone; both experience pain, loneliness, and decreased interest in eating. Not only does the separation mark a disruption of a significant relationship but also it creates a different, often empty unfulfilling mealtime environment.

The *pursuit of thinness* designates one of the most compelling drives and forces for many young women and some men. It is not the loss of appetite or the diminished interest in food which propels them; it is their relentless determination to be thin. To that end, they jog, exercise, vomit, diet, and work. They want perfect bodies. A young struggling and hopeful ballerina focuses on achieving the optimum figure. Thinness means power, position, and the part.

Control in many forms constitutes a significant personal anorectic dynamic. Some patients have a strong desire to regulate and command all facets of their lives. Diet, as one of these areas becomes a focal point, with all food measured, all meals categorized, and all calories counted. Control of food intake defends against feelings of insecurity, helplessness, and worthlessness. A rigid diet, the pursuit of thinness, and a denial of food provides an identity.

A shy, quiet young boy felt overwhelmed by his father's verbal assaults, helpless to his parents' pending separation, powerless in school, and loneliness in his neighborhood. He rigidly started to control his food intake. As he began to lose weight, he suddenly became the focus of his parents and teachers. Anorexia not only defended against the hopelessness of his plight, but also afforded him a tool to gain power and keep his parents together.

Personal preference, ethnic orientation, and ideologic considerations contribute to diet restrictions and, in certain situations and with particular individuals, may cause anorexia. In the former circumstances, many people choose specific food patterns in accordance with their beliefs: keeping kosher, following a vegetarianism program, or only eating organically grown foods. In the latter, patients adopt extreme eating rituals and codes which ultimately produce weight loss. A 23-year-old schizophrenic college student claimed vitamin E to be the answer for not only himself but also the world. He devoured vast quantities of the vitamin and throughout the campus proclaimed its importance. He required involuntary hospitalization as his weight dramatically dropped and his behavior became increasingly bizzare.

Rejection and avoidance of sexuality represents one of the major psychodynamics underlying anorexia for many patients, especially those in their adolescence. Through a control of diet, denial of food, weight reduction, and hyperactivity, they diminish their sexuality and the emergence of their secondary sexual characteristics. Indeed, one of the cardinal features of anorexia nervosa in women is amenorrhea and in men, impotence.[1] Anorexia provides a way of staying forever young, avoiding the conflicts, struggles, and turmoil associated with sexuality. These powerful dynamics often remain unconscious and violently denied. A 35-year-old anorectic, amenorrheic woman busied herself reading, caring for her sick, widowed mother as the devoted only child, and attending cooking classes. Through psychotherapy, she became aware of her sexuality. She commenced eating and gaining weight. Her breasts enlarged; her periods started. She placed her mother with an aunt, and she started dating.

Defiance through anorexia represents another important dynamic. Children may refuse to eat in rebellion against parental edicts. Hunger protests have been dramatic and occasionally highly effective. In the film *Exodus*, an immigrant ship challenged the British Empire through a hunger strike. Gandhi twice achieved monumental control of riots in India through fasting.

Biologic Explanation

Anorectic mechanisms A number of basic mechanisms account for anorexia.[14] The foundation of all these systems revolves about the hypothalamus. Other components include neurochemicals, glucose, proteins, and the gastrointestinal (GI) tract.

Two interrelated and ineracting centers of the hypothalamus control eating.[15] The ventrolateral nucleus (VLN) is the "feeding center." Lesions there produce aphagia; on the other hand, stimulation there causes consumption. In contrast, the ventromedial nucleus (VMN), the "satiety center," when damaged, leads to hyperphagia. The VLN has predominant control. Anorexia results from VLN lesions.

Several neurotransmitters are involved in anorexia.[16] Amphetamines trigger release of norepinephrine; which in turn produces anorexia through β-adrenergic stimulation of the hypothalamus. Serotonin and tryptophan levels have been observed to be low in patients with anorexia nervosa.[17]

Glucose levels and insulin effects are responsible for loss of appetite and weight reductions. A glucose infusion stimulates the VMN leading to the cessation of eating. In contrast, insulin decreases VMN activity and increases consumption. The opposite occurs in luteinizing hormone (LH) activity: with a glucose infusion LH activity diminishes and appetite decreases; with insulin, LH activity increases and appetite is enhanced.

Three other mechanisms may be involved. The first is related to dietary proteins where, specifically, a high protein consumption diminishes appetite. The second pertains to the GI tract activity. Decreased stomach contractions correlate satiety intake as does gastric distention. Third, two hormones, both peptides—bombesin, mostly found in the stomach, and cholecystokinin, in the intestine—are responsible for reducing food intake.[18]

Starvation process Starvation produces profound body changes, both physiologically and mentally. Starvation generates a number of physiologic changes.[19] First, in order to maintain serum glucose levels to ensure CNS integrity, the plasma insulin falls permitting fatty acids and amino acids utilization from adipose and muscle tissue. Instead of protein synthesis, amino acids are diverted to oxidative metabolism and gluconeogenesis. Second, metabolism decreases and serum T_3 decreases. Third, in this negative balance state, mass is lost, muscles diminish, eg, midarm circumference is decreased, and weight is reduced. The laboratory study best reflecting the starvation effect remains the decreased 24-hour urinary creatinine/height ratio. Fourth, mineral depletion occurs. Fifth, cardiac output declines with a subsequent fall in blood pressure. Additionally, renal blood flow decreases. The heart and kidneys become reduced. Sixth, a normocytic, normochromic anemia develops. Seventh, in terms of immunology, cell-mediated immunity becomes impaired, wounds heal slower, and there are fewer polymorphonuclear cells. Eighth, hypothermia emerges.

A variety of laboratory and physical findings demonstrate these physiologic changes. As cited, the 24-hour urinary creatinine/height ratio is diminished. Decreases occur in serum albumin, serum transferrin, and the hematocrit. Reductions are noted in serum amino acids, urinary urea, and urinary creatinines. Function diminishes in T lymphocytes; glucose tolerance is abnormal as in diabetes; T_3 is lower. Chest films reveal a smaller heart size. Physical manifestation includes bradycardia, hypotension, hypothermia, dependent edema, and lanugo hair.

Starvation also creates a wide range of mental alterations.[2] Initially, patients become preoccupied with thoughts of food, eating, meals, and dining. They crave it and have food illusions.

They dream about food. They display irritability, belligerence and argumentativeness. Often, they may turn to less than honest methods to handle food procurement and its distribution. As starvation progresses, they show lethargy, pathos, withdrawal, inertia, fatigue, and listlessness.

Genetics

Genetic factors relate to anorexia nervosa in two ways: In familial incidences of eating disorders and in family patterns.

Patients with anorexia nervosa have a number of familial correlations with eating disorders. Crisp et al noted that anorexia nervosa patients have many relatives with weight disorders.[20] In that study of 102 anorexia nervosa patients, obesity occurred within the nuclear family in ten cases and definite low weight was found in 29 cases. These 29 cases involved 14 of the mothers, nine of the fathers, six of the sisters, and one of the brothers. Nowlin found in a literature review a concordance for anorexia nervosa of 11 out of 24 (46%) monozygotic women twins.[21]

Certain psychiatric disorders occur at high rates within families of anorexia nervosa patients. Alcohol abuse appears to have a heightened prevalence within those families.[22] Winokur et al found that of the relatives of anorexia nervosa patients, 22% had an incidence of primary affective disorders.[23] The affective disorder included and encompassed 34 relatives with unipolar and nine with bipolar disorder. Although disputed, such work suggests an affective conribution to the etiology of anorexia nervosa.[24]

The major *affective disorders* both account for severe anorexia in certain instances and have strong inheritance patterns; major depression, unipolar depression, and manic-depression depressed phase—all can result in extreme loss of interest in food, not eating, avoidance of meals, and significant weight loss. Patients during a "high," manic phase, often have no time for eating, burn up many calories, and also may lose weight. Genetic vulnerability plays a major role in the transmission of these disorders. A gene located near the gene for color blindness on the x chromosome may be responsible for the bipolar disorders.[25] Chapter 2 details these relationships.

Environment

Concentration camps, prisoner-of-war camps, and labor camps meant anorexia, weight loss, and death.[26,27] These places of incomprehensible brutality not only provide some of the worst moments in human history, but also wretchedly prove the overwhelming destructive crushing affect of the environment. Prisoners lost weight, gave up, and died. The death camps stand as one of pivotal, signed, and traumatic events of the twentieth century.[28]

Conflicts lead to anorexia.[29] An atmosphere heavily laced with altercations, violence, pestilence, anger, and fighting often decreases appetite. When the table becomes the battlefield, family members may avoid meals, eat quickly and run, or sit without consuming. Marital discord may deprive combatants and their children of any relaxed dining opportunities. Parents may chose mealtimes as the time to "control," teach, and train. One little girl refuses all food as her parents attempt to get her to eat her peas! Anorexia is her weapon as many other children and adolescents have used it to fight their parents.[30]

Deprivation triggers anorexia. Anorexia nervosa most commonly occurs in upper-class homes and within the context of "good" families.[2] Yet, a careful dissection of the family's interaction reveals a subtle form of deprivation. It lacks intimacy. According to Bruch, these parents trumpet their children's accomplishments as their own rather than those of the kids.[31] Mother and infant fail to establish basic attachment and trust. An 18-year-old girl vomits, loses weight, and fears "she has anorexia nervosa." Her mother, although pleasant and "concerned," only talks about herself, her achievements, and goals. In actuality she has no communication, connection, or understanding of her daughter.

Rebellion accounts for anorexia. In the political arena, prisoners have often resorted to hunger strikes to protest conditions, to gain popular support, and to challenge governments. In the family, children and adolescents may use not eating to challenge their parents. One common thread in anorexia nervosa is where a girl pursues thinness to fight against her domineering mother and her passive father.[32]

A *demand for thinness* characterizes not only a general Western societal expectation but also a specific requirement in certain settings. Members of gymnastics groups, ballet companies, and other athletic teams must adhere to particular weights. These groups place huge pressures upon their participants to be thin and thusly foster anorexia.

Differential Diagnosis

Nonpsychotropic drugs Digitalis toxicity accounts for anorexia in two ways. First, these cardiac glycosides affect the smooth muscles of the GI tract with nausea, vomiting, and diarrhea as the result.[33] Second, digitalis stimulates the chemoreceptor trigger zone.[34]

Xanthines, CNS stimulants, have marked anorectic properties and potential. Of particular interest are theophylline and caffeine, both methylated xanthines, with a dioxypurine as the basic xanthine structure.

Theophylline, an important bronchodilator, causes anorexia. Oral administration often leads to gastric irritation. Gastrointestinal distress symptoms, nausea, and vomiting are related to its plasma levels.[35] Pulmonary functions improve in the 5-20 mg/L range; the 15-20 mg/L level produces nausea, vomiting, abdominal distress, and anorexia.[36]

Caffeine has long been recognized for its appetite appeasement qualities. Caffeine is found in coffee, tea, cola beverages, aspirin compounds, "cold" medications, and as part of analgesic preparations. In excessive amounts, often above 1000 mg/day (a cup of brewed coffee contains 100-150 mg caffeine), it produces violent gastric distress, epigastric nausea, vomiting, and heartburn. The heartburn results from gastroesophageal reflux.[37] Caffeinism also produces insomnia, rapid speech, anxiety, restlessness, jumpy legs, and palpitations.[38]

An interplay of caffeinism and anorexia nervosa has been reported by Sours.[39] Not infrequently, these patients consume a remarkably large amount of caffeine-containing beverages. For example, one 16-year-old girl anorectic daily has between four to six quarts of diet cola after running 6 miles.

Sympathomimetic drugs have been particularly noted for their anorectic qualities. Amphetamines, methamphetamine, phenmetrazine hydrochloride and methylphenidate hydrochloride depress appetite and the effect historically led to their use and abuse as dieting agents. Amphetamines like ephedrine act in the CNS to release stored catecholamines—especially norepinephrine.[40]

Antibiotics not uncommonly are responsible for anorexia in a number of ways. First, their oral administration produces GI distress. For example, oral penicillin causes nausea without vomiting and diarrhea.[41] Second, superinfection resulting from the treatment of a primary infection leads to medical debilitation and appetite loss. Oral gentamicin sulfate can produce an overgrowth of *Candida*.[42] Third, inflammations about the mouth follow in the wake of some antibiotics. The combination of trimethoprim and sulfamethoxazole commonly results in glossitis and stomatitis.[43] Fourth, major untoward reactions, eg, drug fever, hepatitis, and aplastic anemia destroy appetite, interest in food, and desire to eat.

Cancer chemotherapy produces anorexia through a variety of mechanisms. Cancer chemotherapy affects the GI tract. The alkylating agents, for example, nitrogen mustard, interfere and interrupt mitosis. The greatest disruptions occur in the most rapidly growing tissues, eg, the GI tract. The clinical result is nausea and vomiting. The antimetabolites, eg, pyrimidine and purine analogs, cause anorexia, weight loss, and diarrhea through cytotoxic actions at the GI cellular level. Cytoplasmic vacuolization occurs within the intestinal epithelium mucosal cells.[44]

The cancer drugs have emetic effects. Nausea follows within thirty to sixty minutes after administration of mechlorethamine.[45] Pretreatment with a phenothiazine decreases this phenomenon. The "smell" of the clinic and a resultant sense of nausea often accompany cancer chemotherapy. Patients develop a pseudohallucination of the odors of the clinic and the taste of the medication following receiving their drugs. They know the experiences are not real, yet they still find them quite compelling. For some it produces nausea, appetite loss, and anorexia. Nesse et al suggest the pairing of the clinic odors and the drug administration causes a conditioned perception reflex and produces this phenomenon.[46]

The circumstances of cancer chemotherapy may precipitate anorexia. The confrontation with the disease and death, the alopecia produced by some drugs, and the GI distress induced by some medications all cause depression and may lead to loss of appetite. Additionally, Silberfarb et al suggest cognitive impairment can be engendered by cancer drugs.[47]

Drugs producing depression, eg, antihypertensive medications, are reviewed in chapter 2.

Psychotropic drugs *Lithium toxicity* accounts for eating disturbances as well as other distressing symptoms. The usual therapeutic blood level range for lithium carbonate remains between 0.5 and 1.5 mEq/L. Above this level and certainly in the clearly toxic level of above 2.0 mEq/L patients experience nausea, vomiting, diarrhea, and anorexia.[48] Additionally, patients may develop fatigue, dysarthria, muscle twitching, a course tremor, trouble concentrating, and ataxia. Toxic levels result from excessive consumption of lithium, as well as concomitantly occurring dehydration, or the use of diuretics.

Abrupt neuroleptic discontinuance precipitates episodes of nausea and vomiting.[49] These GI disturbances erupt usually during the first week after withdrawal. Other symptoms also occurring in that period include restlessness, increased motor activity, stomach pains, headaches, dizziness, numbness, rhinorrhea, and nightmares. Although not dose-related, these withdrawal events are much more commonly experienced on the discontinuance of drugs with marked autonomic properties (usually the aliphatic neuropletics). The phenomena may represent an anticholinergic rebound effect.

Minor tranquilizer withdrawal also is marked by anorexia. Patients display little interest in eating during this period. Additionally, throughout this withdrawal phase which may last up to 5 weeks for diazepam addicts, patients exhibit agitation, insomnia, diaphoresis, anxiety, and myoclonus.[50]

Alcohol

Alcohol abuse leads to anorexia, eating disturbances, and weight loss through a variety of mechanisms. Some revolve about the toxic effects of the substance on vital organs. Others emerge as a result of lifestyle. Still others reflect vitamin deficiencies.

Gastritis, hepatitis, and pancreatitis often follow in the wake of alcohol abuse.[51] Patients develop abdominal pain, bloody emesis, and lethargy. Alcohol directly damages the GI mucosa and produces malabsorption. Further, this destructive process impedes transport of fats, proteins, vitamins, and minerals. Because of disease to the liver and pancreas, malutilization of nutrients occurs and impaired nucleic acid synthesis takes place.

Alcohol may interfere with daily life and eclipse dining patterns. Patients focus their lives on the "next drink," with eating as the casualty.

Chronic alcohol abuse with its incumbent physical, psychological, and social deterioration leads to poor nutritional state. Patients enter into Jellinek's "chronic phase."[52] They will consume anything with alcohol in it including mouthwash and hair tonic. Hepatitis leads to cirrhosis; pancreatitis becomes a chronic condition. Vitamin deficiencies especially of thiamine (vitamin B_1) produce Wernicke's syndrome, polioencephalitis, haemorrhagica superior, marked pathologically by hemorrhages to the superior aspects of the brain, and clinically by memory defects, delirium, and nystagmus and Korsakoff's psychosis.[53] The latter, although it commences as Wernicke's, has a greater and more pronounced memory defect and confabulation.

Alcohol withdrawal also leads to anorexia, often in dramatic ways. In the ensuing agitation, violence, terrifying hallucinations, and disorientation in delirium tremens, patients not only do not eat but also use up a tremendous amount of energy.[54] This may also occur in an attenuated form during alcoholic hallucinosis.

Other Abused Substances

Amphetamine abuse not only clearly produces anorexia but also its very appetite suppression qualities lead to its initial use. One used to hear with alarming regularity how a patient began to lose weight on amphetamines. Chronic amphetamine abuse causes malnutrition. Amphetamines' CNS effects involve the neuronal release of norepinephrine which works in the lateral hypothalamic feeding center to suppress appetite.[55] The patient's major weight loss results from the hypothalamus action rather than their increased activity.

Barbiturate withdrawal accounts for appetite disturbances. The mechanism is similar to alcohol withdrawal. Patients withdrawing experience nausea and vomiting as well as anxiety, insomnia, irritability, tremulousness, and postural hypotension.[56] Severe cases develop seizures, psychosis, and hyperpyrexia.

Cocaine also, like amphetamines, accounts for anorexia. Users experience euphoria, alertness, energy, vitality, freedom from fatigue and diminished appetite. A 26-year-old man came into the emergency department "high" after 24 hours of continually snorting "coke." He talked nonstop, could not sleep, felt "too wonderful," and was scared, yet apprehensive. He not only had no time to eat but also had no desire to. Cocaine works by potentiating the actions of catecholamines yet its mechanism of CNS effects may not be identical to that of amphetamine.[53]

Opiates create major disruptions of appetite and eating. They interfere in all three phases: intoxication, chronic use, and withdrawal. Opiates act at the same sites that the endorphins (endogenous morphine) bind to: in the brain, the nuclei raphes, the locus ceruleus, the periaqueductal gray area, and in the spinal cord, the dorsal horns. All of these sites are involved with the transmission of pain. Opiates reduce the messages and raise the pain threshold.

On the neuronal level, opiates have a number of effects.[57] They interfere with the influx of calcium into the cells, lowering the intracellular calcium and impeding neurotransmitters' release. They also inhibit adenylate cyclase activity. During withdrawal, calcium influx increases and neurotransmitters are released.

Opiate intoxication produces anorexia in two ways. First, it causes nausea and vomiting by stimulating the chemoreceptor trigger zone in the brainstem. Second, it creates a sense of euphoria, a feeling of well-being, and a moment of "all is well." Anxiety disappears; fears evaporate; worries melt; food ceases to be significant.

Chronic use leads to anorexia also in two ways: constipation develops; opiates decrease gastric hydrocholoric acid secretion, diminish large intestine peristalsis, and heighten muscle tone. Consequently, fecal passage slows and the waste absorbs more water. Additionally, chronic abuse leads to a lifestyle precluding interest in eating: periods of euphoria merged with episodes of craving and searching for the next fix.

Opiate withdrawal is marked by dramatic eating disruptions.[58] Patients develop nausea and vomiting. They also display rhinorrhea, diaphoresis, gooseflesh, insomnia, lacrimation, yawning, involuntary muscle movements, chills, weakness. These symptoms usually emerge eight to ten hours after the last fix and can persist for up to ten days.

Medical Illnesses

General In general, anorexia may result from any acute medical illness or from any chronic disease. Being acutely ill abolishes appetite in many ways: distress, discomfort, apprehension, pain, inflammation, fever, fatigue, malaise, anxiety, depression, regression, withdrawal, lethargy, and excessive sleep. Chronic disease for many patients produces anorexia and loss of weight. Although some of the mechanisms may be similar to those involved with acute illness, others prove more reflective of this protracted situation. More specific dynamics of chronic disease include interminal pain, a major curtailment in vocation and recreation, loss of motility, continued reliance upon medications, resignation, financial reverses, and extra expenses. Chronic illness means losses and chronic depression.

A number of *cardiac* conditions account for anorexia. Heart failure, in addition to the more prominent and characteristic features of dyspnea, orthopnea, paroxysmal nocturnal dyspnea, wheezing, pulmonary edema, insomnia, and fatigue, is accompanied by nausea, vomiting, diarrhea, loss of appetite, and constipation secondary to venous distention. In severe and prolonged cases of congestive heart failure, patients develop cardiac cachexia.[59] These patients exhibit significant malnutrition and illness associated with hypoxia.

Myocardial infarctions produce loss of appetite and weight. During the acute phase, the pain, the distress, the apprehension, and the discomfort often preclude eating. The initial anxiety interferes with appetite. Commonly, patients in fear of recurrence of a heart attack finally and successfully commence the diet which may have been recommended for years by their physician.

Dental difficulties and diseases not unexpectedly produce anorexia. When it hurts to eat, people do not eat, eg, pain, sores, or inflammation to the mouth. One frequently overlooked cause of anorexia remains ill-fitting dentures. Also lost, misplaced, or forgotten dental appliances lead to the same result.

Certain *endocrine* diseases manifest themselves through appetite disruptions. In thyroid disorders, an interesting weight-related phenomenon develops.[60] Patients with hypothyroidism experience constipation and a decline in appetite, yet gain weight. In contrast, those with hyperthyroidism exhibit weight loss in the face of a heightened appetite. They also have nausea, vomiting, anorexia, and hyperdefecation. Addison's disease, primary adrenocortical deficiency, has as its hallmark, weight loss. Patients reveal profound asthenia, striking hyperpigmentation, hypotension, and often devastating GI disturbances. They have nausea, vomiting, diarrhea, and occasionally severe, yet ill-defined, abdominal pain. They have pronounced anorexia and significant weight loss. Low to absent 24-hour urine 17-hydroxycorticoids, and 17-ketosteroids and lower to zero serum cortisol values indicate this diagnosis.[61] Juvenile diabetes presents with polydipsia, polyuria, and an increased appetite, yet a weight loss—all within a matter of days.[62]

Gastrointestinal disturbances, not unexpectedly, are often implicated. Gastric outlet obstruction caused by peptic ulcer commonly causes weight loss. Gastric ulcers lead to reduction in weight in 40% of patients. The mechanism is either anorexia, or a strong distaste for eating, secondary to eating-induced discomfort.[63] Certainly, any of the malabsorption syndromes trigger weight loss, diarrhea, and malnutrition. Small bowel disease accounts for anorexia. Crohn's disease (regional enteritis) presents with weight loss, right lower quadrant pain, and diarrhea. Other symptoms may include low fevers, nausea, vomiting, and loss of food interest. Bloody diarrhea, abdominal pain, weight loss, and fever stand as the cardinal features of chronic ulcerative colitis.[64] Hepatic diseases impede, diminish, and eliminate appetite.

Hematologic disorders account for anorexia. Anemia in general leads to fatigue, dyspnea, dizziness, sleeping difficulty, and GI symptoms. These include indigestion, anorexia, nausea, and blood irregularities. The mechanism for these involve blood shunted from the splanchnic bed.[65] Pernicious anemia, vitamin B_{12} deficiency presents through the classic triad of sore tongue, weakness, and neurologic symptoms in the extremities, eg, tingling and numbness.[59] Patients may also exhibit anorexia, diarrhea, a burning feeling in their tongue, abdominal discomfort, constipation, and reduction in weight.

Infections frequently are responsible for anorexia. In the acute phase, they generate fever, malaise, exhaustion, and generalized discomfort. Chronic infections prove remarkably debilitating. They leave in their wake, fatigue, depression, dejection, destruction, and decrease in both appetite and weight. Infections, such as tuberculosis and osteomyelitis cause anorexia. A 40-year-old woman developed chronic osteomyelitis of her right leg following an automobile accident. She lost interest in food, in life, as the infection and hospitalization became prolonged.

Metabolic disorders produce anorexia. Uremia accounts for it, as does mercury poisoning. Mercury causes nerve degeneration in the cortex and basal ganglia.[66] Gaucher's disease, an inherited metabolic disorder caused by a deficiency of glucocerebrosidase, a lysosomal enzyme, and frequently encountered in Jews, may present through severe weight loss. Indeed, its initial manifestations may appear as anorexia nervosa.[67] Uremia commonly produces lethargy, diminished appetite, and fatigue. Metabolic acidosis regardless of etiology, be it renal failure, diabetes, alcoholism, salicylates, or diarrhea, produces both anorexia and fatigue.

Neurologic disorders can either present with or are accompanied by anorexia. In one of the more dramatic manifestations, patients with destruction of the pituitary's anterior lobe secondary to trauma, infection, infarction, or hemorrhage (Simmonds' disease) develop "pituitary cachexia."[66] This syndrome caused by pituitary hypofunction includes extreme asthenia, fat wasting, decreased body temperature, and hypotension. It commonly afflicts women in midlife especially after childbirth and, not uncommonly, has been misdiagnosed as anorexia nervosa. Cerebral vascular events may either prohibit eating or cause patients great difficulty in eating. Any interruption or lesion of the cranial nerves involved with mastication cause eating complications, anorexia, and potentially weight loss. Any chronic debilitating neurologic condition carries with it the possibility of depression and decreased appetite.

CNS tumors can produce an anorectic picture. Both hypothalamic and third ventricle tumors have been implicated in causing the typical anorexia nervosa picture.[68] An infiltrating tumor of the hypothalamus precipitated the clinical manifestations of anorexia nervosa.[69]

Cancer produces cachexia through a variety of mechanisms. A number of observations help to explain and account for the tumor-induced weight loss. First, investigators report abnormal carbohydrate metabolism in cancer patients.[70] These patients have diabetic-like glucose tolerance test results (mainly a heightened glucose level as a diabetic patient would have following glucose challenge), increased glucose turnover, and increased lactate oxidation. Schein et al argue the glucose alterations reflect a significant degree of insulin resistances.[71] Second, Schein et al also suggest the wasting of body fat is caused by the mobilizations of these stores.[71]

Third, other investigators using animal models strongly advance the theory that weight loss results from anorexia. [72] Costa et al have documented this relationship for male cancer patients but not for women.[73] In essence, they found that male cancer patients ate less and lost weight, yet the female patients did not decrease their food consumption.

Fourth, patients may develop certain food aversions during the tumor's growth.[74] Patients then continue this learned response later and sustain a markedly diminished appetite. The tumor's physiology itself may be responsible for the originally generated aversion.

The tumor itself leaves in its wake significant weight loss. Esophageal cancer may present through malnutrition. Pancreatic cancer produces massive decreases in weight in addition to vomiting, nausea, diarrhea, and difficulty eating. Metastatic cancer causes fatigue, debilitation, and diminished appetite.

The various neoplastic therapies yield anorexia as a result. The chemotherapy, as discussed earlier, induces nausea, vomiting, diarrhea, and avoidance of food. Radiation therapy produces GI disturbances. Surgery, as discussed below, clearly may interfere with eating.

In the final analysis, it may be the entire cancer gestalt which causes anorexia. For many patients, cancer has the connotation of "terminal" and death. For many the tumor means pain, embarrassment, shame, and isolation. Not uncommonly, the family shares these views. As a result, they lose their appetite within the context of giving up.

Pregnancy maintains a significant link to appetite disruptions and disturbances. About half of pregnant women in Western societies develop and manifest nausea and vomiting during the first trimester.[75] In extreme cases, the vomiting becomes profound, pronounced, and protracted and results in the serious condition of hyperemesis gravidarum. About 10% of the fathers will also experience GI distresses similar to their pregnant companions including nausea, vomiting, morning sickness, and eating idiosyncracies and peculiarities.[76] These fathers' responses and reactions have been termed the Couvade syndrome.

Respiratory disorders are frequently accompanied by anorexia. In acute situations, such as an asthmatic attack, the distress, the apprehension, the terror, the dyspnea preclude eating. In chronic conditions, bronchitis, emphysema, and airway obstruction, patients exhibit clear evidence of weight loss. For many of these patients, as their lives become centered on breathing and avoiding dyspnea, activities of daily living and appetite shrink.

Immunologic diseases also present with anorectic features. Systemic lupus erythematosus stands as an example of this. Patients develop GI distress, and loss of appetite leading to loss of weight, in addition to the malaise and debility.[77] The chronicity and multisystem involvement of the disease may help to explain the anorexia diarrhea, and avoidance of food. Radiation therapy produces GI disturbances. Surgery, as discussed below, clearly may interfere with eating.

Surgical Complications

The *preoperative reactions* often include anorexia. The anticipation of surgery, the necessity of an anesthetic, and the dread of the actual operation may produce a decided lack of interest in food for many patients. Some preoperative patients will talk about their "last meal"; others will diet prior to surgery, finally following their physician's frequently offered advice.

In the *general postoperative* picture, anorexia frequently occurs for a variety of reasons. Pain precludes any interest in food. Medications, especially opiates, diminish appetite.[78] Opiates activate the chemoreceptor trigger zone producing nausea and vomiting, cause sedation, and result in constipation. Any postoperative infection of fever would certainly account for this as immobilization would for some patients. Abrupt withdrawal from alcohol, barbiturates, or minor tranquilizers would also reduce anorexia.

Surgery designed to create weight reduction commonly leads to appetite disturbances and GI problems. The jejunoileal bypass procedure for morbid obesity has a number of important side effects including frequent bowel movements and liver failure.[79] Additionally, calorie intake diminishes; patients develop a decreased preference for sweets; and malabsorption of fats, nitrogens, calcium, potassium, carbohydrates, and vitamins occurs.[80] In some cases, malnutrition with hypoproteinemia, electrolyte disturbances, and hair loss develops.

The *malabsorption syndrome,* marked by diarrhea, weight loss, steatorrhea, pain in bones, anemia, dermatitis, and neuropathies results as a complication in a variety of abdominal procedures.[81] Fat malabsorption follows esophagectomy and esophagosgastrectomy. Both total and partial gastrectomies account for deficiencies in protein and calorie absorption. Weight loss remains a common experience in patients having had Billroth I or Billroth II anastomosis. Vagatomy frequently produces diarrhea. Small bowel resection leads to malabsorption with a distal resection increasing transient time and a resection of terminal precipating vitamin B_{12} deficiency. The procedure accounts for heightened gastric secretions and sugar intolerance. The blind loop syndrome with weight loss, abdominal pain, vitamin deficiencies, anemia, diarrhea, and steatorrhea occurs when the small bowel becomes trapped. This event sets the stage for intestinal stasis and its consequent infections.

Surgery precipitating depression may also lead to a melancholic constellation including anorexia. Not uncommonly, patients who have undergone severe, disfiguring, and devastating procedures suffer loss of interest in food and eating, eg, amputations, mastectomies, and colostomies.

Physical Trauma

The *general* gestalt of trauma dramatically, strikingly, and compellingly produces anorexia. As patients recoil in emotional numbness and "shock," struggle with immense pain, confront their mutilations, and attempt to orient themselves to an alien intense environment, they do not eat. They do not want to think about food. In the context of their responses of anxiety, depression, guilt, rage, withdrawal, and projection, food often ceases to be of importance.

Metabolic changes induced by trauma lead to weight loss.[82] Following severe injuries, patients enter into a period of nitrogen loss. These patients' initial weight reduction involves 10% to 14% of a protein loss and 18% to 25% of fat loss. Energy requirements for patients with multiple fractures increases from 10% to 25% above normal. Protein metabolism accounts for the nitrogen loss and its metabolism provides carbons for gluconeogenesis Patients have a hyperglycemia both from amino acid breakdown and from catecholamine suppression insulin secretion.

Burns produce a hypermetabolic state which culminates in both weight loss and body mass erosion. Patients sustaining a burn to 40% or more of their body surface develop a metabolic rate of two to two and a half times the normal rate.[83] Consequently, they show evidence of increased metabolism with elevated cardiac output, and general heightened oxygen consumption in addition to a reduction in body weight. Attention to the burn patients' huge nutritional requirement represents a key factor in their survival.[84]

A sequela of *head trauma* may be loss of appetite. In the initial phases, coma, stupor, lethargy, and delirium preclude eating. Resulting organic defects and dementia further interfere with eating organization and efforts. For some patients, frontal lobe trauma blunts and dulls affect, causes disinterest, and leaves them apathetic. Finally, for other patients, depression as a consequence of head injury often yields to an anorectic condition.[85]

Psychiatric Differential Diagnosis

Anorexia nervosa stands as one of the most important psychiatric causes of anorexia with specific diagnosis criteria, particular clinical features, certain laboratory findings, linkages to a variety of other mental and physical illnesses, and a studied course. It has been demonstrated and documented to be increasing in incidence in recent decades.[86] Also emerging has been a unified concept of this diagnosis as representing an underlying deficit of identity and self, resulting from major disturbances in the parent-child relationship.[31] The incidence of this disorder has doubled in the last two decades.[87] Families are overinterested and overdirecting in their interactions with the would-be anorectic child. This focuses that child toward the concerns of others and disrupts inner security.[88]

The American Psychiatric Association has established specific criteria for the diagnosis of anorexia nervosa.[89] First, patients demonstrate an extreme, protracted, severe dread of being fat. Indeed, in spite of weight reduction, they maintain this fear. Second, they exhibit basic distortions in their body images. Commonly, in the face of incredible thinness, they view themselves as "too fat." Third, they have a weight decrease of at least 25% of their body weight. Finally, no physical disease accounts for such a weight reduction.

Yet, those criteria fail to capture the intriguing, fascinating, and amazing features of this illness. Affecting predominantly (90%) women, in their adolescence and young adulthood, these patients relentlessly pursue "thinness." Their total devotion to being perfectly thin and their disdain for obesity eclipses their lives. They manifest no apparent depression in spite of their condition, they run, they vomit, they abuse laxatives, they hide food, they cook, yet they do not eat; they avoid meals. One is always struck by the sight of a 22-year-old coed, "thin as a rail," doggedly jogging down the track and protesting her fatness. Their dissatisfaction with their body image, their extreme hyperactivity, and their seeming indifference in the face of starving to death—all characterize their disease.

Their pursuit of thinness becomes their method to control their internal and external environment and their way to defend themselves against sexuality.

In addition to the laboratory findings associated with starvation, a number of specific results occur in anorexia nervosa patients. They exhibit hypercarotenemia.[8] They have an elevation of low-density lipo-protein cholesterol.[10] They appear to have increased cerobrospinal fluid opioid activity during their weight reduction periods compared with similar activity once their weight has been restored and with normal controls.[90] These observations were based on measurements of CSF endogenous opiate peptides (endorphins). Gerner and Gwirtsman have shown that the majority of anorexia nervosa patients have had abnormal dexamethasone suppression tests.[91]

Their serum cortisol levels remain generally elevated because of both an increase in adrenocortical activity and a decrease in its metabolism.[92]

Gonadotropin secretions are altered in anorexia nervosa. In women, the amenorrhea reflects a return to a prepubertal pattern.[93] There appears to be a hypothalamic or suprahypothalamic etiology for this.[94] In anorectic men, similarly, there occurs a diminished gonadotropin release and a lower testosterone level.[95]

Of great interest, patients with anorexia nervosa despite their starvation continue to maintain their cell-mediated immune system.[96] In contrast, other malnourished patients do not. These anorexia nervosa patients have a normal T lymphocyte population with unimpaired responses to a phytohemagglutinin and concanavalin A challenge, although Kay and Stricker discuss granulocyte bactericidal defects, chemotactic defects, and hypocomplementemia as well as anemia, leukopenia, and mild thrombocytopenia.[7] Anorectics also demonstrate slower and delayed gastric emptying.[97] Their thyroxine (T_4) levels are consistently on the low normal side and their tri-iodothyronine (T_3) levels are generally lower than normal.[98]

Margo and Hawton have recently noted abnormalities in arginine vasopressin in anorexia nervosa patients.[99] The antidiuretic hormone arginine vasopressin's plasma level in normal patients increases in direct response to intravenous (IV) hypertonic saline. However, they noted that anorectic patients' reaction to vasopressin proved to be erratic and unrelated to the plasma sodium level. These differences are also reflected in a reversal of the usual CSF/plasma ratio of arginine vasopressin. The investigation concluded these changes indicate an intrinsic neurohypophyseal defect in anorexia nervosa patients.

Although anorexia nervosa most frequently occurs in young apparently healthy women, it has also been noted in patients with another disease. For example, a number of patients with Turner's syndrome (gonadal dysgenesis, XO syndrome) also develop anorexia nervosa.[100] Similarly, patients with mental retardation have had anorexia nervosa.[101]

Hsu et al reported six anorexia nervosa patients who manifested a schizo-phrenic disorder during their treatment.[102] The association of anorexia nervosa emerging within the context of diabetic patients has been cited.[103]

The course of the disease remains variable. Many patients fully re-cover from their first and only episode. A legal secretary with anorexia nervosa, severe weight loss, and absence of menses following intensive psychotherapy gained weight, began to have periods, developed secondary sexual characteristics, married, and eventually had a child. Others continue to have episodes of anorexia. A number of patients die from starvation; Schwartz and Thompson reported mortality of 6%.[104] Poor outcomes correlate with lower weight, longer illness, troubled childhood and parent relationship, and the presence of vomiting, bulimia, and eating with others anxiety.[105]

A schizophrenic disorder may be manifested through anorexia. Aside from the occurrence of a schizophrenic episode in anorexia nervosa patients or the simultaneous happenstance of both diagnoses, a thought disorder, in and of itself, may account for an avoidance of food. Deter-ioration, the 6-month duration, and prodromal phase, bizarre delusions, somatic delusions, auditory hallucinations, and delusions of persecution characterize the schizophrenic disorder.[89] As a result of these delusions of hallucinations, patients may cease to eat. Examples include the extremely paranoid woman who believes people are about to attack if she goes out and thus never leaves home to obtain groceries; the suspicious man who "knows" his food is poisoned and does not eat; or the grandiose coed who claims her starvation will save humanity from a nuclear war.

A *major depression* often has as its hallmark a significant loss of appetite and weight. Occurring with the constellation of a severe mel-ancholic mood, psychomotor disturbances, fatigue, inability to concen-trate, guilt, worthlessness, self-destructive thoughts and behavior, and sleep disruptions, these patients frequently develop weight reduction.[89] They lose weight without dieting; they complain of no interest in eating; they avoid meals. Indeed, for young children, failure to thrive frequently signals a major depression. Such a depression can appear as solitary episodes, as one of a series of depressions, major depression, recurrent, or as part of a number of depressions in between manic episodes, manic-depressive illness. One 45-year-old woman with recurrent major depres-sion noted each depressive episode was heralded by a loss of appetite and weight.

Anorexia frequently, definitely, and temporarily develops within the context of an *adjustment disorder*. The hallmark of this diagnosis remains a maladaptive response to an identifiable event or stressing situation with an impairment at work or home or an excessive reaction. Besides an expected subsiding of symptoms once the stress has passed, this distress does not meet the diagnostic criteria for other disorders. Clearly and commonly, some patients cease eating, lose interest in food, or miss meals after a separation; ie, job loss, a divorce, significant financial reverse, or being confined.

Organic mental disorders, both delirium and dementia, lead to anorexia.

In delirium, the clouded consciousness, disturbances of perception, interruption of the normal sleep-wake pattern, alterations of activities, memory deficits and disorientation—all contribute to not eating. In dementia, the memory deficits, loss of abstract thinking, and judgment impairment, all may result in patients literally forgetting to eat. In both disorders, the anorexia develops as a result of the CNS disturbances.

BINGE EATING

BINGE EATING Excessive food consumption, massive periodic ingestion, eating too much at one time.

Case report: A 25-year-old woman, pursuing an irresistible craving for something to eat, sneaks into the kitchen at 11:30 pm and devours the refrigerator's contents. Often vomiting and guilt feelings follow this behavior. Her history shows evidence of stealing and she senses herself out of control. Her physician has recently begun her on a drug. She is depressed. A sympathetic interviewer attempts to fathom the dilemma.

Features

Mood Craving, urgency, insatiability, and remorse dominate the emotional picture of the binge eater.[106] These feelings generate a variety of thoughts and propel the individual through a host of activities. Intensity, persistence, and recurrence characterize these enduring emotions which do not readily remit.

Craving sets the emotional tenor. This is the driving force. It says food now! It screams with one loud voice—eat!

Urgency follows. It captures the anxiety, the pressure, the immediacy, and the present. It mobilizes and belies a loss of control.

Insatiability accounts for protracted behavior. It conveys the limitlessness of the experience. No amount satisfies. Nothing is enough. There is no "when"!

Finally, *remorse* often culminates the event. Food has not only fulfilled the craving but also has caused a depression. The individual feels shame, guilt, anger, and defeat.

Thoughts   The binge eaters focus their thoughts on food, on eating, on control, and on their weight. These reach an obsessional level. They become a major, often sole preoccupation, and rule their lives.[107]

These persons *dwell upon food.* Food dominates their thinking; it intrudes into all their thoughts. They fantasize, and center their inner world on it. They are preoccupied with the entire food process: purchasing, preparing, and consuming.

These patients perceive their thoughts and actions toward food as *beyond their control.* They find themselves incapable of stopping the preoccupation or the eating. One patient reports his being "out of control" in the face of food; chaos reigns in their lives.

Many binge eaters represent a subgroup of patients with anorexia nervosa, and these individuals pursue thinness.[108] They have a morbid fear of fatness; they are obsessed with weight.[109] This leads to their vomiting behavior. Yet bulimia with or without anorexia nervosa represents an important marker of psychopathology.[110]

Behavior   A variety of behaviors provides the key ingredients in the description of the binge eater.

Binge eating itself stands as the central feature of this symptom. The individuals, usually alone, on the sly, frequently consume a significant amount of food. They binge-eat.[111]

The eating frequently occurs *in private and on the sly.* These patients prefer a sole binge-eating experience, often late at night when everyone else has gone to bed. They sneak the food even when in more public settings. Observation often inhibits the behavior.

Frequently vomiting follows this binge eating.[106—108,111] It is usually self-induced.[112] It too is done privately. The patient uses it to expel the food and to remove the results of the dietary excesses. This provides a dramatic counterreaction to the eating action. These patients frequently also use and abuse laxatives.

In contrast to binge-eating episodes, many of the individuals also go through periods of *fasting* . They become abstinent. They swing to the opposite extreme.

Alcohol and substance abuse commonly occurs with this symptom.[108] The binge eaters drink to excess also. They use and abuse street drugs. Some become drug addicts.

Individuals who consume food slyly sometimes have a coincident behavior in stealing. Indeed, kleptomania is quite prevalent in these individuals.[107]

These patients involve themselves in a variety of *impulsive acts*. They run away when distressed. They attempt suicide. They mutilate themselves. They strike out. When confronted, trapped, or challenged, they act impulsively!

Some patients follow a seasonal variation in their binging. They will demonstrate significant carbohydrate craving in the winter with its diminished daylight time. Then, the appetite return to normal as the daylight time lengthens.[113]

Physical examination and laboratory findings The *physical examination* of the binge eater demonstrates a number of features which represent sequelae and profound, pronounced, and protracted vomiting. Some patients will show benign bilateral parotid enlargement after several days of emesis.[114] Teeth reflect certain changes produced by vomiting.[3] These involve evidence of dental decalcification and erosions. Additionally, certain women will develop amenorrhea. The patient's body will range from extreme thinness to marked obesity.

A variety of *laboratory findings* are associated with bulimia. Many reflect the changes induced by significant vomiting. Others are related to diagnostic groups of bulimic patients.

Vomiting of a severe nature causes a diminished serum potassium.[106] Patients may develop a hypokalemic alkalosis. Reduced potassium causes pronounced muscle weakness. Their ECGs demonstrate flattened or inverted T waves or V waves and sagged ST segments.[115]

Binge eating is accompanied by several findings. Some patients may have acute gastric dilation.[116] Some bulimic patients will demonstrate EEG abnormalities, eg, 14 and 6 per second positive spiking pattern.[117]

Bulimia has been shown to be associated with two other findings.[118] First, many of these patients have abnormal cortisol suppression tests. They showed during the test a cortisol not suppressed but in the range of 4 to 5 mg/100mL at 4:00 pm. This gives more evidence of the link between bulimia and depression. Second, these same patients also had blunted thyrotropin-releasing hormone (THR) tests with a delay in the raise of thyrotropin (TSH) in response to TRN.

Interviewer's reaction   The interviewer experiences a number of reactions to the binge eater: sympathy, a distant wonderment, and a sense of pathos.

The sympathy stems from the fact that many of us struggle with impulses to eat, yet to be thin. We share their desire to consume, we have eaten to excess, we have enjoyed ourselves; and then we feel terrible.

The interviewer betrays a feeling of wonderment as the patient in a too detached manner describes eating, then vomiting. The predicament strikes one as almost unreal. One hears a sequence out of a textbook, yet blandly presented. The sympathy turns to a remoteness born of disbelief.

Yet, the interviewer catches their pathos, their anger, their depression, their preoccupation with food, their trap, and their dilemma—all are perceived during the interview. One comes away from the encounter with a sense of uneasiness, of pain, of emptiness, and of anguish.

Psychodynamics

Psychodynamics   A wide range of psychodynamically significant events and conflicts lead to and find expression in and through binge eating. The behavior represents a response to these dynamic issues of which the individual may be consciously or unconsciously aware. Engel described bulimia as a conversion reaction.[119]

A *traumatic* event may cause binge eating. A 25-year-old secretary was raped in her apartment by an unknown assailant. She turned to binge eating. Sudden, devastating, unexpected circumstances trigger a major food consumption response. Death, disfiguration, or disaster—all may cause an eruption of eating. This frequently produces what Bruch terms "reactive obesity."[120]

Loss may trigger bulimia. The person responds to a loss of a relationship, a position, an ego ideal, a hope, a future, an activity, or an opportunity through eating. A 45-year-old executive turned to binge eating after being passed over for a promotion for the second time. A 37-year-old woman physician began a massive rapid food binge following the death of her mother.

Separation may lead to binge eating. This commonly occurs when children go away from home for the first time, be it camp or college. An 18-year-old coed began her freshman year at a college some 100 miles from where her parents lived. She had never been away from her home before. She binge-ate for the entire fall semester. By spring, her dietary habits returned to normal. Separation of lovers, spouses, and friends all may initiate binge eating.

Binge eating emerges as one way to handle a *sexual conflict*. To persons fearful of their sexuality or sexual relations, binge eating provides an escape in two ways. First, the activity by its extent and preoccupation avoids sexual opportunities. Second, through the resultant weight gains, they become less likely to be sought after as a date.

Many persons handle *intense emotions* through binge eating. These strong feelings include anger, anxiety, depression, loneliness, boredom, fear, rage, and frustration.[121] One nurse would become enraged at his mother; he would never acknowledge any feeling toward her, but every time he talked to her on the telephone, he would then ingest the contents of the refrigerator.

Binge eating dramatically may represent a *wish to devour*.[121] The patient wants to consume all, to ingest everything, and to incorporate the world. The eating explosion serves to "take the world in" and gain oral control over the universe.

Binge eating may become an escape. These patients find no pleasure in their lives, their relationships, their work, and their leisure. They feel such an emptiness in their lives and themselves and the binge represents a focus.

Binge eating may be part of the anorexia nervosa disorder.[107,108] Here, the behavior reflects the dynamics of that and develops within the constellation of its symptoms.[122] The prognosis for anorexia nervosa patients has been cited as poorer by the presence of bulimia.[105]

Biologic explanation The hypothalamus provides essential control of eating.[123] The interplay and mutual feedback relationship between the ventromedial nucleus (VMH), "the satiety center", and the ventrolateral nucleus (VLN), "the feeding center," govern food consumption.[14] Lesions to the VMN will prove responsible for binge eating.[124]

Glucose and insulin levels influence hypothalamus activity and under certain conditions promote excessive eating.[14] Hyperglycemia increases VMN and decreases VLN electrical activity; hypoglycemia diminishes VMS and heightens VLN stimulation. Low serum glucose leads to eating. Similarly, insulin by glucose reduction will trigger consumption.

Neurotransmitters have a role in generating binge eating. Norepinephrine when injected into the VMH causes a prompt short-lived appetite enhancement. Hoebel speculates an inhibitory function of the norepinephrine.[125] Dopamine has been suggested as motivating or rewarding eating. Blocking of this neurotransmitter decreases intake of sweet solutions by rats, the same as diluting the same liquid would do.[18]

Genetics *Anorexia nervosa* which often includes within its clinical course episodes of bulimia, has a number of genetic correlates outlined in the first section of this chapter.

Affective disorders, major depressions, and manic-depressive illness, which, not infrequently, include excessive eating in their presentations, have strong inheritance patterns as also discussed in the earlier anorexia section.

Bulimic patients' family histories suggest a number of clinical correlations and relationships. First, obesity occurs frequently in relatives of bulimic patients.[106] Further, and more striking, many of these binge eaters have obese mothers.[108] Second, alcoholism and depression are found to have a high prevalence within families of bulimic patients.[106] Third, not uncommonly, patients with bulimia will have other members of their families with binge-eating histories.[106]

Environment In *families* which stress food, prize thinness, and apply great pressure, members are apt to sneak food, binge-eat, and then vomit. They respond to the family dynamics and tensions. A compulsive mother placed high achievement demands upon her daughter. The daughter both feared and loved her mother. She accomplished during the day; she ate and vomited late at night.

Physical exertion leads to binge eating. Individuals and teams after the event, the competition, and the triumph celebrate in food and drink. Exercise promotes consumption for many people.

Weather often prompts binge eating. Hot weather leads to high fluid consumption. Cold weather produces binge-eating to "keep warm." A day of ocean sailing leads not only to too much drinking and eating on the boat, but also a huge appetite and a large meal once on land.

Differential Diagnosis

Nonpsychotropic drugs *Insulin* triggers episodes of binge eating as a result of the induced hypoglycemia.[126] Patients respond to a hyperinsulinism-caused rapid drop in glucose with diaphoresis, hunger, weakness, increased pulse, and an inner sense of trembling. More profound and pronounced effects include convulsions and coma. Oral hypoglycemic drugs, eg, sulfanylureas may also precipitate excessive eating episodes through a similar glucose reduction mechanism.

Any *drug* which *induces a depression* has the potential of causing binge eating as a response to the dysphoria. Chapter 2 details these medications.

Any *drug* which *precipitates anxiety* has the capacity to trigger excessive eating as a reaction to that anxious state. Chapter 1 outlines these medications.

Psychotropic drugs All *phenothiazines* will both enhance appetite and produce weight gain. Of interest, haloperidol does not appear to have these properties.[127] Chlorpromazine is particularly marked for its eating augmentation as well as its ability to diminish neurohypophyseal hormone secretion. It will cause satiated rats to eat.[14] It has been used effectively to promote eating for patients with anorexia nervosa.[128]

Antidepressant medications may produce increased appetite, gains in weight, and cravings for food. Although appetite enhancement may occur with tricyclic, tetracyclic, and MAO antidepressants, the effects of amitriptyline hydrochloride have been particularly noted. Paykel et al report that not only does amitriptyline use lead to weight gain but also it produces a remarkable and striking craving for carbohydrates.[129] This side effect proved of such a discomfort and concern that some patients stopped the medication. Kupter et al point out that treatment with amitriptyline is associated with weight gain, but actual mechanisms are complex and as yet not clear.[130]

Alcohol *Alcoholic* patients not infrequently exhibit binge drinking. Episodic massive consumption represents a key feature in the alcoholism consellation. Jellinek argues the loss of control in the face of and following the first drink constitutes the crucial third phase in the evolution of a person becoming an alcoholic.[52] Uncontrollable alcohol ingestion parallels part of the bulimic phenomenon: huge rapid consumption, then guilt and remorse.

Binge drinking occurs in the diagnostic criteria of both alcohol abuse and dependence.[89] The criteria for *alcohol abuse* involve a pathologic alcohol use pattern with daily need for it, inability to stop, failed attempts to halt it, intoxication-induced amnesia (blackouts), drinking despite physical consequences, and binges—intoxication during the day for at least two days. Two other criteria are social or work impairment and at least 1 month of disturbance. For *alcohol dependence*, there must be in addition to the pathologic pattern and impairment, either tolerance or evidence of withdrawal.

Bulimic patients frequently have problems with alcohol.[108] This is another area where their control difficulties and impulsivity shows. A 25-

year-old separated woman developed a bulimic pattern each night after work when she was alone. She would ingest up to 4 lbs of food and then vomit. Additionally, she would binge to intoxication a couple of times a week to handle her depression, loneliness, and sleeping difficulty.

Other abused substances *Cannabis* use not infrequently produces an enhancement of thirst and appetite.[48] Such a heightened consumption comes in the context of a marijuana elevation of senses. Patients under the influence of cannabis note an accentuation of tastes and smells.[53] They crave certain foods and drinks.

Medical illnesses

Hematologic disorders *Iron deficiency anemia* is often dramatically present as a result of a perverted appetite, or *pica*.[131] Pica may take a variety of forms: a craving for earth or clay (geophagia), for starch (amylophagia), or for ice (pagophagia). One woman complained to her family physician about her constant drive to eat newspapers. She always carried shredded newspapers with her in her pocketbook. Following diagnosis and treatment of her iron deficiency anemia, her desire and behavior disappeared. Other symptoms of this anemia include headaches, easy fatigue, pallor, edema, and tachycardia. Laboratory studies show a hypochronic microcytic anemia, serum iron decreased in the range of 75 mg/100mL (mild) to 25 mg/100mL (severe) with normal 100 mg/100mL and the iron binding capacity increased in the range of 300 mg/100mL (mild) to 600 mg/l00mL (severe) with normal of 300 mg/100mL.

Endocrine disorders *Reactive hypoglycemia* may trigger an episode of intense hunger.[132] Other hypoglycemic symptoms include sweating, tachycardia, palpitations, weakness, confusion, blunted affect, headaches, clouded vision, tremor, anxiety, and in extremes, seizures and loss of consciousness. This syndrome is also referred to as postprandial hypoglycemia. It is caused by alimentary hyperinsulinism. A glucose tolerance test with a serum glucose lower than 50 mg/100mL between two and five hours has some diagnostic potential; the definitive diagnosis involves a serum glucose below 50 mg/100mL accompanying the development of the above symptoms.

Fasting hypoglycemia may generate similar binge eating.[132] Here the causes are either due to an underproduction of glucose, eg, hypopituitarism, glucose 6-phosphatase deficiency, liver disease, or alcohol or glucose overutilization, eg, insulinoma. Diagnosis is made by a fasting plasma glucose in men below 50 mg/100mL or in women lower than 40 mg/100mL with accompanying hypoglycemic symptoms.

Cushing's syndrome may be encountered in patients demonstrating massive eating. Gifford and Gunderson report a 33-year-old woman with bilateral adrenocortical hyperplasia with an insatiable appetite.[133] Buffalo hump, moon facies, hypertension, easy bruisability, osteoporosis, and impaired glucose tolerance are found with this syndrome. Elevated cortisol and urinary 17-hydroxycorticosteroids prove diagnostic.[134]

Neurologic electroencephalographic (EEG) abnormalities have been related to compulsive eating. Green and Rau report EEG findings in these patients involve 14 and 6 per second positive spikes occurring in the temporal and occipital regions.[135] This observation correlates with episodic somatic complaints, eg, headaches and impulsive behavior. Their study further suggests neurologic dysregulation as a cause of compulsive eating and provides evidence these patients' consumption activities are limited by phenytoin.

Huntington's disease may first present through binge eating.[136] This mendelian dominant genetic disease affects bilaterally the caudate nucleus and putamen and these patients' brains demonstrate deficiencies in both glutamic acid decarboxylase and gamma-aminobutyric acid (GABA).[137] Choreiform movements and involuntary motions, eg, grimacing, typify this disease as does dementia.

Parkinson's disease may be associated with bulimia. Rosenberg et al report on a number of patients who had Parkinson's disease and also exhibited massive bulimic eating.[138] In these cases, treatment of their disease with appropriate antiparkinsonian medications, eg, levodopa, amantadine hydrochloride, or trihexyphenidyl hydrochloride led to an abatement of their various appetites.

Kleine-Levin syndrome may prinicipally manifest itself through bulimic episodes.[139] Other symptoms include hypersomnolence. The sleep may last for several days. It occurs in adolescent boys and they will show massive excessive appetite especially for sweets. Following periods of hypersomnia and overeating, they will exhibit depression, insomnia, and anemia.[140]

Klürer-Bucy syndrome not only provides a vivid example of excessive eating, but also offers further evidence of CNS control of eating behavior. In the classic study, the investigator removed from laboratory monkeys bilaterally the temporal lobes, uncus, hippocampus, amygdalae, and tail of the caudate nucleus. The animals then exhibited hypersexuality, aggressive behavior, and profuse eating.

Medial hypothalamic lesions produce binge eating. Celesia et al discuss the case of a 28-year-old man who rapidly developed a massive prodigious appetite attributable to a midline glioblastoma multiforme.[123] The tumor destroyed the right ventromedial hypothalamic nucleus (VMN) and the posterior hypothalamic nucleus. This further supports the control of the VMN in feeding; namely, that destruction of this nucleus leads to hyperphagia and obesity.

Pulmonary disorders Pickwickian syndrome involves massive obesity and hypoventilation.[141] Patients develop voracious appetites and achieve huge weights. Additionally, they have polycythemia, hypersomnolence, and right ventricular hypertrophy. Although the underlying defect may be idiopathic hypoventilation, these patients demonstrate marked improvement with weight reduction.[142]

Surgical complications Alimentary surgery may produce postprandial hypoglycemia which in turn precipitates episodes of binge eating. The common procedures responsible for this hypoglycemic situation include gastrectomy, gastrojejunostomy, pyloroplasty, and vagotomy. The mechanism involves a prompt gastric emptying with a rapid glucose absorption followed by insulin release.[132]

Not uncommonly some patients respond to the threat of surgery or the consequential changes as a result of surgery with either anxiety or depression.[143] The fear, the challenge, the pain, and the discomfort of any procedure proves quite disquieting to many patients. Some may handle the event and its sequelae with binge eating.

Physical trauma *Head trauma*, which results in damage to the ventromedial nucleus (VMN), may trigger binge eating.[123] This again demonstrates the hypothalamic control of eating.

Trauma leads to a host of intense emotions, eg, anxiety and depression.[143] These feelings often cause the patient to eat excessively. A 45-year-old separated woman received significant facial lacerations as a result of an automobile accident. In her horror over her appearance, she began to eat massively, proclaiming herself to be ugly. She wondered about eating herself to death.

Psychiatric differential diagnosis Bulimia constitutes a major psychiatric diagnostic category and has gained recent prominence and definition.[144] Classified by the DSM-III under adolescent disorders, it is found commonly in women with onset during adolescence or early adulthood.[89] Criteria involve episodes of binge eating defined as huge consumption in less than two hours and include three of the following:

ingestion of high calorie food; secretive consumption; binge halted by abdominal pain, social intrusion, sleep, or vomiting; many failed weight reduction attempts by diet, vomiting, or cathartics; and weight alterations of more than 10 lbs due to binging or fasting. These patients are aware of the abnormality of their eating behavior and sense that it is beyond their control. Additionally, binges lead to depression and self-deprecation. Finally, the bulimia does not occur within the context of anorexia nervosa or a medical cause.

Looking at a group of patients with bulimia, Pyle et al made a number of observations.[106] The women commenced binge eating at the same time they were dieting and they initiated it following a particularly traumatic event, eg, a separation from a significant individual. Most of the patients, although attempting to lose weight, were thin. They binged at home. Usually food craving, uncontrollable appetite, unhappiness, inability to sleep, or hunger preceded the binge. Guilt, worry, feeling full, hunger, satisfaction, or revulsion followed it. Their family histories included alcoholism and obesity. Frequently, they engaged also in stealing. Mitchell et al studied 40 patients with bulimia and found that these patients ate on the average for 1.18 hours with a range of from 15 minutes to eight hours, consumed an average of 3415 calories per day with a range of from 1200 to 11,500 calories per day, and did so on the average of 13.7 hours per week with a range of from 30 minutes to 43 hours.[111] They ate a lot quickly and often.

Bulimic patients have two other significant correlations. First, they appear to have a high incidence of depression.[145] The bulimia may represent a manifestation of a major depression. Many of these patients demonstrate an abnormal cortisol suppression test.[146] Second, the bulimic patients often show impairments in their life adjustments. Although not as impaired as the anorexia nervosa patient, they have been found by Johnson and Berndt to have an adjustment similar to that of alcoholic women.[147]

Bulimia can represent an all-encompassing problem. A 20-year-old woman came for therapy because of her binging and vomiting. She became depressed following the indifference of and then rejection by her boy friend. She worked in an office, had an overbearing, depressed, obese mother, jogged 6 miles a day, and had a dread of being fat. Since the rupture of the relationship, she consumed up to 6 lbs of sweets every night, then vomited it all up, and felt guilty, depressed, and empty. In psychotherapy, she talked about her unhappiness, the loss, the wish to vomit away her boy friend, and her lack of direction. She improved on imipramine hydrochloride and recognition of her profound contributing dynamics.

Anorexia nervosa patients may display bulimic behavior. These patients all meet the criteria for anorexia as outlined earlier in this chapter—fear of obesity, body image disturbance, at least 25% of initial body weight lost, refusal to return to normal weight, and no medical cause for the weight reduction.[89] Casper et al in looking at this bulimic subgroup, found that they appeared more extroverted, had stronger appetites, and were older than fasting anorexic patients.[107] They found this subgroup experiences very compelling hunger, intense affect of depression, guilt, and anxiety, and noted a poor prognosis for bulimic subgroups, eg, longer illness duration, lower social adjustment, and more hospitalizations than did the fasting type of anorectic patient. Garfinkel et al also observed a high incidence of impulsive behavior for this bulimic subgroup.[108] Activities include kleptomania, drug and alcohol abuse, suicide attempts, and self-mutilation.

Pica represents a rare binge-eating extreme classified in the DSM-III as a disorder of infancy, childhood, or adolescence.[89] The criteria involve the repetitious eating for at least a month of a nonnutritive substance and is not associated with either a mental or physical disorder. Infants may persistently eat plaster, hair, paint, or cloth; children, sand, paper, pebbles, or leaves. Neither group has a food aversion and the pica, although usually remittent, may continue into adolescence or adulthood.

Within the context of a *major depression,* binge eating may present as the principle feature. The dysphoria generates a strong desire to eat, to consume, to escape into food, and to devour. The patients meet the criteria for a major depression; a persistent dysphoric mood, and at least four of the following each day for two weeks; weight gain or loss; sleep disturbances; psychomotor alterations; loss of pleasure; fatigue without energy; unworthiness feelings; inability to concentrate, and preoccupation with death. Additionally, in the absence of depression, the picture must not be dominated by incongruent delusions or hallucinations nor by bizarre behavior, nor can the depression be superimposed upon schizophrenia, a paranoid disorder, an organic mental disorder, or uncomplicated bereavement.[89]

The binge eating occurs in the constellation of a significant depression. That depression may be a single episode—major depression or a series of depressive, major depressant or recurrent depression. Or the major depressions may be intertwined with manic episodes—bipolar disorders or manic-depressive illness. Chapter 2 explores this diagnosis.

Adjustment disorder wih depressed mood may feature binge eating. Patients responding to an identifiable stress may eat massively. Criteria include a clear stress followed within 3 months by a maladaptive reaction of either functioning impairment or excessive symptom. The response does not represent an underlying mental disorder, will diminish with the absence of the stress, or if the stress continues, a better level of adaptation will be achieved. Many people under pressure, stress, conflict, loss, or tension eat to excess.

Schizophrenia may reveal itself through binge eating. Patients may indulge excessively in response to bizarre messages, commands, or ideas. A belief that eating all the apples in the world will lead to peace may trigger such a craving. The diagnosis is made on the criteria for schizophrenia outlined in chapter 3.

A *posttraumatic stress disorder* may have as a cardinal feature binge eating. The excessive eating becomes a method of responding to the traumatic event. A young girl was raped by her uncle. For fear of him, she could not tell anyone. Each time she thought about the incident, she became enraged and ate. She vouched to become so big no man would ever touch her again. The criteria involve a significant distress reexperienced by recurrent recollections, dreams, or abreactions, a responsive numbness marked by lost interest, detachment, or affect construction, and two of the following symptoms: hyperalertness, disturbed sleep, survivor guilt, memory impairment, avoidance behavior to things which would cause trauma recall, and heightened symptoms when confronting something symbolizing the trauma.[89] The disorder may be acute, occurring within 6 months of the event, or chronic, persisting longer than 6 months, or delayed with onset at least 6 months after the traumatic event.

Bulimia may occur within the constellation of a seasonal affective disorder. Here the carbohydrate craving appears only during the winter along with symptoms of depression. Then these patients sleep too much, have low energy, and are dysphoric. In contrast, in the spring and summer they demonstrate high energy, are active, and become elated.[148]

REFERENCES

1. Halmi KA: Pragmatic information on the eating disorders. *Psychiatr Clin North Am* 1982;5:371-377.
2. Dally P: *Anorexia Nervosa.* New York, Grune & Stratton, Inc, 1969.
3. Stege P, Visco-Dangler L, Rye L: Anorexia nervosa: review including oral and dental manifestations. *JAMA* 1982;104:648-652.

4. Khuri R, Gehi M: Psychogenic amenorrhea: an integrative review. *Psychosomatics* 1981;22:883-893.

5. Hasler JF: Parotid enlargement: a presenting sign in anorexia nervosa. *Oral Surg* 1982;53:567-573.

6. Halmi KA: Anorexia nervosa: recent investigations. *Annu Rev Med* 1978;29:137-148.

7. Kay J, Stricker B: Hematologic and immunologic abnormalities in anorexia nervosa. *South Med J* 1983;76:1008-1010.

8. Dally PJ: Carotenaemia occurring in a case of aneorexia nervosa. *Br Med J* 1959;2:1333.

9. Wallach J: *Interpretation of Diagnostic Tests,* ed 3. Boston, Little, Brown & Co, 1978.

10. Mordasini R, Klose G, Greten H: Secondary type II hyperlipoproteinemia in patients with anorexia nervosa. *Metabolism* 1978;27:71-79.

11. Halmi KA: Anorexia nervosa and bulimia. *Psychosomatics* 1983;24:111-128.

12. Kohlmeyer K, Leha K, Uhl G, et al: Computed tomography of anorexia nervosa. *AJNR* 1983;4:437-438.

13. Lindemann E: Symptomatology and management of acute grief. *Am J Psychiatry* 1944;101:141-148.

14. Garfinkel PE, Coscina DV, The physiology and psychology of hunger and satiety, in Zales MR (ed): *Eating, Sleeping, and Sexuality.* New York, Brunner/Mazel, 1982, pp 5-42.

15. Olefsky JM: Obesity, in Isselbacker KJ, Adams RD, et al (eds): *Harrison's Principles of Internal Medicine,* ed 10. New York, McGraw-Hill Book Co, 1983, pp 440-446.

16. Kaye WH, Ebert MH, Raleigh M, et al: Abnormalities in CNS monoamine metabolism in anorexia nervosa. *Arch Gen Psychiatry* 1984;41:350-355.

17. Kennedy S, Garfinkel PE, Anorexia nervosa, in Hales RE, Franceo AF (eds): *American Psychiatric Association Annual Review,* Washington, American Psychiatric Press, Inc, 1985, vol 4, pp 438-463.

18. Gibbs J, Smith GP: The physiology of hunger and satiety, in Hales RE, Frances AI (eds): *American Psychiatric Association Annual Review.* Washington, American Psychiatric Press, Inc, 1985, vol 4, pp 406-418.

19. Rudman D: Protein and energy undernutrition, in Isselbacher KJ, Adams RD, Braunwald E, et al (eds): *Harrison's Principles of Medicine,* ed 10. New York, McGraw-Hill Book Co, 1983, pp 436-439.

20. Crisp AH, Hsu LKG, Harding B, et al: Clinical features of anorexia nervosa. *J Psychsom Res* 1980;24:179-191.

21. Nowlin NS: Anorexia nervosa in twins: case report and review. *J Clin Psychiatry* 1983;44:101-105.

22. Goodwin DW, Guze SB: *Psychiatric Diagnosis,* ed 2. New York, Oxford University Press, 1974.

23. Winokur A, March V, Mendels J: Primary affective disorders in

relatives of patients with anorexia nervosa. *Am J Psychiatry* 1980;137:695-697.

24. Attshuler KZ, Weiner MF: Anorexia nervosa and depression: a dissenting view. *Am J Psychiatry* 1985;142:238-242.

25. Lipton MA: The evolution of the biological understanding of affective and schizophrenic disorders, in Zales M (ed): *Affective and Schizophrenic Disorders.* New York, Brunner/Mazel, 1983, pp 5-28.

26. Dawidowicz LS: *The War Against the Jews 1933-1945.* New York, Bantam Books, 1975.

27. Solzhenitsyn AI: *The Gulag Archipelago 1918-1956.* New York, Harper & Row, 1973.

28. Frankl VW: *The Unheard Cry for Meaning.* New York, Simon & Schuster, 1979.

29. Yager J: Eating disorders introduction, in Hales RE, Frances AF (eds): *American Psychiatric Association's Annual Review.* Washington, American Psychiatric Press, Inc, 1985, vol 4, pp 401-405.

30. Groen JJ, Feldman-Toledano Z: Educative treatment of patients and parents in anorexia nervosa. *Br J Psychiatry* 1966;112:671-681.

31. Bruch H: Anorexia nervosa: therapy and theory. *Am J Psychiatry* 1982;139:1531-1538.

32. Amdor MJ, Tucker GJ, Detre J, et al: Anorexia nervosa: An interactional study. *J Nerv Ment Dis* 1969;148:559-566.

33. Greenblatt DJ, Shader RF: Digitalis toxicity, in Shader RI (ed): *Psychiatric Complications of Medical Drugs.* New York, Raven Press, 1972.

34. Katzung BG, Parmley WW: Cardiac glycosides and other drugs used in the treatment of congestive heart failure, in Katzung BG (ed): *Basic and Clinical Pharmacology.* Los Altos, Calif, Lange Medical Publishers, 1982, pp 124-137.

35. Rall TW: The xanthines, in Gilman AG, Goodman LS, Gilman A (eds): *Goodman and Gilman's The Pharmacological Basis of Therapeutics,* ed 6. New York, Macmillan Publishing Co, Inc, 1980, pp 592-607.

36. Boushey HA, Holtzman MJ: Bronchodilators and other agents used in the treatment of asthma, in Katzung BG (ed): *Basic and Clinical Pharmacology.* Los Altos, Calif, Lange Medical Publishers, 1982, p 205.

37. Cohen S: Pathogenesis of coffee-induced gastrointestinal symptoms. *N Engl J Med* 1980;303:122-124.

38. Lutz EG: Restless legs, anxiety and caffeinism. *J Clin Psychiatry* 1978;39:693-698.

39. Sours JA: Case reports of anorexia nervosa and caffeinism. *Am J Psychiatry* 1983;140:235-236.

40. Hoffman BB: Adrenergic receptor-activating drugs, in Katzburg BG (ed): *Basic and Clinical Pharmacology.* Los Altos, Calif, Lange Medical Publishers, 1980, pp 72-81.

41. Mandell GL, Sande MA: Penicillins and cephalosporins, in Gilman AG, Goodman LS, Gilman A (eds): *Goodman and Gilman's The*

Pharmacological Basis of Therapeutics, ed 6. New York, Macmillan Publishing Co, Inc, 1980, pp 1126-1161.

42. Sande MA, Mandell GL: The aminoglycosides, in Gilman AG, Goodman LS, Gilman A (eds): *Goodman and Gilman's The Pharmacological Basis of Therapeutics,* ed 6. New York, Macmillan Publishing Co, Inc, 1980, pp 1162-1180.

43. Mandell GL, Sande MA: Sulfanamides, trimethoprim-sulfamethoxazole, and urinary tract antiseptics, in Gilman AG, Goodman LS, Gilman A (eds): *Goodman and Gilman's The Pharmacological Basis of Therapeutics,* ed 6. New York, Macmillan Publishing Co, Inc, 1980, pp 1106-1125.

44. Calabresi P, Parks RE: Antiproliferative agents and drugs used for immunosuppression, in Gilman AG, Goodman LS, Gilman A (eds): *Goodman and Gilman's The Pharmacological Basis of Therapeutics,* ed 6. New York, Macmillian Publishing Co, Inc, 1980, pp 1256-1313.

45. Salmon SE, Sartorelli AC: Cancer chemotherapy. in Katzung GD (ed): *Basic and Clinical Pharmacology.* Los Altos, Calif, Lange Medical Publishers, 1982, pp 629-664.

46. Nesse RM, Carli T, Curtis CC, et al: Pseudohallucinations in cancer chemotherapy patients. *Am J Psychiatry* 1983;140:483-485.

47. Silverfarb PM, Philibert D, Levine PM: Psychosocial aspects of neoplastic disease: II Affective and cognitive effects of chemotherapy in cancer patients. *Am J Psychiatry* 1980;137:597-601.

48. Slaby AE, Lieb J, Tancredi LR: *Handbook of Psychiatric Emergencies,* ed 2. Garden City, NY, Medical Examination Publishing Co, 1981.

49. Lacoursiere RB, Spohn HE, Thompson K: Medical effects of abrupt neuroleptic withdrawal. *Compr Psychiatry* 1978;17:285-294.

50. Mellor CS: Diazepam withdrawal syndrome: its prolonged and changing nature. *Can Med Assoc J* 1982;127:1093-1096.

51. Jamburro CH: The nutritional management of alcoholism, drug addiction and acute toxicity syndromes, in Halpern SL (ed): *Quick Reference to Clinical Nutrition.* Philadelphia, JB Lippincott, 1979, p 370.

52. Jellinek EM: Phases of alcohol addiction. *Q J Stud Alcohol* 1952;13:673-678.

53. Snyder SH: *Biological Aspects of Mental Disorder.* New York, Oxford University Press, 1980.

54. Victor M: The alcohol withdrawal syndrome. *Postgrad Med* 1970;47:68-72.

55. Weiner N: Norepinephrine, epinephrine and the sympathomimetic amides, in Gilman AG, Goodman LS, Gilman A (eds): *Goodman and Gilman's The Pharmacological Basis of Therapeutics,* ed 6. New York, Macmillan Publishing Co, 1980, pp 138-175.

56. Wesson DR, Smith DE: Managing the barbiturate withdrawal syndrome, in Bourne PG (ed): *Acute Drug Abuse Emergencies.* New York, Academic Press, 1976, pp 99-104.

57. Way WL, Way EL: Narcotic analgesics and antagonists, in Katzung BG

(ed): *Basic and Clinical Pharmacology*. Los Altos, Calif, Lange Medical Publishers, 1982, pp 309-322.

58. Hollister L: Drugs of abuse, in Katzung RG (ed): *Basic and Clinical Pharmacology*. Los Altos, Calif, Lange Medical Publishers, 1982, pp 323-334.

59. Jefferson JW, Marshall JR: *Neuropsychiatric Features of Medical Disorders*. New York, Plenum Medical Book Co, 1982.

60. Ingbar SH, Woeber KA: Diseases of the thyroid, in Isselbacher KJ, Adams RD, Braunwald E (eds): *Harrison's Principles of Internal Medicine*, ed 10. New York, McGraw-Hill Book Co, 1983, pp 614-634.

61. Williams GH, Oluhy RG, Thorn GW: Diseases of the adrenal cortex, in Isselbacher KJ, Adams RO, Braunwald E (eds): *Harrison's Principles of Internal Medicine*, ed 10. New York, McGraw-Hill Book Co, 1983, pp 634-657.

62. Foster DW: Diabetes mellitis, in Isselbacher KJ, Adams RO, Braunwald E (eds): *Harrison's Principles of Internal Medicine*, ed 10. New York, McGraw-Hill Book Co, 1983, pp 661-679.

63. McGuigan JE: Peptic ulcer, in Isselbacher KJ, Adams RO, Braunwald E (eds): *Harrison's Principles of Internal Medicine*, ed 10. New York, McGraw-Hill, 1983, pp 1697-1712.

64. LaMont JT, Isselbacher KJ: Diseases of the small and large intestine, in Isselbacher KJ, Adams RO, Braunwald E (eds): *Harrison's Principles of Internal Medicine*, ed 10. New York, McGraw-Hill Book Co, 1983, pp 1752-1765.

65. Bunn HF: Anemia, in Isselbacher KJ, Adams RO, Braunwald E (eds): *Harrison's Principles of Internal Medicine*, ed 10. New York, McGraw-Hill Book Co, 1983, pp 282-292.

66. Merritt HH: *A Textbook of Neurology*, ed 3. Philadelphia, Lea & Febiger, 1963.

67. Erman MK, Murrary GB: A case report of anorexia nervosa and Gaucher's Disease. *Am J Psychiatry* 1980;137:858-859.

68. Weinberger DR: Brain disease and psychiatric illness: when should a psychiatrist order a CAT scan? *Am J Psychiatry* 1984;147:1521-1527.

69. Weller RA, Weller EB: Anorexia nervosa in a patient with an infiltrating tumor of the hypothalamus. *Am J Psychiatry* 1982;139:824-825.

70. Holroyde CP, Richard GA: Carbohydrate metabolism in cancer cachexia. *Cancer Treat Rep* 1981;65(suppl 5): 55-59.

71. Schein PS, Kinner D, Haller D, et al: Cachexia of malignancy. *Cancer* 1969;43:2070-2076.

72. Guitani A, Recchia M, Carli M, et al: Walker carcinoma 256: a model for students on tumor-induced anorexia and cachexia. *Oncology* 1982;39:173-178.

73. Costa G, Bewley P, Aragon M, et al: Anorexia and weight loss in cancer patients. *Cancer Treat Rep* 1981;65,(suppl 5):3-7.

74. Bernstein IL, Sigmundi RA: Tumor anorexia: a learned food aversion? *Science* 1980;209:416-418.
75. Fairweather DV: Nausea and vomiting in pregnancy. *Am J Obstet Gynecol* 1968;102:135-138.
76. Trethowan WH: The Couvade syndrome: some further observations. *J Psychosom Res* 1968;12:107-115.
77. Hall RCW, Stickney SK, Gardner ER: Psychiatric symptoms in patients with systemic lupus erythematosus. *Psychosomatics* 1981;22:15-24.
78. Cooperman LH, Wellman H: Preparation of the patient for anesthesia, in Dudrick SJ, Bave AE, Eiseman B, et al (eds): *Manual of Preoperative and Postoperative Care,* ed 3. Philadelphia, WB Saunders Co, 1983, pp 213-225.
79. Kuldau JM, Barnard G, Kreutziger S, et al: Psychosocial effects of jejunoileal bypass for obesity. *Psychosomatics* 1979;20:462-472.
80. Bray GA, Benfield JR: Intestinal bypass for obesity. *Am J Clin Nutr* 1977;30:121-127.
81. Shingleton WW, Grant JP: Malabsorption syndromes, in Sabiston DC (ed): *Davis-Christopher Textbook of Surgery.* Philadelphia, WB Saunders Co, 1981, pp 1035-1044.
82. Kinney JM, Gump FE: The metabolic response to injury, in American College of Surgeons (eds): *Manual of Preoperative and Postoperative Care,* ed 3. Philadelphia, WB Saunders Co, 1983, 15-37.
83. Pruitt BA, Treat RC: The burn patient, in American College of Surgeons (eds): *Manual of Preoperative and Postoperative Care,* ed 3. Philadelphia, WB Saunders Co, 1983, 697-726.
84. Bingham HG, Krischer JP, Schuster JJ, et al: Effects of nutrition on length of stay and survival for burned patients. *Burns Incl Therm Inj* 1981;7:252-257.
85. Ross ED, Rush J: Diagnosis and neuroanatomical correlates of depression in brain-damaged patients. *Arch Gen Psychiatry* 1981;38:1344-1354.
86. Willi J, Grossmann S: Epidemiology of anorexia nervosa in a defined region of Switzerland. *Am J Psychiatry* 1983;140:564-567.
87. Herzog DB, Copeland PM: Eating disorders. *N Engl J Med* 1985;313:295-303.
88. Yager J: Family issues in the pathogenesis of anorexia nervosa. *Psychosom Med* 1982;44:43-60.
89. American Psychiatric Association: *Diagnostic and Statistical Manual of Mental Disorders,* ed 3. Washington: American Psychiatric Association, 1980, pp 67-69.
90. Faye WH, Pickar D, Nabar D, et al: Cerebrospinal fluid opioid activity in anorexia nervosa. *Am J Psychiatry* 1982;139:643-645.
91. Gerner RH, Gwirtsman HE: Abnormalities of dexamethasome suppression test and urinary MHP6 in anorexia nervosa. *Am J Psychiatry* 1981;138:650-653.

92. Boyar RM, Hellman LD, Roffwarg HP, et al: Cortisol secretion and metabolism in anorexia nervosa. *N Engl J Med* 1977;296:190-193.

93. Boyar RM, Katz J, Finkelstein JW, et al: Anorexia nervosa: immaturity of the 24-hour luteinizing hormone secretory pattern. *N Engl J Med* 1974;291:861-865.

94. Marshall JC, Kelch RP: Low dose pulsatile gonadotropin-releasing hormone in anorexia nervosa: a model for human pubertal development. *J Clin Endocrinol Metab* 1979;49:712-718.

95. Wheeler MJ, Crisp AH, Hsu LKG, et al: Reproductive hormone changes during weight gain in male anorectics. *Clin Endocrinol (Oxf)* 1983;18:423-429.

96. Doerr P, Fichter M, Pirke KM, et al: Relationship between weight gain and hypothalamic pituitary adrenal function in patients with anorexia nervosa. *J Steroid Biochem* 1980;13:529-537.

97. Golla JA, Larson LA, Anderson CF, et al: Immunological assessment of patients with anorexia nervosa. *Am J Clin Nutr* 1981;34:2756-2767.

98. Holt S, Ford J, Grant S, et al: Abnormal gastric emptying in primary anorexia nervosa. *Br J Med* 1981;308:1117-1123.

99. Margo JL, Hawton KE: Anorexia nervosa and Turner's syndrome. *Br Med J* 1978;1:15-16.

101. Mohl PC, McMahon T: Anorexia nervosa associated with mental retardation and schizoaffective disorder. *Psychosomatics* 1980;21:602-606.

102. Hsu LKG, Meltzer ES, Crisp AH: Schizophrenia and anorexia nervosa. *J Nerv Ment Dis* 1981;169:273-276.

103. Powers PS, Malone JI, Duncan JA: Anorexia nervosa and diabetes mellitus. *J Clin Psychiatry* 1983;44:133-135.

104. Schwartz DM, Thompson MG: Do anorectics get well? Current research and future needs. *Am J Psychiatry* 1981;138:319-323.

105. Hsu LKG, Crisp AH, Harding B: Outcome of anorexia nervosa. *Lancet* 1979;1:61-65.

106. Pyle RL, Mitchell JE, Eckert ED: Bulimia: a report of 34 cases. *J Clin Psychiatry* 1981;42:60-64.

107. Casper RC, Eckert ED, Halmi KA, et al: Bulimia. *Arch Gen Psychiatry* 1980;37:1030-1035.

108. Garfinkel PE, Moldofsky H, Garner IM: The heterogeneity of anorexia nervosa.*Arch Gen Psychiatry* 1980;37:1036-1040.

109. Fairburn CG: *Binge eating and bulimia nervosa.* Garden City, NY, SKF Publications, 1982.

110. Garner DM, Garfinkel PE, O'Shaughnessy M: The validity of the distinction between bulimia with and without anorexia nervosa. *Am J Psychiatry* 1985;142:581-587.

111. Mitchell JE, Pyle RL, Eckert ED: Frequency and duration of binge eating episodes in patients with bulimia. *Am J Psychiatry* 1981;138:835-836.

112. Rich CL: Self-induced vomiting. *JAMA* 1978;239:2688-2689.
113. Rosenthal NE, Sack DH, Carpenter CJ, et al: Antidepressant effects of light in seasonal affective disorder. *Am J Psychiatry* 1985;142:163-170.
114. Levin PA, Falko JM, Dixon K, et al: Benign parotid enlargement in bulimia. *Ann Intern Med* 1980;93:827-829.
115. Levinsky NG: Fluids and electrolytes, in Isselbacher KJ, Adams RD, Braunwald E, et al (eds): *Harrison's Principles of Internal Medicine,* ed 10. New York, McGraw-Hill Book Co, 1983, pp 220-230.
116. Mitchell JE, Pyle RL, Miner RA: Gastric dilation as a complication of bulimia. *Psychosomatics* 1982;23:96-97.
117. Johnson RE, Sinnott SK: Bulimia. *Am Fam Physician* 1981;24:141-143.
118. Gwirtsman HE, Roy-Byrne P, Yager J, et al: Neuroendocrine abnormalities in bulimia. *Am J Psychiatry* 1983;140:559-563.
119. Engel GL: Psychological aspects of GI disorders, in Reiser MF (ed): *American Handbook of Psychiatry.* New York, Basic Books, 1975, vol 4, pp 653-690.
120. Bruch H: *Eating Disorders.* New York, Basic Books, 1973.
121. Alexander F: *Psychosomatic Medicine.* New York, WW Norton, 1950.
122. Lowenkopf EL: Anorexia nervosa: some nosological considerations. *Compr Psychiatry* 1982;23:233-240.
123. Celesia CG, Archer CR, Chung HD: Hyperphagia and obesity. *JAMA* 1981;246:151-153.
124. Hetherington AW, Ranson SW: Experimental hypothalamo-hypophyseal obesity in the rat. *Proc Soc Exp Biol Med* 1939;41:465-466.
125. Hoebel BG: Neurotransmitters in the control of feeding and its rewards, in Stunkard AJ, Stellar E (eds): *Eating and its Disorders.* New York, Raven Press, 1984, vol 62, pp 15-38.
126. Larner J: Insulin and oral hypoglycemic drugs: glucagon, in Gilman AG, Goodman LS, Gilman A (eds): *Goodman and Gilman's The Pharmacological Basis of Therapeutics,* ed 6. New York, Macmillan Publishing Co, Inc, 1980, pp 1497-1523.
127. Baldessarini RJ: Drugs and the treatment of psychiatric disorders, in Gilman AG, Goodman LS, Gilman A (eds): *Goodman and Gilman's The Pharmacological Basis of Therapeutics,* ed 6. New York, Macmillan Publishing Co, Inc, 1980, pp 391-447.
128. Halmi KA: The diagnosis and treatment of anorexia nervosa, in Zales MR (ed): *Eating, Sleeping, and Sexuality.* New York, Brunner/Mazel, 1982, pp 43-58.
129. Paykel ES, Mueller PS, De La Vergne PM: Amitriptyline, weight gain and carbohydrate craving: a side effect. *Br J Psychiatry* 1973;123:501-507.
130. Kupfer DJ, Cable PA, Rubenstein D: Changes in weight during treatment for depression. *Psychosom Med* 1979;41:535-544.
131. Lee GR, Wintrobe MM, Bunn HF: Iron deficiency anemia and the sideroblastic anemias, in Isselbacher KJ, Adams RD, Braunwald E, et

al (eds): *Harrison's Principles of Internal Medicine,* ed 9. New York, McGraw-Hill Book Co, 1980.

132. Foster DW, Rubenstein AH: Hypoglycemia, insulinoma, and other hormone-secreting tumors of the pancreas, in Isselbacher KJ, Adams RD, Braunwald E, et al (eds): *Harrison's Principles of Internal Medicine,* ed 9. New York, McGraw-Hill Book Co, 1983, pp 682-689.

133. Gifford S, Gunderson JG: Cushing's disease as a psychosomatic disorder. *Medicine* 1970;49:397-409.

134. Williams GH, Dluhy RG, Thorn GW: Diseases of the adrenal cortex, in Isselbacher KJ, Adams RD, Braunwald E, et al (eds): *Harrison's Principles of Internal Medicine,* ed 10. New York, McGraw-Hill Book Co, 1983, pp 634-657.

135. Green RS, Rau JH: Treatment of compulsive eating disturbances with anticonvulsant medication. *Am J Psychiatry* 1974;131:428-432.

136. Whittier JR: Mental disorders with Huntington's chorea, in Reiser MF (ed): *American Handbook of Psychiatry.* New York, Basic Books, 1975, vol 4, pp 412-436.

137. Richardson EPJ, Adams RD: Degenerative diseases of the nervous system, in Isselbacher KJ, Adams RD, Braunwald E, et al (eds): *Harrison's Principles of Internal Medicine,* ed 10. New York, McGraw Hill Book Co, 1983.

138. Rosenberg P, Herishanu Y, Beilin B: Increased appetite (bulimia) in Parkinson's disease. *J Am Geriatr Soc* 1977;25:277-278.

139. Orlosky MJ: The Kleine-Levin syndromes: a review. *Psychosomatics* 1982;23:609-621.

140. Williams RL, Derman S, Karacan I: Disorders of excessive sleep and the parasomnias, in Zales MR (ed): *Eating, Sleeping, Sexuality.* New York, Brunner/Mazel, 1982, pp 150-185.

141. Burwell CS, Robin ED, Whaley RD, et al: Extreme obesity associated with alveolar hypoventilation, a Pickwickian syndrome. *Am J Med* 1956;21:811-818.

142. West JB: Disorders of ventilation, in Isselbacher KJ, Adams RD, Braunwald E, et al (eds): *Harrison's Principles of Internal Medicine,* ed 10. New York, McGraw-Hill Book Co, 1983, pp 1586-1592.

143. Henker FO: Body-image conflict following trauma and surgery. *Psychosomatics* 1979;20:812-820.

144. Hoon GF, Brown LB: Bulimia: the emergence of a syndrome. *Aust NZ J Psychiatry* 1984;18:113-126.

145. Johnson L, Larson R: Bulimia: an analysis of moods and behavior. *Psychosom Med* 1982;44:333-354.

146. Gwirtsman HE, Roy-Byrne P, Yager J, et al: Neuroendocrine abnormalities in bulimia. *Am J Psychiatry* 1983;140:774-777.

147. Johnson L, Berndt DJ: Preliminary investigation of bulimia and life adjustment. *Am J Psychiatry* 1983;140:774-777.

148. Rosenthal NE, Sack DA, Gillin JC, et al: Seasonal affective disorder: a description of the syndrome and preliminary findings with light treatment. *Arch Gen Psychiatry* 1984;41:72-80.

7 Sleep Disturbances: Insomnia and Excessive Sleep

Stephen M. Soreff

The great rejuvenator, relaxer, and reflector river of sleep divides into the turbulent stream of insomnia and the deceptively too quiet brook of hypersomnia. The two disturbed tributaries may flow separately and unrelated or may move along interlaced, at times indistinguishable. Sleep remains a potent barometer of the state of the person. It rapidly changes to display alterations in the psyche, the soma, and the environment. Sleep difficulties bring the patient for help, provide major diagnostic clues and furnish focal points in therapy.

INSOMNIA

INSOMNIA Difficulty falling asleep, staying asleep, and early morning awakening.

Case report A 35-year old man asks for help so he can sleep. He has great difficulty in falling asleep, and when he does, frequent wakings interrupt his slumber. He appears depressed, worried, and weary. At night he tosses, coughs, and snores; during the day he often naps. The concerned interviewer wonders where to begin.

Features

Insomnia makes the day unending and the night interminable. It results from a vast host of causes. Once begun, it pervades the patient's life. It can be protracted, devastating, and always compelling.

Mood   The patient with insomnia may show a number of moods. These either have contributed to the sleep difficulty or have been the results of the sleeping problem, or both.

Many patients experience anguish about sleep. This mood combines the painful affects of dread and apprehension and the sense of conflict and turmoil. They crave the sleep, yet fear the night. They want, but cannot find, relief.

Depression remains a frequent mood among patients with insomnia.[1] They are sad, melancholic, and "blue." They may feel down, pessimistic, defeated and trapped.

Some patients express anger. They are frustrated by their insomnia. One woman bitterly complained her husband had no difficulty sleeping while she was "obsessed" all night. They are annoyed by their burden.

Still other patients exhibit a sense of resignation. Their protracted struggle with insomnia has left them weary, exhausted, defeated, and apathetic. With dejection, without emotion, and with no end in sight, they feel overwhelmed and victimized by insomnia.

Thought   The thought content both reflects the insomnia and contributes to it.

Insomniac patients are frequently preoccupied with a series of concerns. At the causative end, many worry about work, school, tests, advancement, taxes, death and life. These, in turn, keep them awake. A 32-year-old woman, obsessed about her health, worried about cancer, heart disease, and her appearance. This preceded sleep. On the other hand, many worry about their insomnia. They spend their day pondering whether they will be able to sleep that night.

Some patients with insomnia report hypnagogic hallucinations. These are hallucinations which occur just as the individual drifts off to sleep and while the person is in a semiconscious state.

Finally, patients may experience painful recollections which interfere with sleep. The grieving person remembers vividly the dead loved one; the accident victim relives the trauma; the veteran recalls combat; and the insecure worker sees all the day's mistakes. The interjection and intrusion of these memories into awareness preclude sleep.

Behavior   Patients with insomnia exhibit a variety of behaviors, either during troubled sleep or in response to not being able to sleep.

Snoring is a frequent finding in people with sleep disturbances. Most often it is the bedmate who complains about snoring. Indeed, in certain cases, the neighbors register the complaint.

Tossing and turning remains another hallmark of sleep problems.

The patients may twist and turn throughout the night. Their beds may appear in the morning like a battlefield.

Sleepwalking, or somnambulism, may occur during sleep. The patient may carry out a complicated series of behaviors during the night. Infrequently this walk can terminate abruptly. In other situations, the individuals may injure or bruise themselves in one of these episodes.

Some patients with insomnia seek a chemical solution. They may obtain a variety of drugs from their physicians to promote sleep. Not uncommonly, they may have tried or are using a variety of over-the-counter as well as prescribed preparations. Some turn to alcohol. One woman has two cans of beer before retiring each evening. Others may use other abused substances. One man with insomnia would buy "black beauties," a barbiturate, from his street friends to get a good night's sleep.

One major effect of insomnia remains sleeping during the day. They fall asleep at work. They require naps during the day. They exhibit fatigue, perpetual tiredness, and a lack of energy and enthusiasm.

In response to insomnia, patients develop a whole series of activities. They may pace. They may eat. They may "count sheep." They may read; some people seek particularly boring books at night. Some watch television or listen to the radio. One woman unable to sleep stays up till 3:00 AM watching television.

Physical examination and laboratory findings The patient with a sleep disorder often demonstrates a number of significant physical findings. No proper evaluation of the patient is complete without a rigorous examination. Salient changes include irregular pulse, elevated blood pressure, and heightened temperature. Body inspection may reveal evidence of a hyperthyroidism (a fine tremor), congestive heart failure (pedal edema), cancer (cachexia), and uremia (the "frost"). Special emphasis must be applied to the pharynx, the lingual muscles, and to evidence of obstruction, (posterior displacement of the tongue), chest (wheezes and rales), abdomen (obesity), and heart (tachycardia and arrhythmias). Similarly, the neurologic and musculoskeletal systems should be closely evaluated.

A thorough assessment includes a wide range and variety of laboratory studies: urinalysis; CBC; chemistry tests including BUN, serum creatinine, serum proteins, folic acid, T_3, T_4, TSH, glucose; radiologic studies including chest films, upper GI studies, facial roentgenograms; and special studies including ECG, EEG, and nocturnal penile tumescence (NPT).

Interviewer's reaction The interviewer has a sense of "where to begin" when listening to a patient with insomnia. The reaction itself has two aspects. First, the interviewer often does not comprehend the magnitude of the problem. The medical setting misses the anguish, pathos, and immediacy which the patient experiences that night, and each night. One patient once called one of the authors at 3:00 AM just so "he would hurt as he hurt." Second, insomnia represents clinically a very complex and important signal.

Pathogenesis

Psychodynamics Personal and interpersonal events, struggles, fears and conflicts represent powerful causes of insomnia. Depression, losses, life changes, control issues, dream concerns, personality factors, and daily activities — all provide explanations for sleep difficulty. The day's drama continues and dominates sleep time.

Depression produces sleep disturbances. Feelings of sadness, melancholia, worthlessness, hopelessness, and uselessness may find expression in insomnia. Indeed, early morning waking remains one of the cardinal signs of an endogenous or manic depression depressed phase.[2] Futile days become futile nights. The seemingly endless anguish of depression stands as the single most significant psychodynamic factor in insomnia.

Loss, the central precipitant of depression, causes insomnia. The loss may be imagined or real. In the former, people set imagined, impossible, ideal goals for themselves. The nonachievement of these goals constitutes a loss to them. Death, divorce, departure, a relationship's rupture, a financial setback, unemployment, and poor health remain significant losses. A recently widowed woman could not sleep. She missed her husband; she complained of feeling "empty"; *their* bed had become only *her* bed.

Life changes produce sleep disturbances. People may react to major alterations in their lives with insomnia. The possible changes include graduation, a new position, marriage, a trip, a vacation, a new home, pregnancy, a new child, or a new pet. A couple could not sleep for weeks before their first child was born.

For some, insomnia may result from a control issue. They fear surrender to sleep as a loss of control. In sleep they see helplessness, assault, or death., A woman whose apartment had recently been broken into could not sleep for fear the burglar would return. For others sleep represents death. They fear they will not awake. The prayer, "Now I lay me down to sleep... if I die before I wake, I pray ..." captures this predicament.

Dreams and nightmares both disturb the sleep and make the would-be sleeper want to avoid sleep. Vivid, painful, terrifying dreams may cause persons to awake with fear, sweat and terror. They are afraid to return to sleep. Combat, war experiences, and witnessing the effects of battle produce this situation in veterans and other participants. [3,4] Vietnam remains with anguish in many nightmares. Any traumatic event, eg, automobile accident, fall, ski mishap, fire, or near-drowning, may lead to protracted painful dream intrusion as part of the posttraumatic stress disorder. [5] In other situations, brutal, conflictual, traumatic childhood events may surface through nightmares. A young man who had witnessed as a child the death of his father had difficulty sleeping because of this event recurring in his dreams. Eventually, he attempted to avoid sleep so he would not dream. Difficult, shameful, anxiety-provoking daily occurrences may be replayed that night in dreams and nightmares. The sleep is disturbed and sleep becomes feared.

Personality factors may contribute to insomnia. The obsessive, worrying, insecure individuals may experience sleep difficulty as they carry their day's preoccupation to bed with them. They dwell endlessly about tests, reports, health, cancer, the world, and relationships. Their inner debate keeps them awake or wakes them.

Finally, some people are so involved in life that they are reluctant to sleep even for a while. They find their lives so exciting, busy, eventful, meaningful, and creative, they deny the need for sleep and resist it. In an extreme, they may be experiencing a manic episode.

Biologic explanation   Sleep stages: An understanding of insomnia requires an appreciation of normal sleep. Sleep involves both rapid eye movement (REM) sleep and nonrapid eye movement (NREM) sleep. It progresses through four stages of NREM sleep and one phase of REM sleep every 90 minutes. [6]

Persons awake have an EEG marked by a fast alpha 8-12 c/s, low-amplitude pattern, full eye movements, and high muscle tone. As they descend into sleep, stage I, their EEG continues a low-voltage fast-frequency pattern, their eyes roll slowly from side to side, and their muscles relax. Stage II sleep has two characteristic EEG findings: sleep spindles, 12-14 c/s pattern and K complexes, high-amplitude waves with an initial sharp negative phase, then a positive component and lasting greater than 0.5 second; also, eye movements have ceased and good muscle tone maintained. Stage III sleep is characterized by a high-voltage slow-wave delta 1-2 cps EEG pattern. In Stage IV sleep, more than half the EEG record is dominated by the 1-2 c/s pattern and growth hormone secretion occurs.

After the initial four stages of sleep, which take between 70 to 100 minutes, sleepers have their first episode of REM sleep. This phase is also called paradoxical sleep and activated sleep. The period between sleep commencement and this initial REM is called sleep latency. During REM sleep, dreaming occurs, the heart rate increases, and trunk muscles are slack. In healthy men of all ages nocturnal penile tumescence (NPT) occurs in REM sleep. Moreover, tension increases in jaw muscles. The EEG is desynchronized, with a low amplitude pattern of both theta and beta frequencies. REM constitutes 20% to 25% of the full sleep time.

Throughout the night an orderly series of cycles occurs: awake, stages I, II, III, IV, --- III, II, REM, --- II, III, IV...[7] With age, the interval between the onset of sleep and the first REM (sleep latency) decreases. Stages III and IV also diminish. Various EEG changes and findings will be discussed under the different diagnostic categories.

Sleep control   Anatomy and biochemistry of CNS provide an organization for and regulation of sleep.[8] Serotonergic neurons occupy the medial tegmentum through the medulla, pons, and lower brain with projections to the hypothalamus, the thalamus, and the orbital frontal and medial temporal cortex. A factor S activates them, suppressing the reticular formation, producing slow wave-sleep.[9] Destruction of these neurons and projections or serotonergic antagonists will cause insomnia.

Another CNS mechanism involves norepinephrine and dopamine neurons. These noradrenergic neurons are located in the lateral tegmentum in the medulla, pons, and locus ceruleus. Norepinephrine has been demonstrated to cause REM sleep; dopamine appears to be less involved with sleep; its major role is in maintaining arousal.[10] REM sleep appears to prime the NREM sleep of serotonergic neurons with both sleeps closely linked.

Genetic factors   There may be an underlying genetic predisposition for sleep apnea.[11] The fact that men have this disease in significant disproportion to women, ranging from 6:1 to 15:1, suggests such a contribution. Further evidence comes from the work by Arkinstall et al.[12] They reported that between 80% to 90% of ventilatory response difference to inhaled CO_2 could be accounted for by genetic factors, pointing toward an inheritance pattern to ventilation regulation and control.

Sleepwalking (somnambulism) and night terrors have been shown to be clinically related and follow a similar inheritance pattern. Both occur during stage III and IV sleep, interfere with sleep, and reflect CNS immaturity. They affect men and women equally. Kales et al studied families of 25 persons with sleepwalking and 27 persons with night terrors.[13] His group found a ten times greater incidence of these disorders in first-degree relatives than in the general population and concluded the two share a common genetic predisposition and adhere to a multifactorial inheritance mode.

In both phases of manic-depressive illness insomnia features prominently. During mania, patients may remain up throughout the entire night. In the depressed phase, patients report early morning awaking. It occurs 25 more times in siblings of patients than in the average population. Winokur et al advance the view of a dominant X-linked transmission pattern for manic-depressive illness.[14] Further perspectives come from the work of Sitaram et al.[15] Patients with bipolar illness had increased cholinergic sensitivity and significantly higher density of eye movements during the first REM sleep, in response to acetylcholine challenge, than did normals.

Environment A noisy environment does not promote sleep. Although people can accommodate to a consistent loud background, eg, living near a busy highway, high-decibel, abrupt, piercing noises cause insomnia.[16] Examples include an airport at dawn, a railroad track only intermittently used, a building being demolished, the people in the next apartment fighting, and the neighbors nailing a new roof at first light. A siren at night, thunder, a dog barking, a car backfiring — all strike at the heart of sleep.

Schedule alterations and variations lead to insomnia. The most common experience involves shift rotation. Persons working different changing time frames, eg, 3 PM to ll PM, then ll PM to 7AM, have difficulty adjusting and adapting to them. They cannot fall asleep during the day "because the sun is out," the whole neighborhood is active, and there are things to do. Frequent shift movements intensify and accelerate the problem. The author recalls the sleep problems attendant to commencing his internship's emergency department rotation.

Similarly, yet more dramatically, rapid changes precipitate sleep disturbances. The classic example involves long airplane trips through many time zones. On an extended passage from east to west, the journeyers encounter a lengthened day. Going west to east, one frequently flies toward the rising sun and experiences a "lost" day. In contrast to rapid changes, slower, more global alterations, such as the hours of daylight, produce less effect upon sleep. Indeed, in those settings, eg, living at the South Pole, group activities and norms dominate the sleep pattern.[17] Persons observe the same sleep sequence as those in temperate zones.

Conditions of the immediate environment — the bed, the bedmate, the room temperature, and the presence of certain irritants — may interfere with sleep. Many people sleep best on particular types of beds, eg, beds with a hard, firm mattress. Or, as Goldilocks said, "This one is just right." They cannot sleep if the bed is "too soft," "too lumpy," "too short," or "too narrow." One bed partner's activities may disturb the mate's sleep: snoring, eating in bed, reading late, or watching television. Many people have strong preferences for nighttime room temperature, and cannot tolerate or sleep in a room if the temperature is too hot or too cold. Dual control electric blankets have proved useful in some of these situations. Finally, certain irritants, such as dripping water or a loudly ticking clock, have disturbed the sleeper.

Intensive care units promote sleep problems. A host of intrusive devices, including monitors, IV recordings, and respirators dominate the environment. The immediate and protracted confrontation with death is always present. The activity around the clock, the lack of privacy, and the medical condition itself — all may interfere with sleep.

Optical stimulation promotes efficient sleep. This represents a theory that each person requires an optimal sensory information flow and load.[18] A low flow and load causes sleep problems; too rapid cadence and too heavy demands lead to insomnia. In the former situation, persons faced with boring, monotonous, uninspiring, or unstimulating environments may have sleep difficulty. In the latter, people confronting too many responsibilities, too much information, too many conflicts, too many stresses become overloaded and cannot sleep. Efficient sleep involves the correct match of sensory input and the person's optimal level of processing. A new young mother was overwhelmed by her "always" hungry baby, the family finances, her mother's impending cancer surgery, and her husband's absence because of his job assignment out of state. She could not sleep.

Overcrowding may lead to sleep problems. This occurs in tenements, in prison, at camp, and sometimes at college. The presence of others, their closeness, their intrusion, their activities, and their noise, as well as the lack of privacy, the violations of personal space, and the inability of individuals to "get away" from others can preclude sleep.

Differential Diagnosis

Nonpsychotropic drugs A host of nonpsychotropic drugs cause insomnia. Most often the sleep disturbance represents a side effect.

Sometimes it signals an excess of the drug. Occasionally, it emerges as a paradoxical effect. The description below offers a survey of the most commonly used medical drugs which either prevent or disrupt sleep.

Adrenocorticosteroids rank as a major precipitant of sleep disturbance.[19,20] These commonly include cortisone, adrenocorticotropic hormone (ACTH), prednisone, and hydrocortisone. These drugs are used to reduce inflammatory processes, eg, ulcerative colitis, treat collagen disease, check multiple sclerosis, and diminish transplanted kidney rejection. A young man received a cadaver kidney and was begun on prednisone. He immediately developed intractable insomnia, pacing, and racing thoughts. He complained of being perpetually energized.

Insomnia develops from the use of certain antiarrhythmic drugs. Specifically, lidocaine and propranolol hydrochloride (Inderal) have been implicated.[21] Lidocaine administered IV has proved useful to treat ventricular arrhythmias. With its lipid solubility, it rapidly enters the CNS and may cause a mild agitation leading to sleep difficulty. Propranolol, a β-adrenergic blocking drug employed to treat hypertension, angina pectoris, and supraventricular arrhythmias, eg, atrial fibrillation and atrial flutter, produces insomnia.[22]

Antihistamines, commonly employed to treat allergic diseases and "head cold" symptoms, often produce sedation. However, not infrequently, they may cause insomnia.[22] The paradoxical response has been noted frequently in children.[21]

Dextrothyroxine sodium (Choloxin) has been used to reduce serum lipids and cholesterol.[22] As an antilipemic and hypocholesterolemic agent, it shares with other thyroid preparations the hypermetabolic effects which include insomnia.

Two antineoplastic drugs, fluorouracil (5-fluorouracil, 5-FU) and procarbazine hydrochloride (Matulane) have been associated with sleep disturbances.[21] Fluorouracil is an antimetabolite which interferes with the biosynthesis of pyrimidine nucleotides and is used to treat cancers of the breast, stomach, colon, pancreas, ovary, bladder, and the head and neck. Procarbazine is a treatment for Hodgkin's disease.

Central nervous system stimulants produce sleep disturbances. By their very action, they cause CNS excitement and lead to insomnia. Amphetamines and their derivatives, eg, dextroamphetamine sulfate (Dexedrine) and phendimetrazine sulfate historically have been employed for weight reduction. They are also currently used to treat narcolepsy. Xanthines (caffeine) represent another group of stimulants well known to coffee and tea drinkers as a stimulant and sleep destroyer. The theophylline derivatives, eg, aminophylline (component of Quinamm), dyphylline, and theophylline represent major drugs that cause bronchial dilation and promote breathing. Not infrequently, one of these CNS stimulants is combined with other medicines, eg, Tedral, which contains both theophylline and ephedrine hydrochloride, or certain aspirins, also have caffeine added to them.

Estrogens have been associated with sleep disturbances. Combined with progestins, they play a major role in oral contraceptives. They have also been used to treat some of the symptoms of menopause, eg, hot flashes and other symptoms of vasomotor activity. They produce paroxysmal EEG activity suggestive of a role as a CNS excitant.[21]

Sympathomimetic drugs cause insomnia. As a group, these drugs mimic the effects of sympathetic nervous system stimulation and produce increased heart rate, myocardial contraction, and myocardial conductivity, dilation of muscle vasculature, constricted vessels to skin and viscera, CNS excitement, relaxation of bronchi, intestine, and bladder smooth muscles, and sphincter constriction. The sympathic system includes both α_1, α_2 and β_1, β_2 receptors and the naturally occurring activating compounds are epinephrine, norepinephrine, and dopamine.

A number of sympathomimetic drugs have been commonly associated with sleep disturbances. The majority are used as bronchial dilators. They include ephedrine compounds, epinephrine, isoproterenol hydrochloride, phenylephrine hydrochloride, phenylpropanolamine hydrochloride, and pseudoephedrine. A woman started on asthma medicine started to breathe easier but found herself more jumpy and sleeping with more difficulty.

The use of thyroid preparations can lead to insomnia. Generally, these drugs are used to treat hypothyroidism (myxedema) and simple goiter; but occasionally in the past they have been employed for weight reduction. Preparations include levothyroxine sodium, liothyronine sodium, thyroid desiccated, and thyrotropin. Sleep difficulty develops if the thyroid is given too rapidly or prescribed in excess.

Psychotropic drugs

Antipsychotic drugs produce akathisia, which leads to disturbed sleep.[23] Akathisia, a dyskinesia, represents motor restlessness and is characterized by an irresistible urge to move about. [22] Patients complain of an inability to sit still. They note their legs will not stop moving at night when they lie down.[23] They report feelings of "wanting to jump out of their skin."[24] This side effect occurs with all antipsychotic drugs; phenothiazines, especially the piperazine group; haloperidol; and to some extent the thioxanthenes. The antidopaminergic effects of these drugs in the basal ganglia account for this reaction. Akathisia also leads many patients to discontinue their antipsychotic drugs.

Additionally, abrupt withdrawal of the neuroleptic drugs causes insomnia. Patients complain of increased activity, restlessness, nightmares, and sleep difficulty. These symptoms represent medical signs of withdrawal rather than an exacerbation of the schizophrenia.[25]

Antidepressants may account for sleep disturbance. The tricyclic drugs increase stage IV sleep and markedly decrease REM sleep. However, not infrequently the initiation of imipramine treatment is accompanied by difficulty in falling asleep. Tricyclic antidepressants may also trigger a manic episode in patients with manic-depressive illness. The monoamine oxidase inhibitors cause insomnia.

The drugs used to treat hyperactivity often lead to sleep disturbance. Common drugs include dextroamphetamine, methylphenidate hydrochloride, and pemoline. All represent CNS stimulants and produce insomnia by CNS excitement and activation.

Sedatives and hypnotic drugs lead to insomnia in several ways. Withdrawal of hypnotic drugs produces less total sleep with shortened NREM sleep in stages II, III, and IV, and decreased stability during sleep.[26] Indeed, withdrawal of sleeping medicine is often accompanied by insomnia.[27] In another form, the patients may experience sleep disturbance because of partial drug withdrawal during the night as the sedative, through long-term administration, looses its efficiency. Kales et al describe this as drug dependency insomnia.[28] With chronic use, tolerance develops and patients have sleep patterns marked by frequent awakenings, diminished REM and NREM sleep, and an EEG with beta wave activity.[29] Finally, patients taking benzodiazepines report frightening, disturbing dreams which interfere with sleep.

Alcohol   Alcohol in all three phases of use can produce insomnia.

Acute alcohol consumption may lead to sleep disturbances.[30] Its major effect is to reduce REM sleep.[31] Many persons after a few drinks experience difficulty falling asleep and staying asleep. Alcohol also causes an increase in hydrochloric acid secretion. In turn, gastric acid excess leads to gastritis and peptic ulcers, which interrupt sleep because of the resultant abdominal pain and discomfort.

Chronic alcohol use may result in insomnia. Many persons with long histories of alcohol use and abuse report restless sleep, frequent awakenings, disturbing dreams, and sleep difficulty. Their EEGs demonstrate decreased stage IV sleep and fragmentation of the sleep pattern.[32] The fragmentation indicates many frequent changes in sleep stages throughout the night. Of interest, these alterations of sleep persist for up to at least 1 to 2 years of abstinence. Another cause of insomnia in chronic alcoholic use develops out of nutritional deficiencies.

Alcohol withdrawal is often accompanied by explosive, dramatic, and threatening sleep disturbances. In mild forms, patients complain of needing a drink to sleep . In the severe form, the patient, although agitated, physically exhausted, is unable to sleep. The major finding of withdrawal sleep remains the excessive amount of REM sleep. REM sleep at 100% of the sleep record constitutes a precursor of delirium tremens.[33] Due to a severe snowstorm, a man with a long drinking history could not get a drink. Within three days, he complained of insomnia, after tossing and turning all night. He reported terrifying nightmares and threatening visual images. He became disoriented and his temperature rose.

Other abused substances   Amphetamines rank as a predominant sleep disrupter with the insomnia reflecting their CNS excitement, stimulation, and arousal effects. Indeed, "dexies," "uppers," "bennies," or "speed" is taken for these reactions. They produce a marked decrease in REM sleep while at the same time promoting heightened body activity and movement during sleep.[34] During chronic use, the REM sleep returns to it normal proportion.[35] And during withdrawal, there is a dramatic increase in REM sleep. A man took "black beauties" (amphetamine) for the high. He could not sleep for three days and nights. He reported he was "flying."

Insomnia follows as a result of barbiturate withdrawal. Within 36 hours to 1 week of abrupt barbiturate termination, drug-dependent persons will show signs and symptoms not unlike delirium tremens.[36] Because of the additional danger of convulsions and status epilepticus, the barbiturates should be tapered during discontinuance, and the patient closely observed.[37]

Cocaine use results in euphoria, decreased sleep, and insomnia. Patients like the elation, the "rush," the heightened awareness, and the high. Often they combine cocaine with amphetamine and heroin. A man was brought by friends to the emergency department. He had been inhaling fine cocaine. He could not sleep; he could not stop talking; and he felt "too good."[37]

Disturbed sleep results from opiate withdrawal, especially if done abruptly. The patients pass through the initial phase of rhinorrhea, yawning, and perspiration within 12 to 14 hours. This is followed by gooseflesh and dilated pupils. Within 36 hours they develop cramps, muscle twitches, intense restlessness, and an inability to sleep, along with an elevated pulse and blood pressure.

Medical illness A host of medical illnesses present as insomnia.

Sleep apnea constitutes a major medical cause of insomnia. The definition is at least 30 apneic episodes during seven hours of sleep in both REM and NREM sleep and with a number of apneic episodes in sequence during REM sleep.[38] This syndrome occurs much more commonly in men than in women. Many symptoms accompany sleep apnea: excessive motor activity during sleep, eg, agitation, kicking bed partners, or sleep walking; snoring, loud, excessive daytime sleeping; daytime actions done in an automatic way, intellectual diminution, hypnagogic hallucinations, personality alterations, and outbursts; impotence and decreased libido; morning headaches; and nocturnal enuresis.

Sleep apnea has three types of causes: obstructive, central, and mixed. In obstructive sleep apnea, there is a physical impediment in the upper airway at the oropharyngeal level. Due to loss of abductor muscle tone during inspiration, the airway actually collapses. The treatment involves a modified chronic tracheostomy. Central sleep apnea has its origin in problems with the metabolic control system for NREM sleep. The underlying respiratory center malfunction may be due to infections, vascular complications, or neoplasms.[39] A similar disorder with metabolic control of respirations has been suggested for sudden infant death syndrome (SIDS). In the mixed type, central sleep apnea precedes the development of upper-airway obstruction.

A 35-year-old man complained of insomnia. Because of this, he dozed off all too frequently on the job and was fired. He snored and "wracked" the bed each night. Studies showed his breathing ceased many times during the night, his upper airway became obstructed before each episode. A tracheostomy reversed this condition.

Asthma attacks at night constitute another cause of insomnia. In asthma, the tracheobronchial tree has heightened responsiveness to a wide variety of stimuli, eg, allergens, aspirin, air pollutants, infection, and emotional stress, and reacts by generalized narrowing of the air passages. The difficulty in breathing and the wheezing represent reduced expiratory flow rates, hyperinflation, and heightened airway resistance.[40] The wheezing, coughing, and orthopnea—shortness of breath—all interfere with sleep. One 45-year-old woman with severe asthma has not slept for months. Finally, as a result of hospital treatment which controlled the asthma, she slept for up to 20 hours per day for the first week.

Gastroesphageal reflux leads to sleep difficulties.[8] An incompetent lower esophageal sphincter causes this condition. As a result, gastric acid is refluxed into the esophagus producing symptoms of heartburn. Large meals or lying down may aggravate the discomfort. The heartburn may simulate angina pectoris. The presence of low pH (1.5-2.0) fluid in the esophagus helps to confirm the diagnosis. Heartburn, a burning epigastric, or retrosternal pain which spreads upward, may disturb or may actually preclude sleep.

Patients with duodenal ulcers experience sleep disturbances. The abdominal discomfort, the "trip" for milk, in the middle of the night, and pain—all contribute to the disruption. Peptic ulcers result from excess gastric acid secretion. In cases of patients with duodenal ulcers, they have a secretion rate three to 20 times greater than normal during sleep. Further, gastric acid secretion has been correlated with REM sleep.[41] A 50-year-old executive worrier could not sleep for weeks before her son's wedding. A gnawing stomach pain usually three to four hours after eating relieved by mild antacids would wake her up. An upper GI study demonstrated a duodenal ulcer.

Angina, chest pain, wakes up patients at night. This form of angina pectoris has been called angina decubitus referring to pain occurring in the recumbent position.[41] It is similar in quality to exertional pain and has been described as a "pressure," "squeezing," or "tightness" in the chest. Studies suggest dreaming and REM sleep both precede the ECG changes of angina (significant ST segment depression) and correlates with the angina.[42] The angina represents transient myocardial ischemia. These patients have evidence of atherosclerosis. Stress testing with ST depression during typical angina symptoms is diagnostic. Also, coronary arteriography proves the atherosclerotic presence.

Congestive heart failure (CHF) interferes with sleep. Patients with CHF experience paroxysmal nocturnal dyspnea (sudden attacks of shortness of breath) and orthopnea (dyspnea while recumbent). Episodes of coughing, wheezing, and difficulty breathing punctuate their night. They often require several pillows to sleep on. Clinical evidence of heart failure includes basal pulmonary rales, dependent edema, hepatomegaly, ascites, weight loss, and hydrothorax. Roentgenograms reveal an enlarged heart, lung, vascular changes, and pleural effusion. A 35-year-old man could not sleep. He coughed, he had difficulty breathing, and he wheezed all night. When he slipped off the pillow, he had shortness of breath. He had congestive heart failure.

Uremic patients complain of insomnia. Renal failure causes uremia, marked by axotemia, and elevation in serum nonprotein nitrogen, the BUN. This condition leads to sporadic muscle movements which frequently are amplified at night, producing sleep disturbance.[43] Additionally, these patients have less total sleep, less slow-wave (stages II and IV) sleep, and less organized sleep cycles than normal.[41] Uremia also results in a pruritus (itching), which disrupts sleep.

Pain, regardless of the source, ranks as a paramount sleep destroyer. Patients in pain cannot fall asleep; they cannot stay asleep, and they cannot get back to sleep. Acute pain, chronic aching, intermittent, sharp "stabbing" sensations, and dull throbbing experiences — all devastate and devour the night.

Prominent causes of nocturnal pain include duodenal ulcers (discussed earlier), arthritis, cancer, carpal tunnel syndrome, spinal disorders, and headaches.

The chronic pain of rheumatoid arthritis causes disordered sleep. Insomnia, not responsive to the usual treatment as a result of epigastric pain, may be one of the earliest indications of pancreatice carcinoma.[43] In the carpal tunnel syndrome, there is pressure upon the median nerve as it passes between the wrist bones and transverse carpal ligament. This frequently occurs in middle-aged women and has a pain which is characteristically most intense at night. Pain in the spinal area often disrupts sleep. Headaches of all types, eg, migraine, cluster, and tension, destroy sleep.

Allergic rhinitis through its symptoms disorders sleep. Typical presentations of this include rhinorrhea, nasal passage obstruction, conjunctival and pharyngeal pruritus, sneezing, and lacrimation. Wind-borne pollens from grass and trees, mold spores, and dust precipitate this immune-mediated disease. The rhinitis has a seasonal appearance and history. A 38-year-old woman every fall bitterly complained of a runny nose, teary eyes, and constant sneezing which kept her up all night.

Nocturnal myoclonus ranks as a primary sleep disorder and a common cause of chronic insomnia.[44] Patients experience sudden muscle jerks in the lower extremities throughout the night. The repetitive myoclonic activity leads to frequent arousals and protracted fatigue. Their beds look like battlefields in the morning. They kick their bedmates during the night. The myoclonic discharge occurs more in NREM sleep than in REM sleep.[7]

Restless legs syndrome represents another common primary sleep disorder.[44] Patients develop an incredible irresistible desire and urge to walk about. This occurs in the twilight period between awakening and sleep. Deep paresthesias in the lower extremities frequently accompany the condition. It has also been associated with folic acid deficiency and uremia.[43]

Seizures occur during sleep. Most often they do not clinically cause arousal, although they clearly may be observed by the bedmate. Sleep brings out the seizure activity with some only manifesting such activity during sleep. In a study of 645 epileptic patients, 38 had seizures only during sleep.[44]

Drug overdoses lead to persistent insomnia for up to 2 months afterward.[45] Patients complain of restlessness and sleep disturbances following an overdose. The clinical picture observed is a result of hypnotic drug withdrawal. There is also an increase during the postoverdose period in REM sleep. A significant degree of drug tolerance and dependence may occur during an overdose with subsequent signs and symptoms of drug withdrawal, yielding sleep disturbances.

Aging itself accounts for sleep difficulty. With maturity comes insomnia, with a marked decline in stage IV sleep. Persons 60 years of age have only 45% as much of stage IV sleep as those 20 years old.[46] Similarly, the 60-year-olds have 86% more awakenings than the 20-year-olds. These changes reflect the alterations physiologically of brain function processes. However, the clinician must be alert to a concomitant or causative depression in this group.[47]

A 75-year-old man experienced severe chronic insomnia. He had noticed progressive sleep difficulty over the last 15 years. He worried about finances in retirement and napped often during the day. He used hypnotics excessively for a long time. He made frequent trips to the bathroom throughout the night. He feared death. All these factors contributed to the sleep difficulty.

Although aging provides one explanation for insomnia, it should not be assumed youth is protection against sleep difficulty. A study by Price et al reported that 13% of eleventh and twelfth graders experienced severe, chronic sleep difficulty.[48] Worrying, family problems, tension, and negative self-images contributed to this picture.

Hyperthyroidism causes fragmented, shortened sleep. It also increases delta sleep — stages III and IV. Patients may have excessive sweat, tachycardia, dyspnea, heightened appetite, emotional lability, hyperkinesia, muscle fatigability, heat intolerance, a fine tremor, hyperdefecation, and decreased concentration ability.[49] Graves' disease accounts for the most common forms of hyperthyroidism. A 35-year-old woman became hyperactive, supertalkative, complained of being too hot, and could not sleep. She had developed hyperthyroidism. In contrast, in hyperthyroidism, sleep is increased and stage III and IV sleep is decreased.

Diabetes contributes to sleep disturbances. The cardinal clinical signs of polyuria, polydipsia, and polyphagia all disrupt sleep. Pruritus may interfere with the night's rest.

Nutrition influences sleep. In the simplest example, infants when hungry at night awaken and cry. Once fed they return to sleep. Decreased nutritional intake and the resultant weight loss cause sleep disruptions. This is observed in the sleep disturbances of patients with anorexia nervosa. The basic formula emerges: weight loss correlates to reduced sleep duration, fragmented sleep pattern, and early morning awakening.[50]

Painful nocturnal penile erections disturb sleep. This occurs in the urologic condition, Peyronie's disease.[51] In this disease, there is induration and inflammation of the penis's corpora cavernosa. As a result, the penis becomes painful during erection. The disease usually happens to men in their fifth and sixth decades. Other features of the disease include a "lump" in the penis, penis curvature in erection, and poor ejection beyond the plaque.

Normally, men will experience seven to eight erections during sleep throughout the night. The erections occur during REM sleep.[52] If they have Peyronie's disease, each erection may be painful and may interrupt sleep.

Surgical complications

Preoperative insomnia is an expected, natural occurrence.[53] Many patients about to undergo surgery experience sleep disturbances, which represents their anxiety, apprehension, and concerns regarding the impending surgery. Modern operative consent forms often spell out in incredible minute detail the surgical risks and consequences. Each person before surgery faces loss of control, the "knife," and death.

Pain in the postoperative period interferes with sleep. Usually the pain occurs at the incision site. However, it may result from the body's position during the procedure. Certainly, as suggested earlier, any pain may devastate sleep.

Postoperative infection may also interfere with sleep through either pain or fever. A 20-year-old man sustained a fractured left femur which required surgical intervention and traction. He developed osteomyelitis. The pain of the fracture and surgery, the traction, the postoperative infection, and his concerns about his athletic future — all contribute to his insomnia.

The use of opiates in the postoperative course leads to insomnia in two ways. First, the opiate sedation causes sleeping during the day. As a result, the patient goes to bed at night already "well rested," interfering with the day/night sequence. Second, too abrupt tapering off of opiates, eg, morphine, following surgery may lead to opiate withdrawal symptoms.

Alcohol and hypnotic withdrawal in the postoperative period causes insomnia. Often, the surgery is emergent or one physician obtains less than a complete alcohol and drug history. As a consequence patients experience unanticipated or unappreciated signs and symptoms of alcohol or hypnotic withdrawal following surgery.

Physical trauma

Head trauma may result in insomnia. In one study 15% of patients who sustained a concussion had sleep disturbances at 6 weeks.[54] Insomnia, along with oversensitivity to intense stimuli, headaches, vertigo, dizziness, fatigability, decreased tolerance to alcohol, inability to concentrate, and emotional lability constitute the postconcussion syndrome.[2]

Spinal injury produces sleep difficulty. The disturbances depend upon the actual location of the spinal insult. Specially, high cervical lesions cause decreased total sleep, eg, initially to five hours per night, markedly increased light sleep, reduced deep sleep, and diminished REM sleep.[55] In contrast, thoracic lesions do not interfere with sleep.[56] This comparison supports the role of the cervical spinal cord and particularly the possibility of the rostral pontine nuclei in inducing REM sleep.

A posttraumatic stress disorder may lead to sleep disturbances.[57] In this disorder, the patients respond to a recognizable devastation with intrusion and recurrent recall of the actual event, recurrent dreams, "flashbacks," "numbing," hyperalertness, sleep difficulty, avoidance of things which activate recall of the event, memory impairment, and reliving of the event because of things which resemble the initial insult. Traumatic events include automobile accidents, sports mishaps—eg, skiing accidents—falls, rape, electrical or other burns, near drowning, gunshot wounds, and physical assaults. A woman sustained a fractured femur in an automobile accident on a rainy evening. Each rainy day thereafter, she could not sleep that night. During the day she thought of the accident.

After having trouble getting to sleep, vivid, terrifying nightmares woke her. The dreams depicted the accident in "too much detail" and pain.

Psychiatric disorders   Insomnia ranks as a major psychiatric symptom and a cardinal sign of distress. It occurs alone or as a part of a constellation of symptoms. It may be incapacitating or just annoying. It often potentiates or aggravates the condition, eg, a depression. The following diagnoses represent those in which insomnia often plays a critical role. However, sleep disturbances frequently are part of many other conditions.

Delirium   often involves and presents with marked sleep disturbances.[57] It interrupts the day/night cycle. Patients experience difficulty in distinguishing their reality, eg, illusions and dreams, from actual events. Other signs of delirium include clouded consciousness, hallucinations, disorientation, and recall deficits. It develops rapidly within hours to days, and its presentation fluctuates throughout the day. An organic condition is the cause of delirium.

Schizophrenic disorders   During the prodromal phase and the acute phase of the schizophrenic disorders, patients may display evidence of sleep difficulty. They may complain of voices in the head arguing and keeping them awake. They may assume hypervigilant stance which precludes sleep. Or they may become so excited and anxious that they cannot sleep. The presence of bizarre delusions, delusions of grandeur, nihilism, or religion, loose associations, ego observations, auditory hallucinations, and a flat affect with evidence of functioning deterioration within the last 6 months, suggests the insomnia is part of a schizophrenic decompensation process.

A dramatic decrease in sleep ranks as a major sign of a *manic episode* . Patients do not report insomnia and often become indignant at the suggestion that they should "get some rest." Their lives are too full of other things, projects, goals, challenges, and activities to consider sleeping. They sleep a few hours a night and start their adventures very early in the morning. Other signs include heightened activity, restlessness, talkativeness, flight of ideas, grandiosity, distraction, and high level to excess of involvement in many ventures. There is frequently a family history of manic-depressive illness as well as the episode occurring within the context of the individual's background as a bipolar disease.

Insomnia constitutes a key symptom of a *major depressive episode* . The depression may occur in the context of manic-depressive illness or stand as a single episode. In the latter, the major depression happens without a history of a manic episode. Often early morning awakening characterizes this sleep disturbance. Patients exhibit a profound depressed affect, have a poor appetite with accompanying weight loss, feel hopeless, helpless, worthless, complain of no energy or interest, and struggle with guilt. The dysphoric mood permeates and dominates their lives and has been present every day for at least 2 weeks.

In the *cyclothymic disorder*, patients experience sleep disturbances to a lesser degree then in the manic and depressive episodes, within the context of the mood swings and conditions being also less severe. The hypomanic periods are marked by a decreased need for sleep along with high self-esteem, restlessness, involvement excesses, and hypersexuality. The depressive periods have sleep disturbances along with social withdrawal, decreased involvements, lost sex interest, pessimism, lowered productivity, and crying spells.

The dysthymic disorder includes in its depressive periods evidence of insomnia. These individuals have sustained depression symptoms for 2 years but the symptoms are not of sufficient severity to rank as a major depression episode. They involve social withdrawal, periods of crying, thoughts of death, decreased productivity, lost energy, reduced talking, and low self-esteem. Again, a depressed mood dominates their lives.

Sleep disturbances clinically represent a manifestation of adjustment disorders. These disorders designate a maladaptive response to a clear, stressing event, eg, divorce, separation, or a child leaving home. The event has happened within the last 3 months. As patients attempt to integrate the experience, they often have difficulty functioning. Insomnia is one signal of their distress and of their working it out.

Posttraumatic stress disorder profoundly alters sleep. Patients reexperience the actual trauma in the night through nightmares and intrusive recollections. They develop insomnia as well as evidence of psychic numbing. They withdraw from the external world. They avoid situations that might trigger recall. They may have survivor guilt.

Insomnia stands as a compelling, pervasive symptom and sign. It demands a comprehensive evaluation and approach. The alert clinician must explore the psychological, social, and biological dimensions of it. In the psychodynamic realm, depression dominates the etiology.

EXCESSIVE SLEEP   Too prolonged, too excessive, too consuming, too exaggerated, too protracted, too interfering, or too inappropriately timed sleep. In contrast to insomnia where sleep cannot be obtained, here the patient can and does sleep but to an excess or at the wrong time.

Case report A 30-year-old man sleeps too much. Not only does he spend his "life in bed" during the evenings and nights, but also he all too frequently, dramatically, suddenly naps during the day. He has suffered several recent business and personal reverses and there is a family history of excessive sleep. At the interview he appears apathetic; his family is distraught; and his employer, irate.

Features

Mood Excessive sleep occurs within the broad context of a number of emotions. Some of these feelings have contributed to the sleep picture. Others represent the patient's response to sleeping too much.

Depression contributes one of the cardinal features of hypersomnolence. Patients feel sad, dejected, defeated, despondent, and melancholic. Their world stands eclipsed, destroyed, and devastated. Their future appears bleak. Resignation reigns over their affective experience.

Apathy arises as another common experience of patients with excessive sleep. They find themselves indifferent, detached, and uninvolved with their universe. They display a marked and remarkable nonpresence and noncommitment in the face of major life confrontation.

In contrast, *anger* not infrequently emerges as a dominant emotion. Patients may be enraged, embittered, and embattled at the world. They portray clear dissatisfaction with everything, or alternately they may rage at their excessive sleep. Because all they do is sleep, they are deprived of living.

Thoughts One of two contrasting preoccupations predominate the thoughts of patients who sleep excessively. Either they are totally concerned, bothered, puzzled, perplexed, and obsessed by their sleep pattern, or they do not care. In the former, they present as struggling with symptoms, bewildered by the dilemma, and searching for an answer. They ask why is this happening and seek help. In the latter, denial, resignation, acceptance, and avoidance dominate their thoughts. They face a catastrophic situation with an air of intellectual noninvolvement.

Hallucinations may play a role in their thought processes. Some experience hypnagogic hallucinations, occurring during sleep onset, and these are either visual or auditory in character. Others choose a path of sleep to avoid terrifying, overwhelming, and threatening voices or images. A 22-year-old schizophrenic man took to bed as a way to silence the voices shouting and quarreling in his head.

Similarly, *delusions* may present as a precipitator of excessive sleep.

Sleep provides an answer to a world perceived to be filled with danger, demons, devils, and devastation. Sleep offers both an escape and a respite to the delusional patients. They secure a moment of satiety in the slumber world existence.

Disorientation may emerge as a result of excessive sleep. Indeed the American Psychiatric Association glossary includes in the definition of hypersomnia, excessive sleep followed by wakening confusion.[58] Certainly too much sleep can prove to be a disorienting experience. The classic tale of Rip Van Winkle sparkingly emphasizes this phenomenon.

Behavior Excessive sleeping, in and of itself, remains the cardinal behavior, and the principle feature of this condition. The sleep problem may take several forms. First, the patient may simply sleep all day and all night. Second, they may sleep too much at night, namely, to bed at 7 PM and up at 11:30 AM. Third, they may sleep too much during the day. The quiet nap becomes the day's activity. Fourth, the sleep may happen at inopportune and inappropriate times, eg, at work, on the job, or suddenly when active.

Patients may undertake a variety of behaviors to challenge their excess sleep. They may turn to caffeine, using coffee, tea, and colas.[59] They may use stimulants. They may employ thrill events or forced excitement. One college student tried four alarm clocks to break the sleep cycle.

A number of sleep behaviors may be manifest, eg, tossing and turning, loudly snoring, or experiencing moments of apnea.

Physical examination and laboratory findings

Physical examination A number of important findings, within the context of a complete physical examination, have been associated with hypersomnolence. Obesity has been correlated with excessive sleep syndromes. Signs of hypothryroidism—hair loss, dry skin, macroglossia, emotionless face, hoarse voice, and general dullness—may be present. Hyperpigmentation occurs in hypoadrenalism; upper airway obstruction in sleep apnea; narcoleptic patients show ptosis and diplopia.

Laboratory findings A variety of studies are particularly relevant in this workup. The EEG, especially done during sleep, remains one of the most important tests. As discussed in the insomnia section, not only are the characteristics of each stage significant, but also their sequence provides major clues. A blood count is critical. Thyroid studies are quite useful as well as an ECG. Blood gases and electrolytes offer further clues.

Interviewer's reaction Clinicians find themselves with a variety of responses. Some will underemphasize the extension and importance of the excessive sleep because the patient does. These patients may minimize their symptoms. History from family members will often counter this. Some will feel challenged by the phenomenon and almost too aggressively pursue a vigorous workup, not recognizing certain patients' protracted sleep defense. Others will realize the devastation and debilitation of the symptoms and will carefully and compassionately search for an explanation.

Pathogenesis

Psychodynamics Excessive sleep represents a major reaction to a loss and reflects resultant depression. The loss takes many forms: of position, of love partner, of employment, of health, of home, of income, of an aspiration, of hope, of freedom, of options, and of children. Not uncommonly some patients may turn to sleep following the death of an important person. A banker lost his wife of 45 years to cancer. He grieved; he cried; and he slept. He felt incapable of leaving his bed.

Avoidance constitutes a power dynamic behind excessive sleep. Many patients through sleep avoid a remarkable range of discomforting, disquieting situations; meeting people, going to work, leaving the house, making a critical decision, or taking a test. A shy, quiet, physically and socially awkward young man took to bed early each weekday night and all weekend days to avoid any possibility of a social encounter.

Withdrawal provides another dynamic explanation for hypersomnolence. Here patients are withdrawing from known stresses, in contrast to avoiding a future of imagined difficulty. Patients turn to sleep to escape an attacking spouse, a painful environment, a medical disease, or an impossible assignment.

Biologic explanation The driving influence on sleep resides anatomically and physiologically within the brainstem.[60] A complete explanation was presented earlier in the discussion on insomnia. Biogenic amines are responsible for NREMs and REMs cycle and interplay. Within the lower midbrain, pons, and medulla are serotonergic neurons. These neurons project into the hypothalamus, thalamus, and the orbital, frontal, and median temporal areas of the cortex and are triggered by factor S. When these neurons fire, they suppress the reticular formation and produce sleep, hypersomnolence, and diminished consciousness. Through destruction of these neurons or through serotonin antagonist drugs, insomnia develops.

Genetics *Narcolepsy* has a significant genetic component. Between 20% and 33% of patients with this disorder will have other family members also with it.[61] Kessler demonstrated in direct relatives of 50 narcoleptic patients an incidence of narcolepsy of 18% and of excessive sleep disorders of 34%.[62]

Sleep apnea also has a genetic contribution as outlined in the insomnia section.

Major depression runs in families and has been demonstrated to have strong genetic patterns as reviewed in chapter 2. Manic-depressive illness has been linked to a single gene on the X chromosome near the color blindness gene.[63]

Environment *Confinement* generates excessive sleep. Persons finding themselves physically trapped and imprisoned often turn to the bed. Not infrequently, inmates in the county jail respond to their sentences through sleep. The trap yields to despair, depression, resignation, withdrawal, and despondency. Sleep becomes the reaction to boredom and monotony.[64]

Similarly, forced *inactivity* will produce hypersomnolence. The young man in traction following a skiing accident, the executive being monitored in bed following a myocardial infarction, and the pregnant woman placed at bed rest during the last trimester to ensure a healthy delivery, all may experience excessive sleeping. The inactivity leads also to frustration, depression, and dejection.[65] Especially in those prone to physical activity and release of tension through that mode, the lack of action proves to be a burden.

Finally, the addition of *indeterminants* to the sense of confinement and inactivity cause excessive sleep. Many can endure difficult, stressful, and painful situations if they know they will eventually be relieved and helped. The lack of hope dramatically amplifies the predicament, accelerates the despair and leads to the sleep escape. "The light at the end of the tunnel" does keep many people going.

Differential Diagnosis

Nonpsychotropic drugs

Antihypertensive drugs produce sedation. Methyldopa inhibits decarboxylation of dopa and 5-hydroxytryptophan with the subsequent diminishing of CNS and peripheral 5-hydroxytryptamine, dopamine, and norepinephrine. Additionally, methyldopa is broken down into α-methylnorepine-phrine which serves as a false norepinephrine transmitter. The overall re-sults include not only decrease of blood pressure but also an initial tiredness, drowsiness, and protracted lassitude. Clonidine demonstrates α-adrenergic stimulation to the vasomotor centers especially in the medulla oblongata and, as a result, inhibition occurs in peripheral sympathetic activity and blood pressure is lowered. Here too sedation represents a sig-nificant early side effect. Prazosin hydrochloride, an α-adrenergic blocker of smooth vessel musculature, causes fatigue and drowsiness.

Propranolol hydrochloride has, as one of its side effects, hyper-somnia.[66]

This β-adrenergic blocker exercises a profound control over high sym-pathetic cardiac stimulation. It has major clinical application in the treat-ment of hypertension, cardiac arrhythmias, anxiety, and in patients with recurrent myocardial infarctions.[67] The excessive sleep often reflects the propranolol-induced depression.[68]

Anticonvulsants can cause excessive sleepiness.[69] Phenytoin, in excess, precipitates mental status alternations of dullness and drowsiness in addition to nystagmus, diplopia, blurred vision, mydriasis, and ataxia. Initiation of barbiturate therapy yields sedation which diminishes as toler-ance develops. Ethotoin accounts for the drowsiness and primidone toxicity is characterized by sedation along with nystagmus, ataxia, nausea and vertigo, and diplopia. Carbamazepine, employed for both the treat-ment of epilepsy and trigeminal neuralgia, produces similar toxic effects. Ethosuximide is responsible for often contrasting mental and behavioral changes ranging from lethargy and tiredness to agitation and restlessness. Trimethadione, used to treat absence seizures, also has sedation as a major toxic effect. Certainly, any of the benzodiazepines employed as anticonvul-sants trigger somnolence, lassitude, quietness, drowsiness, and tiredness.

Antihistamines often cause hypersomnia. Acting as histamine antagonists, these drugs find wide application for anaphylactic and allergic reactions, for motion sickness, and for control of gastric secretions. How-ever, they also serve as CNS depressants and commonly have sedation as a prominent side effect.

Psychotropic Drugs

The benzodiazepines may produce excessive sleep two ways. As tranquilizers, they may cause tiredness, drowsiness, and apathy. Patients report feelings of being removed, detached, and noninvolved with their environment because of the drug-induced sedation. As hypnotic drugs, some patients will experience too much sleep from the benzodiazepines. Not uncommonly, early morning sleepiness occurs before tolerance develops.[70] The CNS effects of the benzodiazepines include decrease of REM sleep, shortening of stage III and IV sleep, an increase in total sleep, and a diminution of the mesoencephalic reticular formation activity.[71] Alcohol appears to potentiate and heighten these drugs' sedative features.

Neuroleptic drugs may yield excessive sleep as a side effect. Of the phenothiazines, chlorpromazine and thioridazine have the most sedative qualities. Physicians have employed this feature when treating psychotic patients who show marked agitation, anxiety, and disruptiveness.

Certain *antidepressants* possess sedating properties. Amitriptyline hydrochloride and doxepin hydrochloride have been particularly noted for these effects. These drugs are frequently employed to treat the agitated depression. Used at night they not only work to reverse the depression but also as an hypnotic drug.

Overdoses of benzodiazepines, neuroleptics, or antidepressants will trigger excessive sleep, stupor, coma, and in certain situations may be fatal.

Alcohol For some people alcohol has immensely sedating powers. When they drink, they sleep. Excessive sleep may follow in the wake of one or two drinks for certain individuals. For others, drinking to a significant excess leads to sleep, stupor, and a semicomatose condition.

Other Abused Substances

Amphetamine withdrawal has hypersomnia as one of its cardinal features. During the first three days following drug discontinuance, patients exhibit profound sleep. This sleep period lasts from 24 to 48 hours.[72] Patients, in addition to depression, experience REM rebound in response to the amphetamine induced REM deprivation.[73] Clinically, patients report many dreams during this withdrawal period.

Barbiturate abuse commonly produces excessive sleep. Indeed, the street name, "downers," underscores this sedative quality. Patients require more and more barbiturates to obtain the quieting effects as they develop tolerance to these drugs. Additionally, overdoses of barbiturates lead to sleep and coma, and alcohol potentiates their sedative effect.

Cocaine withdrawal is also accompanied by excessive sleep. Cocaine serves as a stimulant, and its discontinuance triggers depression, lethargy, and hypersomnolence. Patients' reactions are similar to those observed with amphetamine withdrawal. A 25-year-old student got high on "coke" for several days; he stopped using it and then promptly "crashed." He slept for two days and then experienced a depression, which only slowly resolved.

The opiate experience, in addition to the sought after euphoria, is marked by drowsiness and apathy.[74] Patients use opiates to gain this sedation, quiet, and emotional distance. As with barbiturates, a protracted involvement leads to dependence and tolerance. Excessive sleep follows in the wake of opiate overdoses.

Medical Diseases

Hypothyroidism leads to lethargy, physical and mental slowness, and diminished appetite with weight gain. In its extreme form myxedema produces hypersomnolence. Myxedematous patients not only exhibit a dull emotionless appearance, cool skin, little hair, and orbital puffiness, but also a large tongue. This macroglossia condition causes an obstructive sleep apnea and the resultant hypersomnia.[74] Thyroxin treatment reversed the myxedema, the tongue enlargement, the sleep apnea, and excessive sleepiness.

Menstruation has been reported as linked to excessive sleep. A 16-year-old developed hypersomnia lasting from 1 to 2 weeks accompanying each period.[75] Laboratory studies demonstrated no hormonal abnormalities, a decreased CSF homovanillic acid (HVA), and 5-hydroxyindoleacetic acid (5-HIAA) during excessive sleep episodes. In contrast to symptom-free times, the EEG during hypersomnia featured alpha activity and occasional spike and slow-wave complexes. Once ovulation was pharmacologically prevented, the excessive sleep is shattered.

Infections account for the hypersomnolence phenomenon. Encephalitis lethargica, also called von Economo's disease and sleeping sickness, represents the first instance in humans of a slow viral infection to the central nervous system.[76] It developed in 1914 and for the 10 years thereafter, the influenza epidemic occurred. A profound sleep and opthalmoplegia constituted the outstanding characteristics of this disease. Tuberculous basilar meningitis also causes hypersomnia.[61]

An infection of the hemoflagellate, *Trypahosoma brucei* , results in African trypanosomiasis or sleeping sickness.[77] Species of tsetse flies transmit the two epidemic forms of *Trypanosoma* to humans: *T brucei gambiense* in tropical western and central Africa and the *T brucei rhodesiense* in eastern Africa. The major manifestations of this fusiform protozoan parasitic infection include a febrile lymphadenopathy followed by a chronic fetal meningoencephalomyelitis. Of the two, the Rhodesian is more severe, leading to death within the year; the Gambian produces intermittent bouts of sickness over a number of years. In both the classic picture of sleeping sickness emerges: an expressionless look, droopy eyelids, loose lower lip, and progressive difficulty in arousability. Anemia, hypermacroglobulinemia, cerebrospinal fluid with mononuclear pleocytosis and heightened concentration of protein, and identification of the trypanosome in blood, lymph node, or CSF provide the diagnosis.

Two metabolic conditions generate the clinical hypersomnolent presentation. Uremia, a syndrome resulting from severe renal failure, in addition to anemia, hypertension, hyperuricemia, hypertriglyceridemia, intolerance to carbohydrates, polyuria with nocturia has as a major feature excessive sleep.[78] As BUN and serum creatine levels rise, the patient's status shifts from lethargy to stupor to coma. Hyperammonemia results in hepatic encephalopathy with its accompanying evidence of organicity, asterixis, and excessive sleep.[79] The two causes of the increased ammonia and other toxic substances usually cleared by the liver remain either portal-systemic venous shunting or hepatic cell failure. Precipitating factors superimposed on either compromised conditions include gastrointestinal bleeding, increased protein ingestion, hypokalemic alkalosis which heightens the available NH_3 ammonia and diminishes the NH_4^+ ammonium ions, infection, or further liver deterioration.

Narcolepsy ranks as an important neurologic disorder resulting in excessive sleep. Features of this disease include: (1) sudden, recurrent irresistible sleep attacks lasting from 30 seconds to over 30 minutes; (2) cataplexy, a loss of muscle tone; (3) sleep paralysis, inability to move voluntarily while awakening or going to sleep; and (4) hypnagogic and hypnopompic hallucinations, hallucinations while falling asleep or awaking.[80] Symptoms first begin in the patient's late teens or early twenties. Patients experience restorative daytime naps.[81] Attacks occur generally during periods of inactivity, but also may happen with eating, sex, talking, or athletic events. Patients experience deep attacks on the average from two to six times a day when untreated. An EEG demonstrating the quick (within ten minutes) onset of REM sleep, proves diagnostic. Sakai et al report an opposite cerebral blood flow pattern in patients with narcolepsy compared to patients with sleep apnea and normals.[82] Narcoleptic patients also have been shown to have decreased dopamine and a tryptamine metabolite, indoleacetic acid, levels in the CSF.[83]

Kleine-Levin syndrome represents another neurologic disorder causing periodic excessive sleep. This rare disease generally afflicts adolescent men, and ultimately, spontaneously and gradually remits. Orlosky describes a 19-year-old man who developed an irresistible urge for sleep and then slept for episodes of four to six days continually.[84] He also exhibited withdrawal, an excessive appetite, especially for sweets, and poor hygiene. He gradually improved. Compulsive eating occurs in this syndrome as do a variety of mental disturbances including muteness, sexual inappropriateness, lethargy, agitation, hallucinations, auditory and visual delusions, amnesia, and thought blocking. During the symptomatic phases, sleep patterns resemble the sleep architecture of patients with primary unipolar depression: reduced sleep time, intermittent awakening, no delta sleep, decreased REM latency and total REM time with heightened REM density.[85] This syndrome may represent a brainstem neurotransmitter imbalance in the serotonergic pathway.[86]

Myotonic dystrophy has been linked to hypersomnia.[87] This hereditary disease's features include progressive alopecia, cataracts, myotonia, muscle wasting, and testicular atrophy. A cellular membrane deficit occurs in muscles, neurons, and red blood cells. The excessive sleep accompanying this disorder has two origins. First, membrane changes affect neurons of the brainstem and hypothalamus causing a central dysfunction and affecting respiration and sleep control. Second, chest muscle weakness leads to sleep apnea and alveolar hypoventilation and the consequential hypersomnia.

Idiopathic CNS hypersomnia accounts for excessive daytime sleepiness.[80] Patients experience bouts of long, daytime sleep, which is not refreshing, and is preceded by drowsiness, and followed by a sense of drunkenness and headache. They experience morning disorientation upon awakening. Patients' EEGs demonstrate shortened sleep latency but, critically, no rapid sleep onset REM activity as in narcolepsy. Patients frequently also have histories of fainting episodes and Raynaud's disease implicating an autonomic dysfunction.

Carbon dioxide narcosis, hypercapnia, is the result of a variety of pulmonary diseases and produces excessive sleep as one of its more salient features.[88] Chronic emphysema, cystic fibrosis, and respiratory center inadequacy may lead to a heightened PCO_2 and decreased arterial PO_2. In addition to drowsiness, stupor, and coma, patients experience severe bilateral frontal or occipital headaches, papilledema, muscle twitching, fast tremor, and intermittent signs of organic mental disturbances. The EEG demonstrates slow-wave activity. A young woman patient with advanced cystic fibrosis becomes intensely sleepy, withdrawn, and quiet as PCO_2 increases.

The *Pickwickian syndrome* remains the classic description of the interplay of aleveolar hypoventilation, obesity, and hypersomnolence.[89] Burwell et al, in 1956, reported an executive with this triad and not only depicted his falling asleep with a winning poker hand, but also drew the analogy to Dickens' character.[89] Further study has demonstrated the upper airway obstruction in sleep leading to sleep apnea as the etiology for the excessive daytime sleeping.[74] Sleep apnea is discussed under "Insomnia" above, and through that mechanism, is one of the commonest causes of excessive daytime sleeping.[90]

Oncology provides a number of mechanisms and explanations for hypersomnia. *Central nervous system tumors* prove responsible for that condition. Cancer in the mesodiencephalic region will account for it. Tumors in the hemispheres may generate intracranial pressure and ultimately brainstem compression to result in excessive sleep.[61] Frontal tumors notoriously present through profound and pronounced apathy, withdrawal, and drowsiness.[91] Malignancies often precipitate depression. This melancholic state is particularly noted with abdominal tumors and especially those of the pancreas.[43] Depression, in turn, not infrequently culminates in hypersomnia. Additionally, the debilitation commonly accompanying wide metastasis may manifest itself through excessive sleep. This proves especially true with metastases to the central nervous system.

The various treatments for the cancer provide other routes and explanations for excessive sleep. Drowsiness, tiredness, fatigue, and exhaustion may follow a bout of chemotherapy. Somnolence has been reported in children who received cranial irradiation for their acute lymphocytic leukemia.[92]

Cerebrovascular disease also offers a method, a mechanism, and an approach to understanding the medical basis for hypersomnia. Strokes account for excessive sleep in three ways. Severe cerebrovascular events with extensive brain damage produce unconsciousness and coma. Specific vascular lesions to the mesodiencephalic region produce hypersomnia.[61] Depression follows a stroke in at least half of the patients.[93] Finally, cerebrovascular disease provides an etiology for dementia. Dementia, in turn, accounts for hypersomnia in some patients.

Surgical complications   Postoperative pain medications, especially *opiates* , cause excessive sleep. Patients receiving morphine, codeine, or meperidine hydrochloride commonly experience tiredness, drowsiness, and sleeplessness. These drugs combined with the effects of the anesthetic, the surgery itself, and the bed rest not uncommonly produce a hypersomnolent state for several days following the operation.

Physical Trauma

Head trauma Head trauma is responsible for hypersomnia in two ways. First, the actual trauma itself may cause loss of consciousness and coma. Often the greater the cranial insult, the longer the period of coma proves a useful clinical index. Second, a *frontal lobe syndrome* may follow the physical injury. The syndrome's features include apathy, personality changes, indifference, and sleep.[94]

Psychiatric Differential Diagnosis

In the *organic mental disorder, delirium* , excessive sleep during the day emerges as important. Lipowski emphasizes the alterations in the day/night cycle and disturbances of the sleep pattern as essential features of delirium.[95] Criteria for this diagnosis include: (1) conscious clouding; (2) at least two of: (a) disturbance in perceptions, (b) incoherent speech, (c) disrupted sleep/wake cycle, and (d) alterations in psychomotor activity, (3) disorientation and memory defects, and the key feature (4) typical onset of symptoms.[57] It has an organic basis.

A *major depression* may feature hypersomnia or the prominent sleep disturbance might be insomnia.[96] The principle quality of this diagnostic category remains a dysphoric mood. Other key criteria include at least four of the following: (a) weight and appetite alterations, (b) sleep difficulty, (c) psychomotor activity, either accelerated or diminished, (d) decreased pleasure, (e) fatigue, (f) worthlessness, guilt, or self-deprecatory feelings, (g) difficulty in concentration, and (h) death or suicide thoughts.[57] Additionally, even without the affect component, patients do not have prominent hallucinations, bizarre behavior, do not have schizophrenia, nor do they have an organic etiology. A major depression may occur in any age group, may happen as a single episode, or may be an episode in a series of such depression (recurrent). In either case, the patients have no history of manic episodes. The major depression constitutes a severe, profound, often incapacitating event with or without psychotic features.

In bipolar disorder, depressed patients not only exhibit all the criteria for a major depression, but also have a history of at least one manic episode. These manic-depressive, depressed phase patients have pasts dominated by huge and protracted mood swings: periods of depression, periods of "highs," and periods of "all-right." Often there also is a family history of this disorder as outlined in the genetic section. A 45-year-old woman bitterly complained about "not being able to get out of bed again!" She had one episode of depression which responded to antidepressants one and a half years ago followed by a 2-month period of "tremendous" energy and activity. Her mother, who died 2 years ago, had had many strong "ugly and blue" periods in her life. The patient slept all the time, not to escape, but because that is all she felt like doing. She knew, the one Saturday morning she could not get out of bed, that her depression had begun again.

A *dysthymic disorder* ranks hypersomnia as a problem. Here, patients will experience a depression for 2 years but the symptoms are not of the severity as to warrant the diagnosis of major depression. During that time period, the depressive symptoms will last for days to weeks but not for months, and will be characterized by a sad mood or loss of interest. Criteria also involve at least three of the following symptoms: sleep disturbance, low energy, feeling of worthlessness, diminished production, inability to concentrate, social withdrawal, reduced interests, anger to excess, living without pleasure, changes in activity level, either an increased or decreased, negative life view, crying, and death or suicide thoughts.[57] Beyond not being psychotic or severely depressed, these patients exist in a protracted dysphoric melancholic world. Excessive sleep provides them with one alternative and momentary respite. It applies to the situation of a chronic depression and also fits the notion of a depressive neurosis.

In contrast to the affective disorders, an *adjustment disorder with a depressed mood* represents a maladaption to an identifiable stress and event within the last 3 months. Here the mood all of a sudden predominates along with impaired functioning and an excessive reaction, but it does not represent a response to underlying mental disorder. Further, it is expected to remit once the stress passes.

Cyclothymic disorder covers the intermittent swings of sadness and feeling high interlaced with normal mood over the last 2 years. Again, it does not have the severity of manic-depressive illness. The depression does appear similar to the dysthymic disorder, but is also accompanied by episodes of hypomania with at least three of the following symptoms: diminished sleep requirements, higher energy, heightened view of worthiness, increased production, creativity, gregariousness, hypersexuality, pleasure seeking without care for the consequences, restlessness, talkativeness, excessive optimism, and inappropriate humor.[57]

Posttraumatic stress disorder may present with excessive sleep. The hypersomnolence may represent a maladaptive but potent reaction to a traumatic event. A 10-year-old-boy was "touched in his private area" by his grandfather. He never told anyone until he was 25 years old. Since the event, he was continually obsessed about it. He had nightmares about it, passively gained weight to protect himself, and when not working, slept all the time. He took to bed to avoid all people, all obligations, and all commitments. Criteria for the diagnosis involve (a) a significant event; (b) re-experiencing of it through recurrent thoughts, dreams, or aberrations; (c) psychic numbing with reduced interest, detachment, or contracted emotions, and (d) at least two of the following not present before the event: hyperalertness, disturbed sleep, guilt, concentrating difficulty, activity avoidance, or memory-evoked responses. The stress disorder may be acute — within 6 months of the event and lasting 6 months, or chronic —lasting beyond 6 months, or delayed — occurring at least 6 months after it.[57]

REFERENCES

1. Kales A, Caldwell AB, Preston TA, et al: Personality patterns in insomnia. *Arch Gen Psychiatry* 1976;33:1128-1134.
2. Kolb LC, Brody HK: *Modern Clinical Psychiatry,* ed 10. Philadelphia, PA, WB Saunders Co, 1982.
3. Friedman NJ: Post-Vietnam syndrome. *Psychosomatics* 1981;22:931-943.
4. David P, Hefez A, Halperin G, et al: Long-term effects of traumatic war-related events on sleep. *Am J Psychiatry* 1979;136:175-178.
5. Horowitz MJ, Wilner N, Kaltreider N, et al: Signs and symptoms of post-traumatic stress disorder. *Arch Gen Psychiatry* 1980;37:85-92.
6. Kales A, Kales JD: Sleep disorders. *N Engl J Med* 1974;240:487-499.
7. Reynolds CF, Coble P, Holzer B, et al: Sleep and its disorders. *Primary Care* 1979;6:417-438.
8. Martin JB: The sleep-wake cycle and disorders of sleep, in Isselbacher KJ, Adams RD, Braunwald E, et al (eds): *Harrison's Principles of Internal Medicine,* ed 10. New York, McGraw Hill Book Co, 1983, pp 118-124.
9. Brown RP, Mann JJ: A clinical perspective on the role of neurotransmitters in mental disorders. *Hosp Community Psychiatry* 1985;36:141-150.
10. Karacan I, Moore C: Physiology and neurochemistry of sleep, in Hales RE, Frances AJ (eds): *American Psychiatric Association Annual Review* . Washington, American Psychiatric Press, 1985, vol 4, pp 266-293.

313

11. Guilleminault C, Dement WC: Sleep apnea syndromes and related sleep disorders, in Williams RC, Karacan I (eds): *Sleep Disorders: Diagnosis and Treatment.* New York, John Wiley & Sons, 1978, pp 9-28.

12. Arkinstall WW, Nirmal K, Klissouras V, et al: Genetic differences in the ventilatory response to inhaled CO_2. *J Appl Physiol* 1974;36:6-11.

13. Kales A, Soldatos CR, Bixler EO, et al: Hereditary factors in sleepwalking and night terrors. *Br J Psychiatry* 1980;137:111-118.

14. Winokur G, Clayton RJ, Reich T: *Manic Depressive Illness.* St. Louis, CV Mosby Co, 1969.

15. Sitaram N, Nurnberger JI, Gershon ES, et al: Cholinergic regulation of mood and REM sleep: Potential model and marker of vulnerability to affective disorder. *Am J Psychiatry* 1982;139:571-576.

16. Soldatos CR, Kales A, Kales JD: Management of insomnia. *Annu Rev Med* 1979;30:301-312.

17. Shurley JT, Pierce CM, Natani K, et al: Sleep and activity patterns at South Pole Station. *Arch Gen Psychiatry* 1970;22:385-389.

18. de la Pena A: Toward a psychophysiologic conceptualization of insomnia, in Williams RL, Karacan I (eds): *Sleep Disorders: Diagnosis and Treatment.* New York, John Wiley & Sons, 1978, pp 101-143.

19. Hall RCW, Popkin MK, Stickney SK, et al: Prevention of the steroid psychoses. *J Nerv Ment Dis* 1979;167:229-236.

20. Laurence DR, Bennett PH: *Clinical Pharmacology.* Edinburgh, Churchill Livinstone, 1980.

21. Hall, CWR (ed): *Psychiatric Presentations of Medical Illness.* New York, Spectrum Publications, 1980.

22. Gilman AG, Goodman LS, Gilman A (eds): *Goodman and Gilman's The Pharmacological Basis of Therapeutics,* ed 6. New York, Macmillan Publishing Co, Inc, 1980.

23. Greenblatt DJ, Shader RI, DiMascio A: Extrapyramidal effects. *Psychotropic Drug Side Effects.* Baltimore, Williams & Wilkins Co., 1970, pp 92-106.

24. Soreff S: *Management of the Psychiatric Emergency.* New York, John Wiley & Sons, 1981.

25. Lacoursiere RB, Spohn HE, Thompson K: Medical effects of abrupt neuroleptic withdrawal. *Compr Psychiatry* 1976;17:285-294.

26. Brezinova V, Oswald I, Loudon J: Two types of insomnia: too much walking or not enough sleep. *Br J Psychiatry* 1975;126:439-445.

27. Kramer PD: Insomnia: importance of differential diagnosis. *Psychosomatics* 1982;23:129-137.

28. Kales A, Malmstrom EJ, Rubin RT: Psychophysiological and biochemical changes following use and withdrawal of hypnotics, in Kales A (ed): *Sleep: Physiology and Pathology.* Philadelphia, JB Lippincott Co, 1969, pp 331-343.

29. Williams RC, Karacan I: Recent developments in the diagnosis and treatment of sleep disorders. *Hosp Community Psychiatry* 1985;36:951-957.

314

30. Yules RB, Lippman ME, Freedman DX: Alcohol administration prior to sleep. *Arch Gen Psychiatry* 1967;16:94-97.
31. Johnson LC, Burdick JA: Sleep during alcohol intake and withdrawal in the chronic alcoholic. *Arch Gen Psychiatry* 1970;22:406-418.
32. Adamson J, Burdick JA: Sleep of dry alcoholics. *Arch Gen Psychiatry* 1973;28:146-149.
33. Greenberg R, Pearlman C: Delirium tremens and dreaming. *Am J Psychiatry* 1967;124:133-142.
34. Valzelli L: *Psychopharmacology.* New York, Spectrum Publications, Inc, 1973.
35. Oswald I: Sleep and dependence on amphetamine and other drugs, in Kales A (ed): *Sleep Physiology and Pathology.* Philadelphia, JB Lippincott Co, 1969, pp 317-330.
36. American Medical Association: *Drug Abuse.* Chicago, American Medical Association, 1981.
37. Slaby AE, Lieb J, Tancredi LR: *Handbook of Psychiatric Emergencies,* ed 2. Garden City, NY, Medical Examination Publishing Co, 1981.
38. Guilleminault C, Dement WC: Sleep apnea syndromes and related sleep disorders, in Williams RL, Karacan F (eds): *Sleep Disorders Diagnosis and Treatment.* New York, John Wiley & Sons, 1978, pp 9-28.
39. Phillipson EA: Control of breathing during sleep. *Am Rev Respir Dis* 1978;118:909-932.
40. Ramsdell JW: Asthma: clinical presentations and diagnosis, in Bordow RA, Stool EW, Moser KM (eds): *Manual of Clinical Problems in Pulmonary Medicine* . Boston, Little, Brown & Co, 1980, pp 200-205.
41. Williams RL: Sleep disturbances in various medical and surgical conditions, in Williams RL, Karacan I (eds): *Sleep Disorders: Diagnosis and Treatment.* New York, John Wiley & Sons, 1978, pp 285-301.
42. Braunwald E, Cohn P: Ischemic heart disease, in Isselbacher KJ, Adams RD, Braunwald E, et al (eds): *Harrison's Principles of Internal Medicine,* ed 10. New York, McGraw-Hill Book Co, 1983, pp 1423-1432.
43. Jefferson JW, Marshall JR: *Neuropsychiatric Features of Medical Disorders.* New York, Plenum Medical Book Co, 1981.
44. Zorick FJ, Roth T, Hartze KM, et al: Evaluation and diagnosis of persistent insomnia. *Am J Psychiatry* 1981;138:769-773.
44. Gibberd FB, Bateson MC: Sleep epilepsy: its pattern and prognosis. *Br Med J* 1974;2:403-405.
45. Haider I, Oswald I: Late brain recovery processes after drug overdose. *Br Med J* 1970;2:318-322.
46. Feinberg I, Carlson VR: Sleep variables as a function of age in man. *Arch Gen Psychiatry* 1968;18:239-250.
47. Reynolds CF, Coble PA, Black RS, et al: Sleep disturbances in a

series of elderly patients: polysomnographic findings. *J Am Geriatr Soc* 1980;28:164-170.

48. Price VA, Coates TJ, Thorensen CE, et al: Prevalence and correlates of poor sleep among adolescents. *Am J Dis Child* 1978;132:583-586.

49. Williams RH (ed): *Textbook of Endocrinology,* ed 4. Philadelphia, WB Saunders Co, 1968.

50. Crisp AH, Stonehill E: Aspects of the relationship between sleep and nutrition: a study of 375 psychiatric out-patients. *Br J Psychiatry* 1973;122:379-394.

51. Bodher H: Conservative medical treatment of Peyronie's disease, in Kaufman JJ (ed): *Current Urologic Therapy.* Philadelphia, WB Saunders Co, 1980, pp 345-346.

52. Karacan I, Williams RL, Derman S, et al: Impaired, sleep-related penile tumescence in the diagnosis of impotence, in Zales MR (ed): *Eating, Sleeping and Sexuality.* New York, Brunner/Mazel, 1982, pp 186-199.

53. Stoelting RK: Psychological preparation and preoperative medication, in Miller RD (ed): *Anesthesia,* New York, Churchill Livingstone, 1981, pp 95-105.

54. Merrett JD, McDonald JR: Sequelae of concussion caused by minor head injuries. *Lancet* 1977;1:1-4.

55. Adey WR, Bors E, Porter RW: EEG sleep patterns after high cervical lesions in man. *Arch Neurol* 1968;19:377-383.

56. Freemon FR: Sleep in patients with organic diseases of the nervous system, in Williams RL, Karacan I (eds): *Sleep Disorders: Diagnosis and Treatment.* New York, John Wiley & Sons, 1978, pp 261-283.

57. American Psychiatric Association: *Diagnostic and Statistical Manual of Mental Disorders,* ed 3. Washington, American Psychiatric Association, 1980.

58. American Psychiatric Association: *A Psychiatric Glossary,* ed 5. Washington, American Psychiatric Association, 1980.

59. Neil JF, Himmelhook JM, Mallinger AG, et al: Caffeinism complicating hypersomnic depressive episodes. *Compr Psychiatry* 1978;19:377-385.

60. Adams RD: Sleep and its abnormalities, in Isselbacher KJ, Adams RD, Braunwald E, et al (eds): *Harrison's Principles of Internal Medicine,* ed 10. New York, McGraw Hill Book Co, 1980, pp 126-131.

61. Roth B: Narcolepsy and hypersomnia, in Williams RL, Karacan I (eds): *Sleep Disorders: Diagnosis and Treatment.* New York, John Wiley & Sons, 1978, pp 29-59.

62. Kessler S, Guilleminault C, Dement W: A family study of 50 REM narcoleptics. *Acta Neurol Scand* 1974;50:503-512.

63. Lipton MA: The evolution of the biological understanding of affective and schizophrenic disorders, in Zales MR (ed): *Affeetive and Schizophrenic Disorders.* New York, Brunner/Mazel, 1983, pp 5-28.

64. Santy P: The journey out and in: Psychiatry and space exploration. *Am J Psychiatry* 1957;140:519-527.

65. Soloman P, Leiderman H, Mendelson J, et al: Sensory deprivation. *Am J Psychiatry* 1957;114:357-363.
66. McNeil GN, Shaw PK, Dock DS: Substitution of atenolol for propranolol in a case of propranolol-related depression. *Am J Psychiatry* 1982;139:1187-1188.
67. Norwegian Multicenter Study Group: Timolol-induced reduction in mentality and reinfarction in patients surviving acute myocardial infarction. *N Engl J Med* 1981;304:801-807.
68. Petrie WM, Malfucci RJ, Woosley RL: Propranolol and depression. *Am J Psychiatry* 1982;139:92-94.
69. Rall TW, Schleiter LS: Drugs effective in the therapy of the epilepsies, in Gilman AG, Goodman LS, Gilman A (eds): *Goodman and Gilman's The Pharmacological Basis of Therapeutics,* ed 5. New York, Macmillan Publishing Co, Inc, 1980, pp 448-474.
70. Harvey SC, Hypnotics and sedatives, in Gilman AG, Goodman LS, Gilman A (eds): *Goodman and Gilman's The Pharmacological Basis of Therapeutics,* ed 5. New York, Macmillan Publishing Co, Inc, 1980, pp 339-375.
71. Kales A, Kales JO: Sleep laboratory studies of hypnotic drugs: efficacy and withdrawal effects. *J Clin Pharmacol* 1983;3:140-150.
72. Wilford BB: *Drug Abuse.* Chicago, American Medical Association, 1981.
73. Schuckit MA: *Drug and Alcohol.* New York, Plenum Medical Book Co, 1979.
74. Orr WC: The biology of sleep, in Zales MR (ed): *Eating, Sleeping and Sexuality.* .New York, Brunner/Mazel, 1982.
75. Sachs C, Persson HE, Hagenfeldt K: Menstruation-related periodic hypersomnia. *Neurology* 1982;32:1376-1379.
76. Kakulas BA, Adams RD: Viral infections of the nervous system: aseptic meningitis and encephalitis, in Isselbacher KJ, Adams RD, Braunwald E, et al (eds): *Harrison's Principles of Internal Medicine,* ed 9. New York, McGraw-Hill Book Co, 1980, pp 1967-1971.
77. Plorde JJ: Trypanosomiasis, in Isselbacher KJ, Adams RD, Braunwald E, et al (eds): *Harrison's Principles of Internal Medicine,* ed 10. New York, McGraw-Hill Book Co, 1983, pp 1196-1199.
78. Brenner BM, Lazarus JM: Chronic renal failure: pathophysiologic and clinical considerations, in Isselbacher KJ, Adams RD, Braunwald E, et al (eds): *Harrison's Principles of Internal Medicine,* ed 10. New York, McGraw-Hill Book Co, 1983, pp 1612-1619.
79. LaMont JT, Koff RD, Isselbacher KJ: Cirrhosis, in Isselbacher KJ, Adams RD, Braunwald E, et al (eds): *Harrison's Principles of Internal Medicine,* ed 10. New York, McGraw-Hill Book Co, 1983, pp 1804-1816.
80. Williams RL, Derman S, Karacan I: Disorders of excessive sleep and the parasomnias, in Zales MR (ed): *Eating, Sleeping, and Sexuality.* New York, Brunner/Mazel, 1982, pp 150-185.
81. Browman CP, Sampson MG, Gujavarty KS, et al: Hypersomnia: diagnosis and management. *Compr Ther* 1983;9:67-74.

82. Sakai F, Meyer JS, Karacan I, et al: Normal human sleep: regional cerebral hemodynamics. *Ann Neurol* 1980;7:471-478.

83. Montplaisir J, deChamplain J, Young SN, et al: Narcolepsy and idiopathic hypersomnia: biogenic amines and related compounds in CSF. *Neurology* 1982;32:1299-1302.

84. Orlosky MJ: The Kleine-Levin Syndrome: a review. *Psychosomatics* 1982;23:609-621.

85. Reynolds CF, Black RS, Cable P, et al: Similarities in EEG sleep findings for Kleine-Levin syndrome and unipolar depression. *Am J Psychiatry* 1980;137:116-118.

86. Koerber RK, Torkelson R, Haven G, et al: Increased cerebrospinal fluid 5-hydroxytryptamine and 5-hydroxyindoleacetic acid in Kleine-Levin syndrome. *Neurology* 1984;34:1597-1600.

87. Hansotia P, Frens D: Hypersomnia associated with alveolar hypoventilation in myotonic dystrophy. *Neurology* 1981;31:1336-1337.

88. Victor M, Adams RD: Metabolic diseases of the nervous system, in Isselbacher KJ, Adams RD, Braunwald E, et al: *Harrison's Principles of Internal Medicine,* ed 10. New York, McGraw-Hill Book Co, 1983, pp 2104-2112.

89. Burwell CS, Robin ED, Whaley RD, et al: Extreme obesity associated with alveolar hypoventilation: a Pickwickian syndrome. *Am J Med* 1956;21:811-818.

90. Kwentus JK, Schulz SC, Fairman P, et al: Sleep apnea: a review. *Psychosomatics* 1985;26:713-724.

91. Wells CE, Duncan GW: *Neurology for psychiatrists.* Philadelphia, FA Davis Co, 1980.

92. Ch'ien CT, Aur RJA, Stagner S, et al: Long-term neurological implications of somnolence syndrome in children with acute lymphocytic leukemia. *Ann Neurology* 1979;8:273-277.

93. Robinson RO, Lipsey Jr, Price TR: Diagnosis and clinical management of post-depression depression. *Psychosomatics* 1985;26:769-778.

94. Blumer D, Benson DF: Personality changes with frontal and temporal lobe lesions, in Benson DF, Blumer D (eds): *Psychiatric Aspects of Neurologic Disease.* New York, Grune & Stratton, Inc, 1975, pp 151-170.

95. Lipowski ZJ: Organic brain syndromes: overview and classification, in Benson DF, Blumer D (eds): *Psychiatric Aspects of Neurologic Disease.* New York, Grune & Stratton, Inc, pp 11-35.

96. Garvey MJ, Mungas D, Tollefson GD: Hypersomnia in major depressive disorders. *J Affective Disord* 1984;6:283-286.

8 Paranoia

Stephen M. Soreff

PARANOIA   A mental position, an emotional stance, and a physical presence dominated by a personal sense of centrality and characterized by persecutory, grandiose, or jealous ideas and delusions.

FEATURES

Case report   A 26-year-old man, a PhD chemistry candidate, suddenly realized people had "turned" on him.   "They are plotting against me," he had come to believe. Already under many stresses, he recently lost his long-time girl friend to his best friend. He had used alcohol and a number of recreational drugs and had complained of headaches and fatigue. He has become mistrustful, distrustful, distant, and afraid.

Mood

The paranoid patients display certain airs, reveal several emotions, and convey a definite presence. These moods may both manifest the paranoia and underlie it.

Suspicion often depicts one of the dominant paranoid airs.[1] Paranoid patients trust few, if any, people. They doubt motives, question concern, and wonder about interest. They remain vigilant in a perceived dangerous, hostile world.

The paranoid patients may cast an *air of distance* . They stand metaphorically remote, aloof, and detached. Despite their discussion of significant material, they frequently do so in a strangely removed manner.

They may maintain an air of *defiance* . They convey the sense of arrogance, challenge, and assertion. It is them against the world. They

318

generate a mood of confrontation. At one time they created the image of the noble warrior; the unsung hero; and the unconquered champion.

Or they may develop the affect of *indignation* as jealous victims. They portray themselves as innocent, uninvolved recipients of others' designs. Someone took something of theirs.

Or they display an *expansionistic* affect. They appear overly involved, all-encompassing, too intrusive, and overwhelming.

A variety of emotions accompany their paranoid productions: hostility, flatness, grandiosity, or depression.

Frequently, the paranoid patients display *hostility* . They demonstrate dramatically anger, frustration, resentment, and annoyance. In response to threats upon them, they threaten others. One paranoid man challenged the clinic staff with stares, verbal assaults, and impatience.

In contrast, some patients show an inappropriate *flat affect* while describing the most dangerous delusion. The patient, in a monotone, discusses the Mafia plan to eliminate him. Or the patient may announce the deliverance of the world in a decidedly flat affect. This flatness presents as a vivid demonstration of a split between affect and thought.

Grandiosity may dominate the presentation. The patients, believing themselves to be God, the Savior, the True Believer, and the Hope, reveal themselves as open, generous, giving, forgiving, and expansive. As the Light, they appear to generate light.

Yet, the paranoid may also convey a sense of *depression* . They feel sad beneath a colorful appearance. There is the melancholy, the loneliness, the loss, and the emptiness. Without the delusion, they are nothing.[2]

Paranoid patients often reveal a definite, unmistakable, and clear presence. Paranoid patients frequently may demonstrate *momentousness* and *immediacy* . They are there!

Above all, paranoid patients present themselves as *important* .[3] They are the object of powerful enemies, they are the answer for humanity. They convey a sense of being key and totally significant. They dramatically assert their centrality.

Thought

First, and foremost, paranoia represents a disorder of thought. The patient's thinking distortions find expression along a number of avenues. These include delusions, hallucinations, ideas of reference, rigidity, certain preoccupations, unique vulnerabilities, and a value upon independence.

Together they constitute the core and focus of the paranoid process and system.

Delusions stand as the hallmark and cornerstone of paranoia. They are false beliefs which the individual maintains against all incontrovertible and obvious proof.[4] Delusions usually present in one of three forms: persecution, jealousy, or grandiosity.

In *delusions of persecution*, the patients see themselves as the object of potential and imminent assault. The enemies range from spouses or neighbors to the CIA or the Russian hordes. They are always after the patient or ones they care about. To these patients the attackers are real, the threat genuine, and the danger immediate. Dynamically, as the target of powerful forces, the patients often derive a reflected importance.

In *delusions of jealousy*, patients suspect others of infidelity. They perceive spouses as cheating on them, lovers betraying them, or champions becoming disloyal. Their central drama and distress remains what was *done to them* .

In *delusions of grandeur*, patients see themselves as marvelous saviors. They announce their presence in all glory as God, Jesus, Napoleon, the President of the United States, or the Answer to Mankind. They proclaim their centrality.

An *erotic* focus may emerge and dominate their thinking. They come to believe a famous person loves and desires them. They find themselves the object of hidden attention, affection, and admiration from these personages. A shy college student became convinced that the campus queen truly, yet secretly, loved him. He found affirmation of this in all her activities and especially in all her contacts with him.

Hallucinations may herald paranoia. Hallucinations involve a sensory perception in which the actual external stimulus is not present.[5] Again, to the patients, their perceptions are real.

In *auditory hallucinations*, the patients hear something of great significance. They listen to the Mafia plotting to kill them. They hear neighbors making bombs or releasing gas into the vents. Voices tell them of the coming danger and command them to save the world.

In *visual hallucinations*, they see something of great consequence. One man reported seeing a large sailing vessel docking in his hospital room and the crew coming for him. Another patient sighted a nurse with a gun and a doctor with a saw. In contrast, other patients have had visions of a perfect world, order, and calling.

Paranoia involves *ideas of reference*. Paranoid individuals abstract certain events, items, and statements out of context and claim each has a special reference to them. The television programs on cancer meant to the patient she had a tumor. The smile from the neighborhood policeman verified to another patient that the CIA had tapped the telephone. Ideas of reference may represent a stage of delusion formation or an isolated phenomenon.

Paranoid patients are often *rigid in their thinking*. They see and accept only one explanation for a phenomenon — theirs. To the jealous spouse, his wife went to the grocery store for an affair. He would not acknowledge she went for milk.

The paranoid patients commonly *focus* their lives on certain issues. Some become obsessed about the law, right and wrong, and the legal system. Others personalize justice and catalog every insult and hurt they have received. Still others worry about their health. They fear heart disease, germs, and cancer. They develop hypochondriacal concerns and endlessly pursue a physical basis for their problems. Many concentraate upon religion. Some of them will study, quote, and follow to the letter, the Bible. Finally, some will develop a preoccupation with what they believe are the unconscious attitudes of other people.[6] Although they deny their own feelings, they readily ascribe certain nefarious emotions and motivations to others. They feel they can detect resentment in those they encounter yet disclaim any anger on their part.

The paranoid patients also have *unique vulnerabilities*. They are supersensitive and extremely easily "hurt." In the vast ocean of events, they find a tiny island of wrong and personal affront. They focus and dwell upon the "possible" insult and remain in pain. They hear only a word and miss the music, the lyrics, and the melody.

Finally, many paranoid individuals highly prize their *independence*. They fear control, closeness, and containment. They value their autonomy and their freedom. They will resist limitations, defeat, or control by others.

Behavior

A variety of often spectacular behaviors both reflect the paranoid thought processes and trumpet the accompanying mood. These activities range from withdrawal to violence, from silence to screaming, and from withholding to demanding. Critical paranoid behavior includes vigilance, muteness, litigiousness, assertion, flight, self-destructiveness, and assaults.

Some paranoid patients maintain a sharp, constant *vigilance*. Remaining forever on the alert, they perpetually scan their environment for signs of dangers or clues of an attack. They are always on guard and on duty.

Not infrequently, paranoid patients elect *muteness* to defend themselves. One man refused to provide any information for fear it would be overheard by the ever present "aliens." Another, a woman, believing she controlled the balance of the universe, would not speak because her voice would destroy the equilibrium. Such a patient might select total isolation or withdrawal for similar reasons.

Paranoid patients may become *litigious* .[7] They use the courts to address perceived personal wrongs and societal situations. They use the legal system to defend themselves and to attack others.

Certain paranoid individuals *assert* themselves. They demand attention. They are impatient. They want their justice and their rights. When they perceive a danger, they tell the world. As saviors, they proclaim their importance and attempt to change the world.

Some paranoid patients *choose flight* . They leave their homes and keep moving to remain ahead of the enemy. They change jobs to avoid closeness. They go from one apartment to another because of the plotting neighbors.

Self-destructive behavior may emerge from paranoia. Often it results when the underlying depression surfaces and the external danger eases. Or they hurt themselves to appease the enemy or to prove the depth of their conviction.

Of great significance, some paranoid patients turn to *violence* . They assault, fight, and kill. In persecution, they attack before their perceived attack. A woman carries a gun "just in case!" In jealousy, they seek revenge. A man kills his wife and her alleged lover. In grandeur, they demand right. A man assaults a group of worshipers because they "failed" to pray with the proper conviction.

Physical Examination

Although paranoia per se does not carry with it any specific physical findings, it does warrant careful physical examination for two reasons. First, a wide variety of medical and neurologic conditions produce paranoid symptoms.[5] Second, a thorough physical examination can serve to re-assure those patients preoccupied with their health.

Laboratory Findings

The following studies are of diagnostic value in evaluating the paranoid patient. Serum: alcohol; barbiturate; bromide; bilirubin; copper; ceruloplasmin; creatinine; BUN; cortisol; electrolytes (sodium, potassium, chloride); Tri-iodothyronine (T_3) uptake; total thyroxine (T_4) assay; thyroid-stimulating hormone (TSH); vitamin B_{12}. Blood: lupus erythematosus (LE) cell test: Anti-DNA antibodies; antinucleoprotein antibody; Venereal Disease Research Laboratories (VDRL) test: fluorescent treponemal antibody absorbed (FTA-ABS); RBC and morphology; WBC count and morphology. Chromosome studies: count; morphology; Barr bodies. Urine: amphetamine; porphobilinogens; 17-hydroxycortico-steroids; 17-ketosteroids. Neurologic tests: computed tomographic (CT) scan; electroencephalogram (EEG).

Interviewer's Reaction

Paranoid patients produce a series of reactions within the interviewer. These reflect both the paranoid dynamics and clinical situation.

Paranoid patients frequently create a sense of *apprehension* within the interviewer. First, the interviewer sees potential violence. Second, the in-terviewer is concerned with legal ramifications of the encounter. The patients may be suggesting suit, or there may be an intended victim to be protected. Third, the interviewer perceives the patient's stress and distress.

Interviewers commonly experience *anger* in the presence of the para-noid patient.[7] Not infrequently, they have been the recipients of the pa-tient's demands, impatience, mistrust, and rage. The patient's stance has the potential to create a hostile environment.

The interviewers also find themselves strangely *remote and distant* from the patient. For example, the patient has remained aloof during the encounter. The patient, by a flat affect, a delusion, and an hallucination, has created and maintained a clinical gulf.

Or, in contrast, the interviewers may themselves be overly involved with the grandiose patients. These expansive, gregarious individuals often prove to be infectious in their enthusiasm and dynamism. A truly religious zealot can be very persuasive. A hypomanic patient can be a super salesperson and quite convincing.

PATHOGENESIS

Psychodynamics

The psychodynamic explanation for paranoia involves an appreciation of four major convergent themes and factors in these individuals' personality development and symptom formation: maturational issues, core feelings, the projection defense system, and current stresses.

First, the developmental history of paranoid patients commonly indicates a lack in *basic trust* .[8] Trust is the foundation upon which the personality is built. Without it, all subsequent maturation emerges as distorted, damaged, and diverted, and the person develops mistrust.

The failure to achieve basic trust stems from two sources: parental humiliation and messages. Paranoid patients have often sustained great humiliation, both physically and emotionally, at the hands of their parents. Their parents have beat them, screamed at them, ridiculed them, attacked them, and insulted them. The individuals designated to develop a sense of security, continuity, and trust have instead caused fear, apprehension, and doubt.

The parents frequently have also delivered a *series of messages* to the child predisposing to paranoid development. One message says, do not trust others. Families perpetuate myths by telling children "everyone is an enemy," "no one is to be trusted," "everyone is out to use or hurt you." Another message involves the child's worth. These parents openly proclaim and predict the youth's failure.

The second major factor involves the patients' *core feelings of inferiority, low self-esteem, and inadequacy* .[5] These often commence from the parental messages, but become more pervasive, and extensive and devastating. These patients view themselves as less capable, less attractive, less able, and less of a person than other people. To them they are not only no good, but also they believe others share this opinion. They consider themselves as sexually inferior and inadequate. These core feelings account for their underlying depression and their need to become important.

Third, an understanding of paranoia requires an examination of *projection,* their major mental defense mechanism. The mechanism involves several *unconscious* steps.[4] Initially, the patients deny any unacceptable feelings and thoughts within themselves. They have no envy, greed, amorous desires, or rage. Then they project these emotions and concepts on to others; they ascribe their conflicts, wishes, fears, and hopes to others. In one case, a man considered himself inadequate sexually and not fulfilling to his wife. But he was not consciously aware of this feeling. Instead, he denied any problems within himself, accused his wife of infidelity, and attacked his neighbor for taking "his woman."

Part of the projection system embraces the classic homosexual dynamic underlying paranoia.[9,10] In this system paranoia stems from unconscious homosexual feelings and involves the following equation: "I love him" — this is unacceptable; "I do not love him," followed by, "I hate him" — this is almost admissible, but it is denied. Then the projection occurs: "He hates me"; and lastly, "He wants to hurt me."

Finally, paranoid patients encounter a variety of *current stresses* which accelerate or propel them into the projection process. They sustain significant losses in finances, in love, in living, and in their health. They encounter anxiety-provoking situations. They move into new positions with high demands. Important people in their lives die. They feel pushed beyond their capacity, capability, and coping mechanisms.

Biologic Explanation

The catecholamines have emerged as the neurochemicals most associated with paranoia. These include epinephrine, norepinephrine and dopamine. Amphetamines have a long history of triggering paranoid episodes.[11] They both cause dopamine release from presynaptic storage residues and block its retake by the same neurons.[12] Kendler and Davis reviewed a number of studies comparing paranoid to nonparanoid schizophrenics.[13] They noted in both the limbic forebrain and in cerebrospinal fluid of the paranoid group there was a significant elevation of norepinephrine. In essence, any drug or condition which increases CNS catecholamine levels may move the patient toward a paranoid response.

An *organic deficit* often provokes a paranoid response. Patients because of a CNS lesion have difficulty integrating sensory input with their own internal organizing system and, as a result, they react through a sense of persecution. Commonly, this may occur with deafness. Or it has been a frequent pattern in Huntington's disease.[14]

Hemispheric dysfunction may account for paranoia. Right hemispheric deficits have been reported as more common in paranoid schizophrenic patients than in the nonparanoid schizophrenic group.[15] The idea of hemispheric imbalance has been supported by the observations of Bear.[16] He emphasizes the role of the right hemisphere in maintaining emotion surveillance. One of this side's functions is to continually scan the various sensory modalities to develop a cognitive picture and position orientation.

A *blood-brain barrier (BBB)* impairment has been implicated in the development of a paranoid psychosis. Axelsson et al studied 25 paranoid psychotic patients.[17] They examined the difference between CSF and serum albumin concentrations and computed the CSF/serum ratio for each.

A significant derivation from age-related normals in the CSF/serum/albumin ratio constituted the criteria for BBB impairment. Abnormal ratios represented and reflected increased CSF albumin concentrations. The BBB group's ratio was 8.9 compared to 5.5 for the normal group. Of the 25, seven of them had evidence of BBB impairment. These seven patients were also much younger than the other 18. The investigators argued this BBB impairment contributed to the emergence of the paranoid psychosis 20 years earlier in these seven patients.[17]

Genetics

Two sex chromosome disorders have been associated with paranoia. *Klinefelter's syndrome* clinically typified by gynecomastia, aspermia, hypogonadism, and a feminine fat distribution pattern has as a genetic basis the XXY sex chromosomes.[18] *Turner's syndrome* (gonadal dysgenesis), physically marked by women of short stature, lacking secondary sexual characteristics, with primary amenorrhea, and many congenital abnormalities, has as its fundamental cause a single X chromosome.[6] Both syndromes result from meiotic nondisjunction. In Klinefelter's syndrome, the sperm carries both X and Y sex chromosomes; in Turner's, the sperm has neither X nor Y sex chromosomes.

Huntington's disease not infrequently initially presents with paranoid features. Patients may feel persecuted, pursued, and pestered. Or they may develop delusional and hallucinatory states either of persecution or grandiosity emerging from a vague, but all-encompassing sense of change in their world and personal reality.[14] This disease strikes usually in adult life. The cause is the inheritance of autosomal dominant gene with high penetrance. The basic lesions involve degeneration of caudate nucleus and putamen.[19] The twin hallmarks of the disorder are dementia and choreiform movements.

Paranoid schizophrenia, although to a lesser degree than schizophrenia in general, does have a genetic component. Schizophrenia itself has a demonstrated inheritance pattern.[20] The evidence in the schizophrenic disorder includes twins and adopted-away studies. In the twin reports, monozygotic twins have a higher concordance rate for schizophrenia than do the dizygotic twins.[21] Children of schizophrenic parents, after adoption by nonschizophrenic parents, retain a significant incidence for the disorder.[22] In applying these studies and reviewing many others to the genetics of paranoid schizophrenia, Kendler and Davis have made several conclusions.[13] First, there appears to be lower genetic loading in paranoid schizophrenics than in nonparanoid schizophrenia. For example, paranoid schizophrenic patients will have fewer family histories for schizophrenia than will nonparanoid schizophrenic families. Second, paranoid schizophrenia tends to breed true with families. It apparently does pass from one generation to another.

In *manic-depressive illness (MDI)* where paranoia often represents the principle manifestation, genetics make a major contribution.[23] For a 45-year-old housewife with MDI, a period of intense jealousy and fears of her husband's infidelity heralded each depressive episode. For a 35-year-old man with MDI, a sense of world savior and glory preceded each manic episode. Evidence includes concordance work and an X chromosome with color blindness linkage. The MDI concordance in monozygotic twins was 72%, compared with 14% in dizygotic twins.[24] Rich and Winokur have argued that MDI is transmitted as a dominant gene on the X chromosome with variable penetrance. Red-green color blindness also is inherited on the same chromosome providing a generational marker.[25]

Regardless of the genetic component, there remains a dramatic, significant, and profound *family impact and contribution* upon the patient's paranoid development which may take many forms. Some parents verbally and physically beat their children. Other parents teach paranoia to the offspring. For example, a wealthy businessman always told his son and daughter that people only wanted them for their money. They were reared to trust no one, doubt everyone, and distance all.

Environment

A number of environments evoke and provoke paranoid responses. Certain *home environments* promote paranoia among their occupants.[26] Alcoholic husbands may beat and spy upon their wives. These wives develop a fear of their spouses. Parents may scream at, hurt, and humiliate their children — or certain of their children. These boys and girls learn terror at home. Families may feel isolated and afraid in a particular neighborhood. The first minority household in a different ethnic area lives with a sense of apprehension and concern.

Work can produce feelings of paranoia. Some highly tense, aggressive companies foster a sense of rivalry and competition among their employees. Persons fighting for the same job find themselves suspicious and alienated from each other. For individuals engaged in criminal activities, life always involves looking over their shoulders. A young drug dealer came to the emergency department in fear. He had informed on another "pusher" and the gang was after him.

Certain *restricted environments* develop, sustain, and increase paranoia. Settings such as jails and prisons are notorious for this. It also occurs in camps, military installations, and in isolated groups.

Group paranoia also occurs. Immigrants often feel isolated, alien, and unwanted in their new land.[27] Refugees frequently have a unique sense of vulnerability and fear.[28] Religious groups find themselves apart from their environments. Whenever a collection of individuals is not part of the mainstream, the society, or the country, they have the potential to develop paranoia.

A monotonous, isolated, ecology often leads to paranoid feelings.[29] The sailor alone at sea, the winter hiker lost in a whiteout, or the person in any other environment of sensory restriction. All are prone to develop a sense of alienation, fear, and projection. A woman walking at dusk started to see demons and monsters in the woods.

DIFFERENTIAL DIAGNOSIS

Nonpsychotropic Drugs

Two *anti-parkinsonian drugs* have been associated with the onset of paranoid symptoms. First and foremost ranks *3,4-dihydroxyphenyl-L-alanine* (levodopa).[12] Levodopa, an amino acid precursor, crosses the blood-brain barrier and is converted mostly to dopamine; a small amount becomes norepinephrine and epinephrine. In addition to the reported delirium, depression, hypomania, and hypersexuality occurring after levodopa administration, some patients developed a paranoid psychosis. The features included paranoid delusions and both visual and olfactory hallucinations.[30] Levodopa appears to have a CNS awakening and alerting effect. *Amantadine hydrochloride* gains its antiparkinsonian efficacy by the dopamine mechanism also.[31] It causes release of dopamine.[32] It too will produce a psychosis with paranoid features.[31]

Amphetamines and their derivatives, eg, methylphenidate hydrochloride and pemoline, have long been known to provoke paranoid responses.[33] Historically much used and abused for appetite appeasement and weight reduction, these drugs now find application only for the treatment of narcolepsy and minimal brain dysfunction.[24] Amphetamine is quite similar to dopamine and norepinephrine and acts by displacing these neurotransmitters from their storage sites.[34]

A host of *sympathomimetic drugs* produce paranoia. These drugs have a wide range of applications: as bronchodilators, decongestants, and in treatment of "flu" or "cold" symptoms. Their basic compound includes dopamine, ephedrine, epinephrine, isoproterenol, phenylephrine, phenylpropanolamine, or pseudoephedrine.[35] Their mechanisms of action resemble that of amphetamine. A 27-year-old man with a history of manic-depressive illness developed paranoia symptoms including ideas of neighbors spying on him, sensations of vibrations within him, and auditory hallucinations of people commenting. These emerged from his abuse of a decongestant which contained pseudoephedrine. Remission commenced with discontinuation of the drug.

Anticholinergic drugs not uncommonly evoke paranoid ideations.[36] These drugs have wide application. Atropine, as a preanesthetic, decreases bronchial secretions. Belladonna, as an antispasmodic and an antacid, is used to treat peptic ulcer disease by diminishing gastric acid secretion. Atropine drugs, as ophthalmologic agents, produce pupillary dilation. Anticholinergics are employed in cardiac disease to reverse bradycardia. The CNS action of the drugs appear to be threefold.[37] At clinical doses, it stimulates both the medulla and higher cerebral centers. The vagus is activated. As the doses approach toxic levels, the excitation becomes restlessness, delirium, and irritability. At yet increased levels, depression, coma, and ultimately respiratory depression occur.

Adrenocortical steroids are responsible for a wide range of paranoid responses.[38] At one extreme, certain patients will develop a depression with psychotic features. They perceive people and the world to be against them; danger is everywhere; nowhere is safe. At the other extreme, some patients will experience a manic reaction with euphoria and grandiosity. Still others will have a schizophreniclike state. These steroid-induced states occur regardless of the point of steroid therapy: upon initiation of the medication, during steady-state administration, or while tapering.[39]

Cyclobenzaprine, a muscle relaxant, has been associated with an exacerbation of paranoid symptoms in vulnerable individuals. This drug relates closely structurally and pharmacologically to the tricyclic antidepressants.[40] As such it may produce the same eruption of projective, delusional, or grandiose type of behaviors as these antidepressants.[41] The author recently treated a 35-year-old compensated schizophrenic man in the emergency department. His physician had begun him on cyclobenzaprine for low back strain and pain. The patient rapidly developed delusions of people being after him and wanting to attack him. He improved on discontinuance of that drug.

Cimetidine, an extremely widely prescribed histamine H_2 receptor antagonist for peptic ulcer disease, may trigger a paranoid psychosis. Alder et al describe a 51-year-old man who, following aortofemoral bypass surgery and the initiating cimetidine therapy, became paranoid and delusional with both auditory and visual hallucinations.[42] Termination of cimetidine led to resolution of the psychosis.

Ibuprofen, a nonsteroidal antiinflammatory analgesic drug, has been associated with the emergence of a paranoid psychosis in susceptible patients.[43] The drug acts as a powerful prostaglandin synthetase inhibitor. That enzyme is responsible for the conversion of fatty acids into thrombaxines and ultimately into prostaglandins. Of interest, Horrobin advanced the notion of schizophrenia resulting from prostaglandin deficiency.[44]

Phenytoin, a very widely used anticonvulsant, has been noted rarely to be associated with paranoid reaction.[45]

Bromides produce paranoia.[46,47] Although obsolete as sedatives and anticonvulsants, they are still found as either over-the-counter preparations or as part of other medications, eg, certain mouthwashes. Toxic signs appear at serum bromide levels greater than 50 mg/100 mL.[39]

Psychotropic Drugs

Antidepressants may cause a paranoid episode in one of several ways. First, they may provoke, exacerbate, or trigger paranoia in schizophrenic patients and in patients with a delusional depression.[41,48] A graduate student, 30 years old, slowly withdrew into an hedonic world. His physician, believing his condition to represent a depression, started him on a tricyclic antidepressant. The student began to develop a delusional system of his roommate plotting against him. He rapidly experienced a schizophrenic psychosis with marked paranoid features. Second, the combination of imipramine hydrochloride and methyltestosterone has proved particularly potent in inducing paranoid reactions.[49] Four out of five patients receiving both drugs for a unipolar depression promptly experienced paranoid delusions, referential thinking, and agitation. Third, antidepressants not uncommonly have propelled manic-depressive patients from depression into mania.

The underlying mechanism reflects the basic therapeutic properties of the antidepressant — to enhance the available neurotransmitter. The actual method is release and reuptake inhibition in the case of the tricyclics and tetracyclics, or in the MAO-inhibitors, to prevent their enzymatic destruction. These drugs, which especially increase amounts of norepinephrine or dopamine, will most commonly induce a schizophrenic reaction.[50]

Alcohol

Alcohol intoxication unleashes, not uncommonly, a torrent of paranoid presentations. Although each person's tolerance and threshold varies, alcohol's clinical effects generally commence above 150 mg/mL serum level.[39] Alcohol appears to have a disinhibiting result. Some patients will develop feelings of persecution; others emerge with strong notions of their spouses' infidelity; and still others display their great prowess, power, and presence.

Prolonged excessive alcohol use and abuse not infrequently finds expression through paranoid syndrome. Delusions of jealousy and infidelity commonly emerge. Kolb and Brody describe this as alcoholic paranoia.[9] It has its genesis in sexual, especially homosexual, conflicts; in failures; in diminished repression; in inability to perform; and in prolonged indulgence. Together these events provide the ingredients of a vicious cycle leading to delusion formation. A 52-year-old mailman drank heavily for years. He feared for his job, he worried about his decreased physical ability, he felt "too close" to his supervisor, and missed his grown, married, and absent children. He developed the delusion that his wife was having an affair with his boss and the boss planned to have him eliminated by the post office.

Alcohol withdrawal accounts for paranoia in two ways. In *alcohol hallucinosis*, the patients, usually within 48 hours after diminishing or ceasing heavy drinking, experience threatening, terrifying hallucinations. These patients have a clear sensorium.[51] The hallucinations are most often visual and threatening in character. One woman saw a herd of cattle coming toward her. In *alcohol withdrawal delirium* (delirium tremens), patients who have stopped their alcohol use three to five days prior to symptoms encounter vivid, overwhelming, attacking, condemning, and damning visual and auditory hallucinations. These patients are disoriented, frequently have temperature elevation, and show symptoms of sympathetic overactivity.

Alcohol may also cause a *paranoid lifestyle* . Aside from the biochemical properties and effects of ethanol, often the users find it produces major alteration in their routine. For the adolescent, there is sneaking alcohol to dances, spiking the punch, obtaining fake identification, and crossing state lines for liquor. For the chronic alcoholic, there emerges a number of struggles, alibis, and deceptions induced by alcohol: hiding the bottle and supply from the suspicious spouse, covering with mints from the boss that midday "belt"; or making excuses for the long way home. In the end, the pursuit of alcohol, the security of the source, and the protection of consumption generates a world of subterfuge, deviousness, and apprehension.

Other Abused Substances

Amphetamines may erupt into frank paranoia. Induced feelings of hypervigilance, hyperacute recall, and total awareness, senses of cleverness, energy, and control, and notions of apprehension, concern, and fear give way to suspiciousness, visual hallucinations, and persecutory delusions.[52]

Other clinical features associated with amphetamines include loquaciousness, diminished appetite, insomnia, and thirst. The characteristics of perceived boundless energy, the nonrequirement of sleep or food, the enhanced athletic ability and endurance, all contribute to amphetamine's use and abuse. Physical accompanying signs are as follows: reactive but dilated pupils, elevated blood pressure, pulse, and temperature; hyperreflexia; tremulousness; and dry mouth.

The biochemical mechanism remains the release of both dopamine and norepinephrine. Animal studies have indicated different functions[12] for each of these neurotransmitters in the amphetamine-induced events.[53] The dopaminergic responses center about stereotypic behaviors, sniffing, and gnawing compulsively. In contrast, the norepinephrinic reactions involve heightened locomotor activity. Urine amphetamine levels remain a very useful method to detect amphetamine use.

Amphetamines may produce paranoia in all three phases of its use. *Intoxication,* not infrequently, triggers major paranoia episodes. The patients suddenly find themselves thrust into a world of no sleep, hyperalertness, too much energy, and fear. *Chronic use* leads to protracted suspiciousness, apprehension, and terror. The amphetamine addiction involves both tolerance and dependence.[24] A young woman, as she increased her amphetamine requirements, became progressively more paranoid about her source and other people. She took to carrying a knife for protection. *Amphetamine withdrawal* may also initiate a paranoid response.[12] A 50-year-old housewife experienced a paranoid psychosis with persecution delusions after her physician "cut off" her diet pill supply. She barricaded herself at home and held off local police for several hours.

Barbiturate withdrawal may be accompanied by evidence of paranoid ideation. These may occur in a cluster of signs and symptoms of autonomic system hyperactivity; hyperreflexia, blood pressure increases, tachycardia, hyperpyrexia, restlessness, visual hallucinations, and delirium. The dreaded complication remains seizure leading to status epilepticus.[39]

Experimentally, 600 mg of phenobarbital daily for 30 days is enough to cause withdrawal seizures.[32] The entire clinical presentation of withdrawal from barbiturates appears similar to the alcoholic's delirium tremens.

Cocaine use may initiate a paranoid response. Common reactions include ideas of reference, feelings of grandiosity, apprehension, hyperalertness, hypervigilance, and a sense of great mental ability.[39] Additionally, and characteristic of cocaine use, are "snow lights" and bugs as visual hallucinations (see Chapter 4). The cocaine experience resembles that induced by amphetamines but the psychosis usually lasts a shorter time. It potentiates catecholamine action.[24] It also serves to block norepinephrine reuptake.[53]

Hallucinogens may account for powerful paranoid experiences. Patients may have persecutory or grandiose delusions. They may have potent vivid visual hallucinations or clear terrifying auditory hallucinations. The visual distortions may be extremely threatening. The hallucinogens may propel the patients into an egoless world and thus produce a sense of individual annihilation, panic, and terror. The drug effect can be immediate or delayed in the form of flashback. It could be transitory and short-lived, or it might be protracted and of longer duration. A young man of 15 years took some LSD. Within the hour he saw men coming at him with knives. In terror he attempted to fight, injuring himself running through the house. The reaction lasted about six hours.

The actual reaction mechanism will vary with the hallucinogen. Mescaline may effect the mesodiencephalic activating system; in contrast psilocybin may function by depressing the amygdala activity.[54] The LSD works by antagonizing the serotonin in neurons within the brainstem's raphe nuclei. As a result, these neuron firings decrease.[53] The raphe nuclei role has been suggested to filter sensory stimulation to the rest of the brain. Thus LSD blocks the filter and the brain experiences a perceptual flood.[24]

Marijuana has been known to cause paranoid episodes.[55] Although rare, it may produce a paranoid psychosis with persecutory delusions. At higher doses it may have an LSD-like effect. The more potent the cannabis, the more intense the reaction appears to be.

Phencyclidine hydrochloride, PCP, has been responsible for a number of paranoid and violent episodes. PCP has the pharmacologic properties of the sympathomimetics, eg, elevated blood pressure, pulse, and reflexes, and of the cholinergics, eg, sweating, drooling, and constricted pupils. It has effects on the cerebellum including incoordination, slurred speech, and nystagmus.[56] Patients have a variety of potent experiences on PCP. They may become acutely paranoid. They may have auditory and visual hallucinations. They may develop delusional thinking with a sense of invulnerability, invincibility, and superhuman power.[57]

Medical Illnesses

Endocrine disorders Both ends of the *adrenal* activity spectrum have been implicated in the production of paranoid symptoms.

Cushing's syndrome may manifest itself through paranoid ideation, although the more common mental changes are depression and insomnia.[6] Other manifestations include hypertension, hirsutism, osteoporosis, amenorrhea, abdominal strain, easy fatigue, and generalized weakness. These represent the essential mechanism of bilateral adrenal hyperplasia in response to ACTH hypersecretion. Diagnosis is based upon increased cortisol, loss of diurnal variation, and increased urinary 17-hydroxycorticosteroids.[58]

Addison's disease (hypoadrenalism) may generate a spectrum of paranoid reactions ranging from suspiciousness to paranoid psychosis and from *apathetic withdrawal* to frank delusions.[59] Indeed, Addison in his original description of the disease commented upon the reclusiveness these patients exhibited.[60] Features of this disease include marked, progressive fatigue, hypotension, pronounced hyperpigmentation, anorexia, weight loss, nausea, vomiting, and occasionally hypoglycemia. Prominent laboratory values which not only prove diagnostic but also provide the etiology for symptoms involve diminished control, reduced urine 17-hydroxycorticosteroids and 17-ketosteroids, and electrolyte changes: decreased sodium, chloride, and bicarbonate and increased potassium.[58] As expected from this hypoadrenal presentation, *hypopituitarism* may also generate a paranoid psychotic picture.[6]

Parathyroid conditions have been responsible for paranoid reactions with the essential ingredient being alterations in calcium.

Hyperparathyroidism may produce a psychosis with paranoid features.[61] Agras and Oliveau reported on a number of patients with hyperparathyroidism and a marked depression with paranoid symptoms.[62] Of interest, these patients had a clear sensorium. Others have stressed that the paranoia, the delusions, the hallucinations, and projection ideation are all manifestations of the organic psychosis.[59] The essential diagnostic studies remain increased serum calcium and parathyroid hormone levels. Other studies reveal renal stones and osteosis fibrosa cystica. Physical findings include muscle weakness, anorexia, and fatigue.

Hypoparathyroidism also may account for a paranoid episode. Here again, the critical determinant is the calcium level, but this time it is markedly diminished. This condition, not infrequently, occurs following surgery and will be discussed under that head.[63]

Thyroid disorders at both extremes may erupt with paranoid symptoms.

Hyperthyroidism may trigger a variety of psychoses with the common and prominent feature being paranoia.[64] The psychotic manifestations include schizophrenia, manic-depressive illness, and involutional melancholia. Other symptoms and signs of hyperthyroidism involve fine tremor, heat intolerance, weight loss, hyperactivity, sweating excessively, and hyperdefecation, evidence of goiter, and palpitations.

Diagnosis is based upon increased T_4, T_3, thyroid radioactive iodine uptake, resin-T_3 uptake, free thyroxine index, and basal metabolic rate.[65] A 35-year-old woman with Graves' disease entered the hospital for thyroid treatment. She demonstrated a wild marked lability of affect, feelings of people plotting against her, pronounced apprehension, extreme activity, flight of ideas, and excessive talking. She required transfer to a psychiatric unit and responded to both treatment of her hyperthyroidism and psychosis.

Several mechanisms have been advanced to account for the relationship between hyperthyroidism and psychosis. One involves the thyroid hormone increases. In this sequence, the excess hormones affect catechloamine metabolism which in turn heightens adrenal cortical activities and function.[64] In another, the psychoses result from electrolyte charges in hyperthyroidism. Namely, the serum calcium is increased and serum magnesium is decreased.[66] Still another theory revolves about the fact that hyperthyroidism causes dopamine receptor hypersensitivity.[67]

Hypothyroidism may generate paranoid ideation, thinking, delusions, and hallucinations. These are commonly the persecutory type.[6] Myxedema has been associated with a cluster of paranoid features, including delusions of persecution, regression, abstracting difficulty, and auditory hallucinations.[59] In extreme cases, the presentation is an organic psychosis. Other features include fatigue, a generalized slowing in both mental and physical activities, cold intolerance, and menorrhagia. Diagnosis is based upon decreased T_4 and free T_4.[65] The probable mechanism of depression involves a diminution of the available catecholamines.[59]

Of the *hematologic disorders, pernicious anemia* emerges as the one associated with and responsible for paranoid states.[59] Other major mental manifestations include schizophreniform psychoses, depression, dementia, and apathy. The essential lesion remains a vitamin B_{12} deficiency as a result of an absorption defect. Diagnostic features involve dyspepsia, anorexia, sore tongue, peripheral neuropathy, pallor, megaloblastic bone marrow, large oval red cells, no gastric acid, and a Schilling test demonstrating no vitamin B_{12} GI absorption.[68]

A series of *infectious diseases* have been implicated with paranoid productions.

Syphilis causes a distinctive paranoid pattern. *Treponema pallidum* the offending spirochete, following a latent phase of often years produces tertiary syphilis, also called general paresis. General paresis is frequently typified by a hollow, superficial expansive euphoric affect. These patients appear to lack depth, cleverness, and coherence and exhibit poor judgment and dementia. The spirochete attacks the frontal lobes most severely.[24] Serologic tests confirm the diagnosis.

Encephalitis, viral, bacterial, or mycobacterial, may be heralded by paranoid reactions. Physical evidence for encephalitis include fever, headaches, vomiting, and signs of meningeal involvement. Examination of CSF for cell, culture, protein, and glucose provide critical diagnostic information. The author vividly recalls a 45-year-old woman with a pneumococcal emphysema who became acutely paranoid and combative as the first indication of her bacterial encephalitis.

Malaria has been linked to the formation and presentation of persecutory delusions in several patients recovering from *Plasmodium falciparum*.[69] This paranoid reaction represents the cerebral malarial involvement. The hallmark of this disease remains paroxysmal episodes of shaking, chills, fever, headache, and myalgia commencing ten to 16 minutes after a mosquito bite.[70] Diagnosis is made by identification of the ring forms of *Plasmodium falciparum* in a blood smear.

Typhus fever has long been associated with paranoid presentations.[3] The offending organism, *Rickettsia prowazekii* , louse-borne or *typhi* , flea-borne, commonly precipitates an abrupt onset of prostrating fever, headache, and malaise followed by truncal maculopapular rash. Mental changes accompany this course underlined by the disease name (Greek *typhos*, smoke or stupor).[71] Key laboratory studies are *Proteus* OX-19 agglutination, and specific serologic tests.[72]

Trypanosomiasis, African type sleeping sickness, may also generate a mental status change with paranoid features.[3] Other prominent alterations include somnolence, anorexia, mania, coma, and headaches. The trypanosomiasis is transmitted by the tsetse fly and the disease may develop insidiously or acutely. Diagnosis rests upon identification of the organism in the blood.[73]

Toxic shock syndrome may present as a paranoid psychosis. Lewis describes a 35-year-old woman who developed a florid paranoid delusion and behavior and required involuntary hospitalization with the diagnosis of acute paranoid schizophrenia.[74] Ultimately, removal of a tampon and treatment of purulent vaginal discharge led to disappearance of psychotic symptoms. The continued use of tampons has been linked to the syndrome.[75] Also *Staphylococcus aureus* has been associated with toxic shock syndrome and a particular toxin-producing strain linked to its etiology.[76]

Metabolic Disorders

Uremia, especially when progressive and severe, may develop into a delirium with pronounced paranoid features. Early manifestations of renal failure include a pervasive fatigue, withdrawal, mental changes ranging from lability of affect to dullness, slurred speech, memory defects, restless legs and restlessness, decreased appetite and libido, and depression. As the uremic syndrome deepens, a delirium emerges. Anger, further withdrawal, demandingness, and paranoia represent some of the reactions to rising azotemia. Some patients exhibit strong negative and aggressive features and attitudes.[77] Patients with urea above 250 mg/100 mL appear to have the most profound, neuropsychiatric symptoms and disturbances.[78] The manifestations may not only reflect an increased urea but also an increased CNS vulnerability due to its heightened oxygen consumption because of dialyzable endogenous neurotoxins.[79]

Dialysis dementia not uncommonly erupts with episodes of paranoia. The paranoia presents within the context of evidence of dementia, sleep disturbances, stuttering, dysarthria, dyspraxia, and dysphasia, mutism, myoclonus, and seizures.[77] The dementia is thought to be a result of aluminum excess.[80] The syndrome usually develops after patients have been on dialysis for a long time. These patients then follow a progressively fatal course. Their EEGs show a distinctive pattern of bisynchronous delta rhythm with frontocentral spike and slow-wave activity.[81] A 55-year-old salesman who had been on dialysis for 7 years suddenly became suspicious, fearful of going home, and distant. He had several amnesic episodes; within the month further evidence of dementia emerged and the EEG demonstrated marked delta waves. His encephalopathy progressed and he died of complications within 6 months.

Wilson's disease (hepatolenticular degeneration) has been associated with paranoid features and paranoid schizophrenic symptoms.[82] This familiar metabolic disorder is marked by increased copper and amino acid urinary excretion and decreased serum ceruloplasmin. Major effects occur in the basal ganglia, causing tremors and rigidity; in the liver, leading to cirrhosis; and in the cornea, resulting in its greenish-brown pigmentation (Kayser-Fleischer ring).[83] Changes may also be found in the cerebellum and the cerebral cortex. Symptoms commence insidiously between the ages of 11 and 25 years.

Hepatic failure may be accompanied by frightening paranoid delusions and visual hallucinations.[6] Three aspects dominate the precoma period.[59] First, patients develop increasing signs of an organic mental disorder. Second, patients exhibit asterixis, the liver flap. Third, their EEGs display paroxysmal bilateral synchronus slow wave which is actually imposed upon a normal background.[84] Evidence of jaundice and elevated liver function tests prove diagnostic.

Acute intermittent porphyria (AIP) may present as frank paranoia embedded in the constellation of bizarre behavior, abdominal pain, and diverse neurologic symptoms.[85] The psychotic manifestations include delusions, violence, catatonia, and auditory hallucinations. Colic characterizes the abdominal pain along with nausea, vomiting, and constipation. A history of abdominal surgery is not uncommon in these patients. An ascending paralysis, lower extremity peripheral neuropathy, paresthesias, pain, and weakness represent the emerging neurologic picture. As the name implies, these symptoms may develop suddenly and between bouts the patients may be asymptomatic.

An autosomal dominant genetic biochemical lesion accounts for this disease. In the synthesis of porphyrins, the major heme component, δ-aminolevulinic acid synthetase (ALA-synthetase) catalyzes the joining of succinyl-CoA and glycine into δ-aminolevulinic acid (ALA); two ALAs unite to form porphobilinogen (PBG). In porphyria there is an increase of ALA-synthetase. As a consequence, excessive ALA-synthetase leads to overproduction of ALA and PBG.[86] Pepplinkhuizen speculates the accompanying serine-glycine metabolism produces an excess of methyl groups.[87] These methyl groups may lead to a hallucinogenic phenomenon.

A number of other features point toward AIP. It occurs generally in individuals between ages 20 and 50 years and more in women than in men. Patients complain of headaches and urinary frequency. They may have an elevated blood pressure, tachycardia, and fever. Blood studies demonstrate a leukocytosis and a spot test will show diminished activity of the erythrocyte porphobilinogen deaminase (PBG) enzyme.[88] The EEG frequently may show generalized slow activity. Barbiturates, sulfonamides, infection, and alcohol can trigger an attack.

Using these clinical features, Macalpine and Hunter have woven an AIP hypothesis to explain King George III's madness.[89] They note the late onset (50 years), the episodic course, the bouts of colic, and the paresthesia. His bouts of madness included insomnia, excitement, loquaciousness, delusions, and hallucinations. There was eventual organic deterioration. Infections triggered attacks; long symptom-free periods also characterized his illness.

The *menstrual cycle* has been correlated and linked to periodic psychosis with not infrequently paranoid elements in some women. Williams and Weeks emphasize this takes place during the premenstrual phases.[90] Such a psychosis represents an extreme form of the *premenstrual tension syndrome*. Anxiety, insomnia, inability to concentrate, and agitation characterize the syndrome. It occurs 7 to 14 days prior to menstruation, often in 30-to 40-year-old nulliparous women. Its mechanisms may reflect renin augmentation in the latter part of the cycle.[91] The activated angiotensin system causes the release of norepinephrine and aldosterone.

Endo et al advance a different framework for a menstrual cycle related periodic psychosis.[92] He reports on recurring psychotic responses in various phases of their cycles in seven women; not necessarily in the premenstrual phase. The womens' ages ranged from 13 to 23 years and they had histories of developmental conflicts and struggles. Their psychotic symptoms included excitement; heightened appetite; loquaciousness; aggressiveness; belligerence; irritability; hallucinations, auditory and visual; ideas of reference; persecutory delusions; and severe apprehension. The psychosis followed a particular recurring characteristic in each woman, eg, only during menstruation with remission in the rest of the cycle for one 19-year-old woman. Ultimately, each gained full recovery. Endo et al suggest that an interplay of psychological factors and CNS monoamine activities and disturbances generated the periodic psychosis.

Neurologic Disorders

Temporal lobe epilepsy (psychomotor epilepsy) has a strong relationship to paranoia and of all the seizure disorders, this one has the most relevant and compelling association to it. Some patients with temporal lobe epilepsy have paranoid psychotic manifestations. These occur usually after the patient has had the disease for at least a decade.[93]

Four major characteristics depict temporal lobe epilepsy: aura, automatic behavior, autonomic reactions, and amnesia.[94] Patients sense something unusual and different before a seizure. The aura takes many forms: olfactory, gustatory, visual, or auditory hallucinations, a dreamlike state, dèjá vu (being familiar with the unfamiliar), jamais vu (being unfamiliar with the familiar), visceral feeings, forced thoughts, illusions, and a sensation of strangeness. Patients during the seizure engage in a number of fragmented, repeated stereotyped involuntary movements. These automatic behaviors include lip-smacking, chewing, kicking, biting, rubbing, and stamping. Autonomic reactions involve dilated pupils, elevated blood pressure, tachycardia, urinary incontinence, sweating, and altered respirations. Many patients have amnesia for the episode and have to struggle to reorient themselves following one.

Hyposexuality also accompanies temporal lobe epilepsy. Blumer and Walker emphasize the global quality of this hyposexuality.[95] Patients, both men and women, not only lose the performance ability but also the desire. Their finding mirrors the work of Klüver and Bucy, who demonstrated that bilateral destruction of the temporal lobes causes hypersexuality.[96]

The psychosis itself, although appearing in some way similar to schizophrenia, also has a number of significant differences.[97] Many patients displayed paranoid ideations; others developed catatonia; still others evolved into supereligious thinking and behavior. Yet, the same patients remained less bizarre, less withdrawn, more emotionally involved with their environment, and markedly less deteriorated than patients with a schizophrenic disorder. These patients remained affectively available. Additionally, they have negative family histories for schizophrenia.

The relationship between psychosis and temporal lobe epilepsy remains complex. Glaus demonstrated in 1931 the control of the seizures actually led to emergence of the schizophrenialike picture.[98] Yet Jensen and Larsen have shown improvement in some and development of psychosis in others following temporal resection for this disorder.[99] The treatment for the psychosis is one of using neuroleptics in addition to anticonvulsants.

> **Case report** A 40-year-old executive became overtly hostile, accused his wife of having an affair, and was irritable on the job. Although assertive, demanding, and quarrelsome, he continued to be effective and involved with his family and coworkers. An EEG demonstrated a left temporal seizure focus. Further studies, eg, CT scan and a ventriculogram, revealed an arachnoid cyst. Following neurosurgical removal, he returned to normal; he resumed his married life and career.

The EEG remains one of the most useful diagnostic tools, with patients demonstrating seizure activity in the temporal lobes. Often nasalpharyngeal leads help detect these abnormalities and foci. Yet as the work of Jensen and Larsen illustrates and the aforementioned case demonstrates, the role of temporal lobe epilepsy and psychosis continues to be complicated, interwoven, and variable.

Huntington's disease may evolve various paranoid changes in the patient's personality. The constellation of features include the development of suspiciousness, the emergence of excessive religiosity, and the eruption of an inflated self-worth and self-concept of superiority.[100] Patients also display irritability, impulsivity, promiscuity, poor judgment, and signs of dementia. The hallmark of disease remains a dominant inheritance pattern, choreoid movements, and progressive organicity. Various degrees of changes were noted postmortem in the caudate nucleus and the putamen.[101] Spokes has found increased norepinephrine in the striatum and lateral pallidum.[102]

Multiple sclerosis (MS) has been associated with paranoid psychoses.[97] Many mental changes have been linked to MS. These include affective alterations with half the patients demonstrating a depression and the other half showing an inappropriate complacency often termed euphoria; evidence of organicity with short-term memory loss; intellectual diminution; and with chronicity of the disease, apathy, and irritability. Diagnosis rests on increased CSF γ-globulin, a waxing and waning episodic clinical course, and an array of neurologic symptoms and signs, eg, paresthesias, ataxia, nystagmus, visual impairment, slurred speech, incontinence, temporal optic disk pallor, and intention tremors.

Normal pressure hydrocephalus (NPH) may first reveal itself through paranoid manifestations. Price and Tucker describe a 58-year-old man who developed ideas of persecution, people talking about him and out to get him within the context of an 8-month depression.[103] After suicide attempts, not responding to an antidepressant and electroconvulsive therapy (ECT), and increasing dementia, the patients' pneumoencephalography and radioiodinated serum albumin (RISA) scan demonstrated the presence of NPH. They suggest a number of diagnostic clues toward appreciating NPH. First, it may present as a rapidly progressive mental change in an older patient without a history of psychiatric problems, without a family history of such illness, and following a fluctuating course. Second, patients show evidence of dementia and gait disturbances. Third, these patients will exhibit a profound post-ECT delirium. Key NPH features involve unsteady gait, dementia, and incontinence.

Narcolepsy may have paranoid qualities in its presentation.[6] The disorder itself has five diagnostic features: (1) sleep attacks; (2) cataplexy; (3) sleep paralysis; (4) hypnagogic hallucinations; and (5) sleep disturbances.[59] Often the hallucinations — visual, auditory, or tactile — are extremely terrifying and frightening.

Hearing loss is not infrequently accompanied by paranoia.[104] Patients become progressively alienated, distant, and removed from their environment. Some find admitting or accepting hearing difficulty an uncomfortable experience. They silently endure the loss. Some also begin to imagine people making offensive, threatening, or attacking remarks about them. In the absence of communication, feedback, and full dialogue, some patients begin to construct a world dominated by their ideas and concepts.

Immunologic Disorders

Systemic lupus erythematosus frequently leaves in its episodic course moments of paranoia. Lupus is an inflammatory autoimmune process affecting connective tissue in many organs. Although many of mental responses are organic in nature, some present as schizophrenialike or as psychotic depression. Characteristics of these psychoses include insomnia, lability of affect, inability to concentrate, depression, obsessional thinking, and dread.[105] Patients complain of difficulty sleeping and report rapid sudden mood swings. The latter prompts fears of losing their minds. Depression emerges as a common experience of these patients. Patients develop preoccupation, ruminations, and obsessional thinking about their disease, their disability, and their prognosis. Patients also encounter a wide range of other symptoms: pronounced nervousness, hallucinations — visual, auditory, and tactile, projective thinking, flat affect, autism, catatonia, withdrawal, and a sense of quiet.

Lupus itself represents a disease with a strong genetic component and immunologic mechanism. It affects predominantly women in the age range of 20 to 40 years. It follows a variable course with frequent waxes and wanings. Antinuclear antibodies stand as the cornerstone of the illness. The mechanism involves a deficit of T cell activity and a corresponding excessive functioning of B cells.[106] As a result, many antinuclear antibodies are overproduced and they are deposited in various organs, eg, kidney, CNS, and joints.

Meeting four or more of the following 14 symptoms determine the disease's diagnosis according to the American Rheumatism Association criteria: patients have facial erythema (butterfly rash); hematologic disorders—hemolytic anemia, leukopenia, or thrombocytopenia; false-positive syphilis tests; loss of hair; seizures or psychosis; cellular casts; profound proteinuria; nasopharyngeal ulcerations; presence of LE cells; arthritis without ensuing deformation; pericarditis or pleuritis; discoid lupus; photosensitivity; and Raynaud's phenomenon.[107] Laboratory diagnostic studies and results include the following: LE cells (present in two thirds of cases), antinuclear antibody (95% of cases), elevated antibodies to DNA, depressed serum complement, hyper-γ–globulinemia, positive Coombs test, and false-positive syphilis serology. The EEG and CT scan may also demonstrate CNS effects of this disease.

Oncology

The *diagnostic process* and the *diagnosis* of cancer may contribute to paranoid development. The search for a tumor as the origin of symptoms is at once both a comfort and an immense discomfort. It generates apprehension, fear, suspicion, doubt, and concern. An ambiguous cancer diagnosis may prompt a paranoid reaction.[108]

Central nervous system tumors may provoke paranoid reactions. Although these tumors' general presentation has been described by Adams and Victor [100] as "psychomotor asthenia" with decreased mental activity, lack of spontaneity, apathy, inertia, irritability, and lability of affect, in some instances the paranoia dominates the clinical appearance.

Krauthammer and Klerman present a series of patients with mania secondary to CNS tumors.[109] Here, the patients exhibited classic manic symptoms of hyperactivity, pressured speech, grandiosity, diminished sleep needs, distractibility, and flight of ideas. The offending neoplasms included parasagittal meningioma, diencephalon glioma, spheno-occipital bone benign tumor, and a third ventricle craniopharyngioma. Additionally, patients with tumors of the limbic system may present as delusional.[110]

Other tumors through their endocrine disturbances generate paranoid psychoses. The paranoid presentations themselves follow the descriptions outlined in the endocrine section. The evoking neoplasms are of two types. First rank the tumors of the endocrine system: thyroid adenomas producing hyperthyroidism and pituitary basophilic adenomas and adrenal neoplasms causing hyperadrenalism. Second involve diffuse tumors manufacturing hormones: oat-cell carcinoma of the lung, thymoma, islet-cell tumor, and bronchial carcinoid producing ACTH, and choriocarcinoma, epidermoid carcinoma of the lung, and mesothelioma producing thyrotropin.[111]

Pulmonary Disorders

Sleep apnea may lead to paranoid reactions and psychosis. The chapter on sleep problems dealt in detail with this diagnosis. The principle mechanism appears to be related to sleep deprivation.[112]

With aging, paranoia represents a frequent occurrence. Roth in 1955 put forth the term *paraphrenia* to depict this phenomenon.[113] It has come to encompass a paranoid disorder developing within the elderly; it is similar to the DSM-III paranoid disorder, discussed below under "Psychiatric Differential Diagnosis," and it emerges as distinct from patients who have been diagnosed earlier in their lives as paranoid schizophrenic or schizophrenic.[114]

Several features characterize this paranoia of the aged. The delusions are either sexual in nature and follow bizarre concepts or revolve about the spouse's infidelity. Patients have referential thinking and frequently see themselves as objects or victims of nefarious schemes. If hallucinatory experiences occur, they are usually auditory. Patients hear neighbors plotting against them or people outside their door. Not infrequently, the patients live alone, are women, actually are in good health, and have a clear sensorium.

Case report A concerned son brought his widowed 78-year-old mother to the emergency department after she had suddenly been obsessed with a number of sexual indiscretions by her minister. She accused him of not only an affair but also a nonreligious interest in her. Beyond her preoccupation and her insomnia, she was well oriented, had an unremarkable physical examination, and easily maintained herself living alone. She responded to low doses of haloperidol, psychotherapy, and day hospitalization.

A constellation of factors converge to cause paranoia with aging.[115] First, some patients may have been genetically predisposed. Second, two particular personality patterns contribute to this occurrence, paranoid and schizoid. The popular notion of personality attributes becoming exaggerated with aging, lends support and experience to this phenomenon. Third, medical illnesses as well as diminished hearing and seeing capacity play a role. Fourth, social isolation, decreased mobility, loss of family and friends, and restricted economic resources — all critically affect the elderly.

Surgical Complications

Preoperative anticipation may provoke an acute paranoid episode. Patients fear the impending loss of control, submission, "being put to sleep," going "under the knife," pain, discomfort, scars, and the disruption of their lives. Surgery not only threatens their ego boundaries and defenses, but also actually for some represents an assault on their body and its integrity. A 20-year-old college senior became overwhelmed by terror as she faced the extraction of two wisdom teeth. She had insomnia, a sense of herself as a victim, crying spells punctuated by silly, laughing periods, and stopped going to classes. During several crisis intervention sessions, she revealed that surgery meant total loss of control, power, destiny, and herself. It recapitulated a time in her life when she was beaten by her stepfather. Patients in surgery confront potential disfiguration, pain, losses, and death.

The *general* conditions of surgery and the immediate postoperative period may promote a paranoid reaction in some patients. The anesthetic, the pain, the loss of control, the frequent taking of vital signs, the intensive care unit, the pain medications, and the loss of sleep — all contribute to the stress. Generally, the elderly, the medically compromised, and the patient with alcohol problems are more prone to develop postoperative paranoia.

Following *cardiac surgery* a paranoid psychosis may erupt. Current literature and clinical observations stress the delirium and organic presentation in the postoperative period.[116] Although preoperative anxiety and depression did correlate with this complication, the most important factor proved to be the patient's prior medical condition. Yet earlier reports emphasized psychotic responses in patients with a clear sensorium.[117] One explanation remains: closed heart surgery produces fewer psychiatric complications and sequelae than open heart surgery does. A 56-year-old businessman erupted in a paranoid rage four days after triple cardiac bypass surgery. His psychosis proved ego-alien and came after several days of lucid thinking. He accused nurses of trying to poison him and people of trying to kill him. He responded to haloperidol. Later during that hospitalization, he apologized to the staff and thanked them for their help.

Eye surgery provokes paranoid psychotic reactions. Mania, delusions, and auditory and visual hallucinations may emerge following cataract surgery.[118] Although often described as black-patch delirium, the disorientation facets may be a minor part of the bizarre, disruptive presentation. The loss of sensory input and the mind's attempt to fill the information gap helps to explain the phenomena. Of interest, some patients actually develop visual hallucinations because of the cataracts.[119] They experience seeing children, bright colors, and terrifying scenes. Cataract surgery halts these hallucinations.

Postoperative electrolyte changes and medications generate paranoid psychoses. The alterations in the electrolyte balance, distribution, and concentrations influence the CNS. For example, fluctuations in serum calcium and magnesium levels as well as differences between their intracellular and extracellular concentrations may account for *postparathyroidectomy psychosis*.[120] Following this surgery, the serum calcium is low; the phosphate, high. Patients experience tetany with muscle cramps, carpopedal spasms, seizures, wheezing, difficulty breathing, vision changes with photophobia and diplopia, and abdominal cramps.[121] Postoperative medications trigger paranoia, especially the use of steroids and opiates. A 30-year-old dialysis patient received a cadaver kidney. He also was started on prednisone postoperation. He became uncontrollably anxious, suspicious, fearful, and filled with the dread of death on the steroids. The higher his steroid medication requirement, the greater his disorganization and bizarre behavior.

Substance abuse may account for a postoperative paranoid event. The abrupt surgically induced termination of alcohol, barbiturates, or minor tranquilizer use may plunge the patient into a severe withdrawal reaction. Often in the rush of the emergency surgical situation, the patient's alcohol and medication may be overlooked, or patients may minimize or deny the substance use. A 72-year-old woman required urgent operative intervention for a fractured hip. Two days postoperation she erupted with screaming, inappropriate incoherent discourse, and belligerence. Careful history from her husband then revealed a secret pattern of diazepam abuse of up to 50 mg a day.

Physical Trauma

One of the many *reactions to physical trauma* may be paranoia. Certainly, the pain, the disruption, the violence, the suddenness, the scars, the losses, the memory, and the anguish which accompany a traumatic event generate a host of disquieting feelings.[122] Moreover, for some individuals the search for the etiology and the meaning of the accident leads them into paranoid thinking. In certain cases, the patients will pursue a cause, a culprit, a villain, or a force behind the scene. They blame the company, the machine, the state highway department, the hospital, or their spouses. They may turn to litigation; they sue; they demand redress and compensation. A 45-year-old woman cab driver made a wrong turn and caused a serious automobile accident in which she sustained a fractured pelvis. She blamed her company for not repairing her vehicle's brakes. She directed all her rage at her employer. In other instances, patients having survived serious trauma develop an inflated sense of self-worth, of redemption, and of glory. They feel chosen.

Head trauma specifically has been associated with paranoia. Two different causes may account for this phenomenon. First, the trauma can produce organic mental deficits. The patients, to compensate for their consciously unappreciated cognitive loss, use a paranoid defense system. Instead of acknowledging they do not recall where they placed something, they accuse those about them of stealing the objects. They cover their defects by blaming, by attacking, and by quarreling. Second, head trauma may lead to patients becoming overly sensitive.[123] As such, they are predisposed to a paranoid stance.

Psychiatric Differential Diagnosis

Paranoia stands as one of the cardinal mental positions, reactions, and defenses. It constitutes a key symptom in a variety of psychiatric diagnoses. It also occurs as part of, and within the constellation of, an even larger number of psychiatric disorders. This section focuses upon the major diagnostic groups and entities.

Within the context of *organic mental disorders* paranoia makes a frequent occurrence and can be explained by two mechanisms. First, as cited earlier, the paranoid symptoms result from organic deficit. The patients, unable to comprehend a situation, perceive a loss, or appreciate a change, develop a paranoid answer: "I did not misplace the keys; someone stole them." Additionally, a deficit may provide a basis for the patient to become overwhelmed, deluged, and inundated by too much information, material, or stimulation. As a consequence of this "too-much" situation, the patients resort to a projective defensive reaction: "I do not feel too much is happening; I am being attacked."

The deficit accounts partially for the paranoia in *delirium* and significantly for it in *dementia*. [124] The delirium criteria include a clouded consciousness and lack of environmental awareness with two of the following: perceptual disturbance, occasional incoherent speech, sleep-wake disturbance, or alterations in psychomotor activity, disorientation with recall deficits, rapid onset within hours to days and fluctuations during the day, and organic etiologic evidence.[125] The dementia criteria require an intellectual loss leading to functioning impairment, with at least one of: (a) abstract thinking impairment, (b) poor judgement, (c) disturbed cortical functions, and (d) change of personality, consciousness not clouded, and evidence of organicity or exclusion of other diagnoses.

Second, paranoia emerges as a direct effect of substance, drug, physiologic disturbance, or lesion. *Organic delusional syndrome* has the criteria of predominant delusions, without clouded consciousness, without intellectual losses or major hallucinations, and organic etiologic evidence. This occurs with amphetamines, for example.[114] *Organic hallucinosis* features predominantly hallucinations, without clouded consciousness, without intellectual loss, without delusions or major affective component, and an organic etiologic evidence.[114]

Intoxication or withdrawal states similarly represent either direct substance effects or the aftermath of their discontinuance.

The *paranoid disorders* comprise a major diagnostic constellation focused upon the central feature of persistent delusion of either persecution or jealousy.[126] In contrast to the schizophrenic disorders, these usually commence in mid to late life and do not encompass bizarre delusions, significant hallucinations, disorganization, or loose associations. Unlike those with organic disorders, patients with paranoid disorders neither display disturbance of consciousness, intellect, orientation, or memory nor have an organic etiology for their behavior. The differences with various paranoid groups revolve about the time course or the number of persons involved in the delusional system.

The *paranoid disorder* has a number of criteria.[114] The first and foremost remains the persistence of delusions of either persecution or jealousy. Second, the patient's emotions, reactions, and behavior are consistent and in symphony with the actual delusions. Third, the symptoms last at least 1 week. Fourth, the patients do not meet the criteria for schizophrenia. Fifth, hallucinations do not play a prominent role. Sixth, the delusions do not develop in the context of either a manic or depressed phase. Finally, there is no organic basis for the paranoia.

Kendler, after a literature review, concluded that paranoia as a simple delusional disorder constitutes a distinct valid diagnosis separate from both schizophrenic and affective disorders.[127] Further insight and confirmation of the entity paranoia comes from the work of Oxman et al.[128] They have elegantly shown the actual language and the word usage of paranoid patients as different than those of depressed, cardiac, cancer, and manic patients. Specifically, in the paranoids' verbal self-presentation, they significantly use fewer or avoid certain word classes which depict lower status, sexual themes, natural objects, or family than those other patient groups. For example, the depressed patients often emphasized particular family members: husband, wife, son, or daughter, or focused upon specific locations (eg, Eagle Island), and specific dates and times. The authors put forth that the paranoia patients, through their distancing, nonfocused vocabulary, demonstrate their world alienation and lack of personal connections.

If the paranoia persists for at least 6 months and meets the criteria for paranoid disorder and is not a shared paranoia, then this is called *paranoia* in the DSM-III. If the actual paranoid disorder has lasted less than 6 months, it is termed an *acute paranoid disorder*. If the two or more persons who because of their close relationship develop a delusional system meeting the criteria for paranoid disorder, this is referred to as a *shared paranoid disorder*. This has been called in the past, folie à deux. Two widowed sisters lived in an ancient apartment house on the top floor in a run-down section of town. Each and together, they came to believe in harmful forces in the neighborhood. Ultimately, they refused to venture beyond the front door.

The *schizophrenic disorders* encompass paranoia in two ways. First, moments of projective thinking, episodes of euphoria, attacking voices, thoughts of infidelity, or elements of grandiosity may occur within the context of any of the schizophrenic disorders. Second, in *paranoid schizophrenia* there is a predominance of one or more of four major manifestations of paranoia: delusions of persecution, delusions of grandiosity, delusions of jealousy, or hallucinations of a persecutory or grandiose nature.[129]

The schizophrenic disorders represent a profound psychiatric disturbance. The diagnosis is based upon the symptoms, their duration, and the patient's course. This disorder has a global presentation and impact; patients demonstrate bizarre delusions, striking hallucinations, disorganized thinking and flat affect. Bleuler originally described the disease as the four A's: autism, ambivalence, affect, and association.[129] Autism means self-absorption, inner responding and reflecting; ambivalence, two contrasting ideas held simultaneously; affect, flat; and association, looseness in connection, relationship, and coherence of the thought process.

Schizophrenia remains a devastating disturbance of thoughts and affect and their integration. The thought *disorder* is revealed by looseness of association, thought blocking, concrete thinking, circumstantiality, tranquility, neologism, overly abstract thinking, thought insertion, and thought broadcasting. Additionally there are perceptual alterations, including auditory hallucinations, with one or more voices often condemning or quarrelling or commanding them. Other hallucinations involve somatic, tactile, olfactory, gustatory, and visual experiences. The affect stands as flat, monotonous, and inappropriate. The patient describing the voices in his head arguing and threatening with a flat dull affect typifies the integration failure. These patients struggle with loss of identity, self, and ego boundaries. In the paranoid type, concerns about homosexuality and perceived sexual threats may be paramount.

The disorder usually occurs in adolescence or young adulthood. In the paranoid type, onset is later. Indeed, the diagnosis cannot be made if the symptoms start after 45 years of age. Of interest, onset of symptoms and first hospitalizations for men happen at earlier ages than for women with schizophrenia.[130] Although recently questioned, there remains evidence for a genetic contribution to the disease.[131] The paranoid type appears also to run in families.[114]

Symptoms, duration, and course provide the diagnostic criteria. The symptoms sometime during the illness reflect the disordered thoughts, altered perceptions, and flat affect.[132] They represent a "narrow" definition of schizophrenia. They also encompass the schneiderian first rank symptoms emphasizing thought insertion, control, broadcasting, and withdrawal, a thought disorder, and voices (auditory hallucinations) providing a running commentary about the patient.[133] They emphasize the key position of delusions and hallucinations in the diagnosis.[134]

Of symptoms, the patient must have experienced at least one of the six categories of events during the illness: (a) patients have had bizarre delusions which involve thought control, withdrawal, broadcasting, or insertion; (b) patient has developed delusions with marked grandiosity, religiosity, somatic preoccupation, or nihilistic focus; (c) patient has hallucinations with persecutory delusions; (d) patient experiences auditory hallucinations with two or more voices either commenting or discussing between themselves; (e) the patient has loose associations with flat affect, hallucinations, delusions, or catatonia.

Duration provides another essential part of the criteria. Patients must have had acute symptoms for at least 6 months. Additionally, the symptoms may have been preceded by the prodromal period. Characteristics of this period include isolation, flat affect, bizarre thinking, eg, clairvoyance or referential thinking, decline in hygiene, impairment of functioning, or bizarre behavior. In the paranoid types, gross behavioral disorganization is rare.

The course of the disease is often marked by deterioration. However, in the paranoid type, function may be much longer preserved and maintained.

A 30-year-old male computer operator gradually came to believe his machines were taking over the company, destroying personal relationships, replacing individual contacts, and ultimately influencing his thinking. His mood began to be irate; his behavior bizarre; and his family, estranged. He worried about his sexuality and identity. His older sister, when she was 29 years old, experienced a paranoid schizophrenic episode.

Paranoia represents a pivotal response to the *affective disorders*. Patients at both ends of the manic-depressive illness spectrum may demonstrate marked paranoid reactions. The emergence and eruption of delusional thinking may signal the onset of either mania or depression.

Mania constitutes the principle affective psychosis presenting with the sudden onset of grandiosity. The diagnosis again rests upon symptoms, duration, and course. Euphoria, flight of ideas, and hyperactivity form the key characteristic triad of the illness along with grandiose delusions, although some manic patients display profound persecutory delusions, hostility, and apprehensive suspiciousness. An affective contact with and quality to the patient and a favorable prognosis serve as clinical touchstones of mania.

A mood elevation remains the cornerstone of mania. Patients experience euphoria, present expansively, and demonstrate elation. This leads to delusions of grandeur. In the extreme, they proclaim themselves the president, the pope, the prime minister, or the savior. Their affect is often infectious; people find themselves absorbed and captivated by these individuals. One particularly striking variation of this mood disturbance ranks as patients present with marked irritability. Also, not uncommonly, patients exhibit islands of melancholia in a sea of happiness and joy.

The DSM-III provides a list of seven features of which the diagnosis of mania requires at least three.[114] The symptoms must be in evidence for a week or more or must be of such severity as to necessitate hospitalization. The seven symptom areas involve: (a) hyperactivity; (b) talkativeness and pressured speech; (c) flight of ideas; (d) elated sense of self and self-worth; (e) diminished sleep and the need for it; (f) easy distractibility; (g) expansive, inappropriate overinvolvement in situations with great (but unrecognized by the patient) risks.

The mania reaches psychotic proportions with evidence of delusions, hallucinations, or significantly bizarre behavior. The psychotic qualities may either be congruent or incongruent with the mood.

A number of important clinical and historical clues help to establish the mania as the diagnosis. These involve a differentiation of mania from schizophrenia, an appreciation of the patient's course, an investigation into the family's history, and the use of others to provide critical observations and material.

In evaluating patients with mania and those with schizophrenia, several critical differences emerge. First, a mood remains the central feature and focus of mania. Patients reveal a feeling, a sense of emotion, and moment of affect, be it euphoria, elation, irritability, or even sadness. A disorder of thought serves as the key quality of schizophrenia. Second, flight of ideas and pressured speech typify a manic's verbal production. Here, the interviewer can readily follow the concepts, the evolution of the ideas, and the logic of sequence. In schizophrenia, loss of associations dominates the patient's thinking and speaking. The interviewer experiences great difficulty in pursuing the logic and coherence of the discourse. Third, in mania, the interviewer feels an affective contact with and to the patient. In schizophrenia, one finds a sense of distance, and monotony in the dialogue. Fourth, mania carries with it a good prognosis, a favorable outcome, and a higher level of functioning than schizophrenia.[135]

Mania happens as part of manic-depressive illness (MDI). The first manic episode usually erupts before the patient turns 20 years old. They then follow a cyclical course with periodic highs and lows.

Genetics contribute heavily to the MDI. Patients with bipolar illness (MDI) have strong evidence of hereditary patterns. Many of their first-degree relatives will not only have had a major affective illness, but also specifically had MDI.[55] There has been the suggestion of color blindness linked to MDI inheritance patterns.[136] Patients with mania have relatives with histories of MDI. Many of these relatives may be treated successfully with lithium carbonate.

One particularly useful technique in reaching a diagnosis of mania involves interviewing significant others.[137] They often provide vital information. They report bizarre, inappropriate, expansive, destructive, and out-of-control behavior overlooked or underplayed by the patient.

Major depression with psychotic features constitutes another important paranoia diagnosis. This diagnosis first fulfills all the DSM-III criteria for a major depression and also encompasses the gross disturbances, which moves it to psychotic proportions.[114] Delusions of worthlessness, destruction, and persons against them may be predominant. They may develop a total sense of nihilism. A dominant mood of dysphoria represents the key and central affect of this diagnosis. The sadness, the depression, and the hopelessness is accompanied by at least four of the following: (a) decreased appetite or weight loss; (b) sleep disturbance, either too much or too little; (c) psychomotor effects, either retardation or agitation; (d) diminished interests or loss of libido; (e) decreased energy; (f) sense of worthlessness or out-of-proportion guilt; (g) difficulty concentrating; and (h) preoccupation with death, thoughts of self-destruction, or suicide attempt. These symptoms occur daily for at least a 2-week period. Evidence for psychotic extension involve delusions, hallucinations, or muteness (depressive stupor embracing a degree of impairment to preclude daily functioning). The psychotic features are either congruent or not congruent with the dysphoria.

A number of examples serve to illustrate the psychotic features. Patients experience delusions of total worthlessness and hopelessness. This leads them to believe their families would be better off without them. They sense a feeling of overwhelming guilt for a small indiscretion and believe they are being punished; they live a hell on earth. Hallucinations of voices condemning them or pictures of dead relatives may dominate their thoughts. Some patients become paralyzed by their melancholia; they take to bed and stay there.

The occurrence of major depression may fit into one of several patterns.[138] First, a major depression may occur at any age. Second, mania presents in concert with depressive illness. Third, major depression may happen as an isolated event or in conjunction with a series of recurrent depressive episodes — unipolar depressions. A 50-year-old housewife had a series of major depressions over the past decade. Each episode was heralded by a bout of accusing her husband of infidelity. Again, genetics play a contributory role in major depressions. Chapter 2 amplifies this discussion.

Two laboratory studies offer not only insight into mania and depression, but also provide valuable diagnostic and treatment information. First involves urinary 3-methoxy-4-hydroxyphenylglycol (MHPG), a major metabolite of norepinephrine.[139] Patients with MDI show the following pattern: during the manic phase urinary MHPG is increased, and during the depressed phase it is decreased, more than the remission urinary MHPG levels. Further, MDI patients in the depressed phase have significantly lower urinary MHPG levels than patients with unipolar nonendogenous chronic characterologic depressions. Second, the dexamethasone suppression test yields more clues.[140] In normals, a midnight dose of 1.0 to 2.0 mg oral dexamethasone suppresses ACTH and cortisol for 24 hours. In patients with endogenous depression, eg, MDI depressed phase, the serum cortisol demonstrates an "escape" and an increase during the 16 to 24 hours of the study. This reflects an anxiety underlying the depression.

A *brief reactive psychosis* may have as its hallmark paranoia. This diagnosis is based not only on a recognized clear and immediate stress but also on the absence of an organic etiology, a schizophrenic disorder, or an affective disorder. The criteria involve an acknowledged distress, psychotic symptoms of loose associations, delusions, hallucinations, or marked behavior disturbance either disorganized or catatonic, lasting between several hours to no more than 2 weeks, without a prodomal phase, and not due to another psychological diagnosis.[114]

Paranoia may prove to be the paramount feature of the *posttraumatic stress disorder*. The traumatic event and the circumstances surrounding it may engender feelings of fear, apprehension, and terror. This may be especially true when the actual causative situation is prolonged, protracted, pronounced, profound, cruel, horrible, and perpetually threatening. The soldier's Vietnam war experience often meets this definition. Domash and Sparr present a case of a 30-year-old Vietnam war veteran who developed isolation, anxiety, and extreme suspiciousness following his return to the United States.[141] His violence and hallucinations contribute to the initial diagnosis of paranoid schizophrenia. Further evaluation and treatment demonstrated the diagnosis of posttraumatic stress disorder. Criteria for this disorder include a significant distress, reexperienceing it through recurrent recollections, dreams, or aberrations, numbness characterized by diminished activity, detachment, or narrowed affect, and the addition of at least two symptoms since the trauma: hyperalertness, disturbed sleep, survivor guilt, impaired recall, avoidance behavior, and intense reactions to events triggering a recall of the initial distress.[114]

Paranoia may also play a key or secondary role in a number of *personality disorders*. These personality patterns not only designate an intrapsychic structure and interactional program, but also provide the underlying mechanism and substratum for the previously listed paranoid psychosis. The personalities represent the confluence of inheritance, environment, familial backgrounds and experiences, much of which has been explored earlier in the pathogenesis section.

The *paranoid personality disorder* clearly accounts for the paranoid individuals. These supervigilant persons always anticipate abuse, prove to be hypersensitive, and display basic mistrust. Their suspiciousness is marked by at least three of the following criteria: an expectation they will be hurt, hypervigilance, secretiveness, warranted blame avoidance, loyalty questioning, looking for bias confirmation, searching for hidden motives, or jealousy to the pathologic level. Their lives are restricted and constricted by their unemotionality, pride, lack of humor, and absent compassion.[114] These people often precipitate and find what they profess to dread most.

The *narcissistic personality disorder* designates an individual who generates a sense, stance, and undercurrent of subtle paranoia. The DSM-III criteria suggest such a position.[114] First, these patients display a grandiose self. Second, they are preoccupied with fantasies of their brilliance, prowess, or achievement. Third, they are exhibitionists, yet, fourthly, they are indifferent to others. Finally, interpersonally they behave with entitlement, exploitativeness, alternating between overidealization and devaluation and absence of empathy.

The *Schizotypal personality disorder* encompasses a high degree of paranoid thinking. Although these individuals are not schizophrenic, much of their thought process verges and hovers near it. The criteria involve them meeting at least four of the following eight items: (a) magical thinking; (b) referential ideas; (c) social isolation; (d) recurrent depersonalization, illusions, or derealization experiences; (e) odd speech patterns, eg, circumstantiality; (f) inappropriate affect, (g) suspiciousness, and (h) hypersensitivity or exaggerated social apprehension.[114]

356

REFERENCES

1. Cooper AF: The suspicious patient. *Practitioner* 1978;220:270-275.
2. Roy A: Depression in chronic paranoid schizophrenia. *Br J Psychiatry* 1980;137:138-139.
3. Swanson DW, Bonert PJ, Smith JA: *The Paranoid*. Boston, Little, Brown & Co, 1970.
4. American Psychiatric Association: *A Psychiatric Glossary*. Washington, American Psychiatric Association, 1980.
5. Cameron H: *Personality Development and Psychopathology*. Boston, Houghton Mifflin Co, 1963.
6. Manschreck TC, Petri M: The paranoid syndrome. *Lancet* 1978;I:251-253.
7. MacKinnon RA, Michels R: *The Psychiatric Interview in Clinical Practice*. Philadelphia, WB Saunders Co, 1971.
8. Erikson EH: Growth and crises of the healthy personality. *Psychol Issues* 1959;1:50-100.
9. Kolb LC, Brody HKH: *Modern Clinical Psychiatry,* ed 10. Philadelphia, WB Saunders Co, 1982.
10. Fenichel O: *The Psychoanalytic Theory of Neurosis*. New York, WW Norton, 1945.
11. Brown RP, Mann JJ: A clinical perspective on the role of neurotransmitters in mental disorders. *Hosp Community Psychiatry* 1985;36:141-149.
12. Spokes EGS: Biochemical abnormalities in schizophrenia: the dopamine hypothesis, in Curzon G (ed): *The Biochemistry of Psychiatric Disturbances*. New York, John Wiley & Sons, 1980, pp 53-71.
13. Kendler KS, Davis KL: The genetics and biochemistry of paranoid schizophrenia and other paranoid psychoses. *Schizophr Bull* 1981;7:689-709.
14. McHugh PR, Folstein MF: Psychiatric syndromes of Huntington's chorea: a clinical and phenomenologic study, in Benson DF, Blumer D (eds): *Psychiatric Aspects of Neurologic Disease*. New York, Grune & Stratton Inc, 1975, pp 267-286.
15. Magaro PA, Page J: Brain disconnection, schizophrenia, and paranoia. *J Nerv Ment Dis* 1983;171:133-140.
16. Bear DM: Hemispheric specialization and the neurology of emotion. *Arch Neurol* 1983;40:195-202.
17. Axelsson R, Martensson E, Alling C: Impairment of the brain-blood barrier as an aetiological factor in paranoid psychosis. *Br J Psychiatry* 1982;14:273-281.
18. Swanson DW, Stipes AH: Psychiatric aspects of Klinefelter's syndrome. *Am J Psychiatry* 1982;126:814-822.
19. Wells CE, Duncan GW: *Neurology for Psychiatrists*. Philadelphia, FA Davis Co, 1980.
20. Baron M, Gruen R, Kane J, et al: Modern research criteria and the genetics of schizophrenia. *Am J Psychiatry* 1985;742:697-701.

357

21. Kety SS: Genetic aspects of schizophrenia. *Am J Psychiatry* 1978;135:1333-1339.
22. Kety SS, Rosenthal D, Wender PH, et al: Mental illness in the biological and adoptive families of adopted schizophrenics. *Am J Psychiatry* 1971;128:302-305.
23. Cadoret RT, Tanna VL: Genetics of affective disorders, in Usdin G (ed): *Depression: Clinical, Biological, and Psychological Perspectives.* New York, Brunner/Mazel, 1977.
24. Snyder SH: *Biological Aspects of Mental Disorder.* New York, Oxford University Press, 1980.
25. Rich T, Winokur G: Family history studies V: the genetics of mania. *Am J Psychiatry* 1969;125:1358-1369.
26. Lystad MH: Violence at home. *Am J Orthopsychiatry* 1975;45:328-345.
27. Editorial: Paranoia and immigrants. *Br Med J* 1980;281:1513-1514.
28. Jack RA, Nicassio PM, West WS: Acute paranoia in a Southeast Asian refugee. *J Nerv Ment Dis* 1984;172:495-497.
29. Solomon P, Leiderman H, Mendelson J, et al: Sensory deprivation. *Am J Psychiatry* 1957;114:357-363.
30. Goodwin FS: Behavior effects of L-Dopa in man, in Shader RI (ed): *Psychiatric Complications of Medical Drugs.* New York, Raven Press, 1972, pp 149-174.
31. Hausner RS: Amantadine: associated recurrence of psychosis. *Am J Psychiatry* 1980;137:240-242.
32. Bianchine JR: Drugs for Parkinson's disease, spasticity, and acute muscle spasms, acting muscle relaxants, in Gilman AG, Goodman LS, Rall TW, et al: *Goodman and Gilman's The Pharmacological Basis of Therapeutics,* ed 7. New York, MacMillan Publishing Co, Inc, 1985, pp 473-491.
33. Polchert SE, Morse RM: Pemoline abuse. *JAMA* 1985;254:946-947.
34. Hall RCW (ed): *Psychiatric Presentation of Medical Illness.* New York, SP Medical & Scientific Books, 1980.
35. Leighton KM: Paranoid psychosis after abuse of Actifed. *Lancet* 1982;284:789-790.
36. Shader RI, Greenblatt DJ: Belladonna alkaloids and synthetic anticholinergics: uses and toxicity, in Shader RI (ed): *Psychiatric Complications of Medical Drugs.* New York, Raven Press, 1972, pp 103-147.
37. Weiner N: Atropine, scopolamine, and related antimuscarinic drugs, in Gilman AG, Goodman LS, Rall TW, et al (eds): *Goodman and Gilman's The Pharmacological Basis of Therapeutics,* ed 7. New York, MacMillan Publishing Co, Inc, 1985, pp 130-144.
38. Carpenter WT, Strauss JS, Bonney WE: The psychobiology of cortisol metabolism, in Shader RI (ed): *Psychiatric Complications of Medical Drugs.* New York, Raven Press, 1972, pp 49-72.
39. Slaby AE, Lieb J, Tancredi LR: *Handbook of Psychiatric Emergencies,* ed 2. Garden City, NY, Medical Examination Publishing Co, 1981.

358

40. Soreff S: Psychiatric emergencies: principles and practice. *Drug Therapy* 1983;13:185-196.
41. Nelson C, Bomers MB, Sweeney D: Exacerbation of psychosis by tricyclic antidepressants in delusional depression. *Am J Psychiatry* 1974;136:574-579.
42. Adler LE, Sadia L, Willets G: Cimetidine toxicity manifested as paranoia and hallucinations. *Am J Psychiatry* 1980;137:1112-1113
43. Griffith JD, Smith CH, Smith RC: Paranoid psychosis in a patient receiving ibuprofen, a prostaglandin synthesis inhibitor. *J Clin Psychiatry* 1982;43:499-500.
44. Horrobin DF: Schizophrenia as a prostaglandin deficiency disease. *Lancet* 1970;1:936-937.
45. McDanal CW, Bolman WM: Delayed idiosyncratic psychosis with diphenylhydantoin. *JAMA* 1975;231:1063.
46. Sayed AJ: Mania and bromism: a case report and a look to the future. *Am J Psychiatry* 1976;133:228-229.
47. Nuki G, Richardson P, Goggin MJ, et al: Four cases of bromism. *Br Med J* 1966;2:390-391.
48. Pollock M, Klein DF, Willner, et al: Impramine induced behavioral disorganization in schizophrenic patients: physiological and psychological correlates. *Rec Adv Biol Psychiatry* 1965;7:53-69.
49. Wilson IC, Prange AJ, Lara PP: Methyltestosterone with impramine in men: conversion of depression to paranoid ideation. *Am J Psychiatry* 1974;131:21-24.
50. Feighner JP: Second and third generation antidepressants: a clinical overview, in Zales MR (ed): *Affective and Schizophrenic Disorders.* New York, Brunner/Mazel, 1983, pp 144-160.
51. Soreff S: *Management of the Psychiatric Emergency.* New York, John Wiley & Sons, 1981.
52. Ellinwood EH: Amphetamine psychosis: I Description of the individuals and process. *J Nerv Ment Dis* 1977;144:273-283.
53. Cooper JR, Bloom FE, Roth RH: *The Biochemical Basis of Neuropharmacology,* ed 4. New York, Oxford University Press, 1982.
54. Valzelli L: *Psychopharmacology.* New York, Spectrum Publications, Inc, 1973.
55. Goodwin DW, Guze SB: *Psychiatric Diagnosis,* ed 2. New York, Oxford University Press, 1979.
56. Schuckit MA: *Drug and Alcohol Abuse: A Clinical Guide to Diagnosis and Treatment.* New York, Plenum Medical Book Co, 1979.
57. Wilford BB: *Drug Abuse.* Chicago, American Medical Association, 1981.
58. Williams GH, Dluhy RG, Thornm GW: Diseases of the adrenal cortex, in Isselbacher KJ, Adams RD, Braunwald E, et al (eds): *Harrison's Principles of Internal Medicine,* ed 10. New York, McGraw-Hill Book Co, 1983.
59. Jefferson JW, Marshall JR: *Neuropsychiatric Features of Medical Disorders.* New York, Plenum Medical Book Co, 1981.

60. Addison T: *On the Constitutional and Local Effects of Disease of the Supra-renal Capsules.* London, S Highby, 1855.
61. Alarcon RO, Franceschini JA: Hyperparathyroidism and paranoid psychosis. *Br J Psychiatry* 1984;45:477-486.
62. Agras S, Oliveau DC: Primary hyperparathyroidism and psychosis. *Can Med Assoc J* 1964;91:1366-1367.
63. Mikkelsen EJ, Reider AA: Post-parathyroidectomy psychosis: clinical research implications. *J Clin Psychiatry* 1979;40:352-357.
64. Burch EA, Messerry TW: Psychiatric symptoms in medical illness: hypothyroidism revisited. *Psychosomatics* 1978;19:72-75.
65. Ingbar SH, Woeber KA: Diseases of the thyroid, in Isselbacher KJ, Adams RD, Braunwald E, et al (eds): *Harrison's Principles of Internal Medicine,* ed 10. New York, McGraw-Hill Book Co, 1983.
66. Frizel D, Malleson A, Marks V: Plasma levels of ionized calcium and magnesium in thyroid disease. *Lancet* 1967;2:1360-1361.
67. Swanson JW, Kelley JJ, McCorahey WM: Neurological aspects of thyroid dysfunction. *Mayo Clin Proc* 1981;56:504-512.
68. Wallerstein RD: Blood, in Krupp MA, Chatton MJ, Werdegar D (eds): *Current Medical Diagnosis and Treatment.* Los Altos, Calif, Lange Medical Publications, 1985, pp 303-351.
69. Freeman AM: Delusions, depersonalization, and unusual psychopathological symptoms, in Hall RCW (ed): *Psychiatric Presentations of Medical Illness.* New York, SP Medical & Scientific Books, 1980, pp 75-89.
70. Miller LH: Malaria, in Hoeprich PD (ed): *Infectious Diseases,* ed 3. New York, Harper & Row, 1983, pp 1253-1264.
71. Wisseman CI: Typhus fevers, in Hoeprich PD (ed): *Infectious Diseases,* ed 3. New York, Harper & Row, 1983, pp 908-914.
72. Grossman M, Jawetz E: Infectious diseases: viral and rickettsial, in Krupp MA, Chatton MJ, Werdegar D (eds): *Current Medical Diagnosis and Treatment.* Los Altos, Calif, Lange Medical Publications, 1985, pp 836-857.
73. Marsden PD: African trypanosomiesis, in Hoeprich PD (ed): *Infectious Diseases.* New York, Harper & Row, 1983, pp 1146-1150.
74. Lewis JE: Toxic shock syndrome manifested as psychosis. *South Med J* 1983;76:145-146.
75. Shands KN, Schmid MD, Dan BB, et al: Toxic shock syndrome in menstruating women, associated with tampon use and *Staphylococcus aureus* and clinical features in 52 cases. *N Engl J Med* 1980;303:1436-1442.
76. Tashjian JH, Coulam CB, Washington JA: Vaginal flora in asymptomatic women. *Mayo Clin Proc* 1976;51:556-561.
77. Marshall JR: Neuropsychiatric aspects of renal failure. *J Clin Psychiatry* 1979;40:81-85.
78. Stenbeck A, Hapaned E: Azotemia and psychosis. *Acta Psychiatry Scand Suppl* 1967;43:30-38.

79. Massey SG, Sellers AC: *Clinical aspects of uremia and dialysis.* Springfield, Ill, Charles C Thomas Publishers, 1976.
80. Sideman S, Manor D: The dialysis dementia syndrome and aluminum intoxication. *Nephron* 1982;31:1-10.
81. Chokrorertz S, Bruetman ME, Berger V, et al: Progressive dialytic encephalopathy. *J Neurol Neurosurg Psychiatry* 1976;39:411-419.
82. Hall RCW, Gardiner ER, Stickney SK, et al: Physical illness manifesting as psychiatric disease. *Arch Gen Psychiatry* 1980;37:989-995.
83. Aminoff MJ: Nervous system, in Krupp MA, Chatton MJ, Werdergar D (eds): *Current Medical Diagnosis and Treatment.* Los Altos, Calif, Lange Medical Publications, 1985, pp 581-630.
84. Adams RD, Foley JM, in Merritt HH, Hare CC (eds): *Metabolic and Toxic Diseases of the Nervous System.* Baltimore, Williams & Wilkins Co, 1953, pp 198-237.
85. Massey EW: Neuropsychiatric manifestations of porphyria. *J Clin Psychiatry* 1980;41:208-213.
86. Becker DM, Kramer S: The neurological manifestations of porphyria. *J Clin Psychiatry* 1980;41:208-213.
87. Pepplinkhuizen L, Buinrels J, Blom W, et al: Schizophrenia-like psychosis caused by a metabolic disorder. *Lancet* 1980;1:454-456.
88. Tishler PV, Woodward R, O'Connor J, et al: High prevalence of intermittent acute porphyria in a psychiatric patient population. *Am J Psychiatry* 1985;142:1430-1436.
89. Macalpine I, Hunter R: The "insanity" of King George III: a classic case of porphyria. *Br Med J* 1966;1:65-71.
90. Williams EY, Weeks LR: Premenstrual tension associated with psychotic episodes. *J Nerv Ment Dis* 1952;116:321-329.
91. Benson RC, Greenwood S, Margolis AJ: Gynecology and obstetrics, in Krupp MA, Chatton MJ, Werdegar D (eds): *Current Medical Diagnosis and Treatment.* Los Altos, Calif, Lange Medical Publications, 1985, pp 451-498.
92. Endo M, Daiguji M, Asano Y, et al: Periodic psychosis recurring in association with menstrual cycle. *J Clin Psychiatry* 1978;39:456-466.
93. Pincus JH, Tucker GJ: *Behavioral neurology,* ed 2. New York, Oxford University Press, 1978.
94. Blumer D: Temporal lobe epilepsy and its psychiatric significance, in Benson DF, Blumer D (eds): *Psychiatric Aspects of Neurologic Disease.* New York, Grune & Stratton, Inc, 1975, pp 171-198.
95. Blumer D, Walker AE: Sexual behavior in temporal lobe epilepsy. *Arch Neurol* 1967;16:37-43.
96. Klüver H, Bucy P: Preliminary analysis of functions of the temporal lobes on monkeys. *Arch Neural Psychiatry* 1939;42:979-1000.
97. Wells CE, Duncay GW: *Neurology for Psychiatrists.* Philadelphia, FA Davis Co, 1980.

98. Glaus A: *Ueber Kombinationen von Schizophrenie and Epilepsie. Z Gesamte. Neurol Psychiatry* 1931;135:450-500.

99. Jensen I, Larsen JK: Mental aspects of temporal lobe epilepsy. *J Neurol Neurosurg Psychiatry* 1979;42:256-265.

100. Adams RD, Victor M: *Principles of Neurology,* ed 2. New York, McGraw-Hill Book Co, 1981.

101. Vonsattel JP, Myers RH, Stevens TJ, et al: Neuropathological classification of Huntington's disease. *J Neuropathol Exp Neurol* 1985;44:559-577.

102. Spokes EGS: Neurochemical alterations in Huntington's chorea. *Brain* 1980;103:179-210.

103. Price TRP, Tucker GH: Psychiatric and behavioral manifestations of normal pressure hydrocephalus. *J Nerv Ment Dis* 1977;164:51-55.

104. Editorial: Hearing loss and perceptual dysfunction in schizophrenia. *Lancet* 1981;I:848-849.

105. Hall RCW, Stickney SK, Gardner ER: Psychiatric symptoms in patients with systemic lupus erythematosus. *Psychosomatics* 1981;22:15-24.

106. Engleman EP, Shearn MA: Arthritis and allied rheumatic disorders, in Krupp MA, Chatton MJ, Werdegar D (eds): *Current Medical Diagnosis and Treatment.* Los Altos, Calif, Lange Medical Publications, 1985, pp 499-524.

107. Cohen AS, Reynolds WE, Franklin EC, et al: Preliminary criteria for classifications of sytemic lupus erythematosus. *Bull Rheum Dis* 1971;21:643-648.

108. Sanck B: Reactive paranoid psychosis following an ambiguous cancer diagnosis. *Psychosomatics* 1982;23:439-440.

109. Krauthammer C, Klerman GL: Secondary mania. *Arch Gen Psychiatry* 1978;35:1333-1339.

110. Peterson LG, Perl M: Psychiatric presentations of cancer. *Psychosomatics* 1982;23:601-604.

111. Sherwood LM: Endocrine manifestations of nonendocrine disease, in Isselbacher KJ, Adams RD, Braunwald E, et al (eds): *Harrison's Principles of Internal Medicine,* ed 10. New York, McGraw-Hill Book Co, 1983, pp 741-746.

112. Berrettini WH: Paranoid psychosis and sleep apnea syndrome. *Am J Psychiatry* 1980;137:493-494.

113. Roth M: The natural history of mental disorder in old age. *J Ment Sci* 1955;101:281-301.

114. American Psychiatric Association: *Diagnostic and Statistical Manual of Mental Disorders,* ed 3. Washington, American Psychiatric Association, 1980.

115. Varner RV, Gaitz CM: Schizophrenic and paranoid disorders in the aged. *Psychiatr Clin North Am* 1982;5:107-118.

116. Dubin WR, Field AL, Gastfriend OR: Postcardiotomy delirium: a critical review. *J Thorac Cardiovasc Surg* 1979;77:586-594.

117. Bliss BL, Rumel WR, Hardin-Branch CH: Psychiatric complications of mitral surgery. *AMA Arch Neurol Psychiatry* 1955;74:249-252.

118. Weisman HD, Hackett TP: Psychosis after eye surgery. *N Engl J Med* 1958;258:1284-1289.

119. Levine AM: Visual hallucinations and cataracts. *Ophthalmic Surg* 1980;11:95-98.

120. Mikkelsen EJ, Reider AA: Post-parathyroidectomy psychosis: clinical and research implications. *J Clin Psychiatry* 1979;40:352-357.

121. Camargo CA, Kolb FO: Endocrine disorders, in Krupp MA, Chatton MJ (eds): *Current Medical Diagnosis and Treatment*. Los Altos, Calif, Lange Medical Publications, 1983, pp 664-742.

122. Henker OT: Body-image conflict following trauma and surgery. *Psychosomatics* 1979;20:812-820.

123. Monro A: Paranoia revisited. *Br J Psychiatry* 1982;141:344-349.

124. Trethowan WH: Dementia, in Hart FD (ed): *French's Index of Differential Diagnosis,* ed 12. Bristol, England, John Wright, 1985.

125. Lipowski ZJ: Transient cognitive disorders (delirium, acute confusional states) in the elderly. *Am J Psychiatry* 1983;140:1426-1436.

126. Eaton MT, Peterson MH, Davis JA: *Textbook of Psychiatry,* ed 5. New Hyde Park, NY, Medical Examination Publishing Co, 1985.

127. Kendler KS: The nosologic validity of paranoia (simple delusional disorder). *Arch Gen Psychiatry* 1980;37:699-706.

128. Oxman TE, Rosenberg SD, Tucker GJ: The language of paranoia. *Am J Psychiatry* 1982;139:275-282.

129. Bleuler E: *Dementia praecox, or the Group of Schizophrenias,* Zinkin S (trans). New York, International Universities Press, 1952.

130. Lewine RRJ: Sex differences in age of symptom onset and first hospitalization in schizophrenia. *Am J Orthopsychiatry* 1980;50:316-322.

131. Abrams R, Taylor MA: The genetics of schizophrenia: a reassessment using modern criteria. *Am J Psychiatry* 1983;140:171-175.

132. Haier RJ: The diagnosis of schizophrenia: a review of recent developments. *Schizoph Bull* 1980;6:417-428.

133. Fox HA: The DSM III concept of schizophrenia. *Br J Psychiatry* 1981;138:60-63.

134. Andreasen NC: The clinical differentiation of affective and schizophrenic disorders, in Zales MR (ed): *Affective and Schizophrenic Disorders*. New York, Brunner/Mazel, 1983, pp 29-52.

135. Pope H, Lipinsky J: Diagnosis in schizophrenia and manic-depressive illness. *Arch Gen Psychiatry* 1978;35:811-828.

136. Mendelewicz J, Fleiss TC: Linkage studies with X-chromosome markers in bipolar (manic-depressive) and unipolar (depressive) illnesses. *Biol Psychiatry* 1974;9:261-294.

137. Braden W, Bannasch PR, Fink EB: Diagnosing mania: the use of family informants. *J Clin Psychiatry* 1980;41:226-228.

138. Kupfer DJ: Toward a unified view of affective disorders, in Zales MR (ed): *Affective and Schizophrenic Disorders*. New York, Brunner/Mazel, 1983, pp 225-264.

139. Schildkraut JJ, Orsulak PJ, Schatzberg AF, et al: Laboratory tests for discriminating subtypes of depressive disorders, in Zales MR (ed): *Affective and Schizophrenic Disorders*. New York, Brunner/Mazel, 1983, pp 103-123.

140. Rubin RJ, Marder SR: Biological markers in affective and schizophrenic disorders, in Zales MR (ed): *Affective and Schizophrenic Disorders*. New York, Brunner/Mazel, 1983,pp 53-100.

141. Domash MD, Sparr LF: Post traumatic stress disorder masquerading as paranoid schizophrenia: case report. *Milit Med* 1982;147:772-774.

9 Non-Psychotic Distortions of Reality

Walter R. Christie

Case report A 26-year-old man presents in the emergency room with complaints of feeling "very funny." Specifically, he describes a sense of being "numb and detached from my body." This state is extremely unpleasant to him, and he has increased his alcohol use lately to self-medicate himself. The experiences last only a few minutes, but he has grown so fearful of them that he can no longer function in his work as a security guard. His father had similar experiences a few years before and was hospitalized for depression.

Reality is a complex synthesis of organized perceptions. The basic senses, deeper kinesthetic stimuli, and the associative and integrative aspects of the cortex construct a holographic image of self and world through which we move. Damage to any part of the mind can alter receptive and synthetic functions, or extreme external stress may overwhelm the neural pathways by which reality is constructed. This chapter will examine all the disorders of reality which are not part of the phenomenology of psychosis, although they may precede or coexist with it. The nonpsychotic types of reality distortion include depersonalization, derealization, déjà vu, jamais vu, autoscopic phenomena, out-of-body experiences, etc. Following are brief definitions of each. Some are experienced as pathologic and dysphoric; others such as out-of-body experiences (OBE) are pursued as blissful or exhilirating mystical states.

Depersonalization is a feeling of estrangement from a part or the whole of one's body. The estrangement may be anatomical as disconnection from a limb or the more global symptom of being outside the body watching oneself. It also may be a change in one's sense of coherent physical vitality, thus producing an uncomfortable feeling of being mechanical or dead.

Derealization is a change in one's perception of the outer world. Instinctual connections with reality are lost, but unlike psychosis where a new reality is constructed, no new elements are introduced other than the affective response to the estrangement. In derealization, perception may be altered. Sizes and shapes of objects may change, but new objects are not hallucinated, and the perceptual distortions are not symbolically meaningful. Derealization must also be distinguished from the nihilistic descriptions seen in emotionally estranged adolescents or the despair of chronically unhappy adults.

Déjà vu is the distinct conviction that current experience is a repetition of another identical event. There is no change in perception of self or external reality; but rather the eerie or sometimes pleasant feeling of being a part of a repetitive experience outside of one's memory or consciousness; thus déjà vu may be magical or admonitory depending on one's state of mind and taste for the unusual. *Jamais vu* is the opposite perceptual position. Here a very familiar landscape appears foreign. This is painful, for the supporting thread of familiarity which runs through the patient's life is strongly challenged.

Autoscopic phenomena can be a variant of depersonalization, but specifically they refer to the experience of being above one's body and looking down on it. Autoscopy is a form of *out-of-body experience*. These may be purposefully induced "astral projections" where the person tries to leave the body to travel as an energy essence to a distant spot, or it may be like the experiences reported by patients in near-death situations (accidents, cardiac arrests) where the endangered person watches his body being resuscitated. Mountain climbers who have survived falls describe enormous time compression, a sense of being outside the event, their lives flashing before their eyes, split seconds stretching to minutes to discover a way to survive or be reconciled with death. A great deal of parapsychological research has been devoted to out-of-body experiences. In general, however, we will discuss parapsychological issues only to clarify the mechanisms of symptom formation, and we will confine our focus to dysphoric and maladaptive nonpsychotic changes in reality.

Features

Complaints of alteration in reality require a complete psychiatric examination since the complaint may be only one aspect of a serious mental or medical illness. The findings below are described in relation to a dysphoric, depersonalization experience. Reference is made to other entities when pertinent.

Mood

The patient in a depersonalization episode is very frightened, but often does not project the full extent of his fear. This is an internal event, often difficult to describe, and accompanied by concerns about insanity. The patient therefore may seem withdrawn or hypervigilant; he may be reluctant to describe the episode for fear of being seen as mentally ill. If derealization is part of the picture, the examiner and the setting may be included in the estrangement.

Here special attention must be paid to the flow and continuity of mood. Since depersonalization may accompany or precede mania or depression, the buoyancy of the manic or the deeply retarded sadness of the depressive is important to note. The flattened or inappropriate affect of the schizophrenic is present in a case where depersonalization is part of a generalized time/body/space fragmentation of psychosis. In contrast, the examiner might note the garrulous irritability of the intoxicated substance abuser where marijuana or hallucinogen use has triggered the depersonalization or where self-medication with alcohol is part of the picture.

Thought

The thought content of the depersonalization patient will reflect both the primary experience and the patient's reaction to it. The primary experience[1] may be one of shrinking and expanding objects, estrangement of particular body parts, and/or numbness and sensations of changes in size of these body parts, a feeling of dizziness, floating, or giddiness, a feeling of being "dead," a loss of affective responsiveness, a feeling of calm detachment, "remoteness," or flatness of visual and auditory stimuli and slow, subjective time. Thus, content of thought will reflect both the attempt to acknowledge and describe these phenomena and the various real or imaginary interpretations of the events.

For example, an obsessive individual with a tendency toward body damage fears may focus his complaints on a single limb or organ as a manner of making concretely manageable a complex inner experience. A person with hysterical traits whose personality style is emotional and impressionistic may embellish the experience to a level where it resembles psychosis. A schizoid individual who enjoys the peculiarities of his inner world may capitalize on his imaginative strengths and narrate the experience with an enthusiasm that is counterphobic in nature. Substance abusers may use terms that come from their subculture of consciousness changing. Spiritually oriented persons will describe the experience in terms of unity or lack of it. In essense, each person will use his own frame of reference to describe what nearly defies description.

However, a few generalizations apply in most cases. First, depersonalization and other nonpsychotic reality disorders are not delusional, do not loosen associations, and are not accompanied by hallucinations. The presence of any of these findings suggests that another, more serious disorder coexists or is the cause of this symptom. Second, only people with dysphoria present themselves as patients. The seeker of OBE (out of body experiences) does not present in the clinic or emergency room. If he does, then the reality alteration is not the real reason for the presentation. The patient may be a sociopath seeking drugs, lodging, or protection from the law, or the patient may truly be in pain but using the extraordinary OBE as a way to get attention for a less spectacular and possibly more shameful complaint. Some personality disorders are so psychologically impoverished that they "invent" intrapsychic events to try to get treated, ie, nurtured, protected, stimulated, etc. Great care must be exercised in making a diagnosis of character disorder in the emergency room, however, because what looks like manipulation today may be schizophrenia tomorrow.

Behavior

Behavior is an internal psychological event which cannot be seen or measured. What can be observed is the patient's reaction to the symptom or the disease process of which the symptom is a part. The following are behaviors which might be seen in a depersonalization patient: withdrawal and difficulty communicating, restless anticipatory anxiety, unusual detachment or remoteness, alcohol abuse. A personality disorder patient may present with mutilations or slashed arms. Detailed questioning will reveal that the behavior is not suicidal, but an attempt to restore a feeling of aliveness in the midst of depersonalized numbness or deadness.

Physical Examination and Laboratory Findings

The primary symptom causes no physical changes or laboratory findings. However, blood levels of tetrahydrocannabinal (THC) and other hallucinogens may reveal the cause. An EEG may show temporal lobe spikes in a temporal lobe epilepsy (TLE) patient. Any evidence of fever or systemic illness might lead to a question of encephalopathy. Diagnostic testing for major affective illness is coming of age, and it may well be that in the future all depersonalization patients will have blood drawn for biologic indices of depression. However, this is not yet fruitful.

Interviewer's Reaction

Perhaps the most frequent initial reaction to the depersonalization patient is bewilderment and/or disbelief. The remoteness with which some of these patients present makes empathic contact difficult. Another common reaction is to experience the patient as weird or crazy. This indeed may prove to be the case, but often it is not. In some studies, as many as 10% of normal people have experienced depersonalization.[2] Therefore, the patient who presents in the clinic or emergency ward is part of a subgroup and is probably, on a statistical basis, far more impaired than the general population. Most individuals with depersonalization suffer through with a little help from their friends, and that is the end of their episode and treatment.

PATHOGENESIS

Ideas about the etiology of depersonalization and other nonpsychotic alterations of reality range from conceptualizing it as a variant of an evolutionary adaptive mechanism to a conflict-induced anxiety defense. Freud, who introduced one of the first psychodynamic explanations, experienced a depersonalization episode himself while standing at the Acropolis.[3] He interpreted his experience as a defense against the feelings of having surpassed his father. Freud's explanation is in marked contrast to that proposed by Levitan.[4] Levitan hypothesized that in depersonalization there is a blocking of sensory pathways due to the inhibition of the reticular activating system (RAS).

The rate of elaboration of fresh aspects of images, a function moderated by the RAS, is disturbed in depersonalized patients, and the physiological constancy required to maintain coherent reality leads to the peculiarities of perception and the affective response to that perception. Below are a variety of ways which investigators have tried to explain the etiologic mechanisms of nonpsychotic distortions of reality.

Psychodynamics

Psychodynamic explanations use a developmental-conflictual model to explain phenomenology. Since the symptoms partially alter reality, analytic writers tend to look at early developmental problems for explanations. The following are examples of this type of formulation: Jacobson[5] has associated depersonalization symptoms with "narcissistic personalities," "passive-feminine characters" and individuals with "oral strivings." Guntrip,[6] too, has seen depersonalization as evidence of schizoid character formations. Feigenbaum,[7] Searl,[8] and Stewart[9] have proposed that depersonalization is a primitive defense designed to deny needs by representing the situation as unreal. Bird[10] and Stewart[9] have proposed that depersonalization is a defense which only emerges as higher defenses fail. Some writers have moved toward complexity, others toward simplicity. Bergler,[11] Jacobson,[5] Nunberg,[12] and Oberndorf[13,14] have described complex layering of defenses against particular impulses, reactions to conflicting identifications within the ego, or experiences of loss which are viewed as equivalent to loss of part of the self. Stamm's[15] views, however, are much simpler. He sees depersonalization as a partial regression in which one part of the ego maintains contact with reality while the other regresses to fantasy. Oberndorf and West[16] emphasize that depersonalization serves to protect the individual from even more frightening affects, that is, the remoteness is the desired affect of the defense. Blank[17] suggests that the anxiety associated with depersonalization is because the defense itself is so inadequate.

Biologic Explanation

Levitan's[4] theory about depersonalization as malfunction of the RAS has been described above. Investigators such as Milner[18] feel that we know too little about integrated neural functioning to localize the origins of the symptoms. The search for biologic explanation is challenging since a concept of consciousness itself defies simple experimental models. Jaynes[19] in a significant scholarly work focusing on linguistics and cultural history, examined the possibility that the RAS is the agent of consciousness and concluded that although the multiconnected organization of that system supported its role in arousal, it could not explain higher levels of consciousness activity. The RAS is too ancient to be the whole explanation.

Currently, for diverse cultural and intellectual reasons, there is great interest in Karl Pribram's[20] theory that the brain operates like a hologram, an optical storage system where each part contains the whole. Pribram's theory is under scrutiny by many investigators, but if it does have validity, the question becomes: What neuromechanism disrupts the hologram and splits a part from the whole? Such a lesion would tend to be more generalized or a disorder simultaneously at many levels of neural organization rather than at one site. Because depersonalization is seen in temporal lobe epilepsy where a lesion can be found, and as a precursor to major mental/affective illness where there is growing suggestion of specific neurotransmitter disorders, it is very tempting to look for a specific locus or a unitary biochemical explanation for depersonalization. To date, however, nothing has been found.

Genetics

General currents of developmental research suggest that children enter the world with considerable neural programming. Genetic contributions to schizophrenia and manic-depressive illness are widely accepted, and work to study genetic patterns of anxiety and certain personality traits are receiving attention. It is probable that some genetic/familial predisposition to depersonalization will be discovered, particularly since it is such a widely prevalent symptom among the general population.

Environment

Noyes and Kletti[21] investigated depersonalization in response to life-threatening danger and concluded that "the interpretation of depersonalization as a defense against the threats of extreme danger or its associated anxiety seems inescapable...detachment appears to be a major adaptive mechanism, which in the depersonalized state, is seen in bold relief." These investigators studied 101 persons who had experienced life-threatening danger. Sixty-six (65%) reported depersonalization during the time. However, as previously mentioned, this symptom differs from the depersonalized patient who appears in the emergency room. Noyes and Kletti's subjects experienced an adaptive split between participating and observing self. The participating self felt time, thought, and action greatly speeded, but the observant self used detachment to slow thinking and action in hopes of finding a method of survival. The phenomenology of both danger-induced and idiopathic depersonalization is the same, but the intra-psychic experience and adaptive usefulness is quite different.

Cumulative changes in the environment or in one's experience of the environment have also been cited as participants of depersonalization. McKellar[22] reported a case of a 16-year-old boy with prolonged depersonalization who left Lebanon during the civil war in 1975 to attend school in France. The new environment and the stress of civil war were hypothesized to be the cause of the his symptoms. Although both biological and analytical writers might have additional thoughts about the case, certainly the boy did feel like a "stranger in a strange land" after the Heinlein novel.

Experience of the environment can change internally as well as externally. Meditation and hypnosis have both been implicated. Kennedy[23] reported two cases where meditation induced the symptom. In one, a 37-year-old businessman pursued a new fascination with yoga and meditation and developed out-of-body experiences and autoscopic phenomena which were dysphoric and gave him trouble for several months after he stopped the meditation procedures. In the second, a 24-year-old man developed severe derealization performing Arica meditations for several hours daily. These meditations, like many other techniques used by those on spiritual paths, view the ego as an enemy to be overcome in one's spiritual attunement.

Wineburg and Straker[24] reported a case of a subject selected as a "normal" to demonstrate hypnotic techniques to a class of psychiatrists. Following the trance induction she developed a self-limited depersonalization syndrome which her hypnotist did not predict pretrance and which could not entirely be explained retrospectively.

Simpson[25] studied the appearance of "makyo" or Zen-illness. Here the subject on the path to enlightenment tries to pass through successive satoris, where unconscious material is integrated. In the process there may be overvaluation of inner images and feeling states leading to self-induced delusions and occasionally psychoses. He warns that "individuals with hysterical personalities may be more prone to develop dissociative states in relationship to ASC (altered states of consciousness), and those with borderline states may also find ASCs disturbing." Fewtrell found that seven out of 40 (18%) anxious patients treated with a progressive relaxation technique reported depersonalization.[26]

Thus, changing the environment by overwhelming acute stress, cumulation of chronic stress, or by altering responsiveness to external environment through hypnosis, meditation, sleep, or sensory deprivation may induce a symptom complex of similar phenomenology but different meaning. For the examiner the question of environmental inducement becomes: What change in the experience of the environment will also correspond to the inner conditions necessary to precipitate the symptom?

DIFFERENTIAL DIAGNOSIS

A recent article by Gabbard, et al[27] summarizes the differential diagnosis.

Nonpsychotropic Drugs

Any medication which momentarily alters reality testing might, in a vulnerable individual, induce depersonalization. Drugs like reserpine or the β-blockers which induce depression could compromise ego function and release a number of symptoms, depersonalization included. As a general rule, if the onset of the symptom coincides with the introduction of the drug, the drug must be considered the offending agent until proved otherwise.

Psychotropic Drugs

Depersonalization and other nonpsychotic distortions of reality are not typical side effects or reactions of the currently acceptable psychotropic drugs. However, any psychotropic drug which compromises the balance between inner and outer world could cause a syndrome. Antidepressants, for example, which energize the psyche, can cause a range of agitation symptoms from low-grade restlessness to mania. Determining what is the primary syndrome and what is medication effect can be difficult. Liebowitz et al[28] reported two cases of mania which occurred during the treatment of depersonalization syndromes with stimulants and antidepressants. Without long-term follow-up they were unable to determine whether the patients had undiagnosed bipolar disorders, undiagnosed unipolar depressions presenting as depersonalization disorders, primary depersonalization neuroses with secondary depressive features, or drug-induced manic psychoses.

The general rule is that if you induce or worsen any depersonalization syndrome with medication, you must do a long-term follow-up to establish the diagnosis. If psychotropic drugs cause or worsen the symptom, this may be due to an effect on the primary syndrome or to a shift in an undiagnosed underlying disorder.

ALCOHOL

Alcohol abuse among patients with anxiety disorders is a common complication. When a patient presents with depersonalization-derealization as with phobic/anxiety/panic syndromes, a history of alcohol use is extremely important. Alcoholism may lead to personality deterioration and regression with a release of symptoms, or symptom release may lead to self-medication with alcohol. Regardless, alcohol use is extremely problematic in the treatment of the symptom. The rule is that if alcohol abuse is part of the clinical picture, it must be treated first before any other changes will occur. This may confuse the patient who finds (at least temporarily) that alcohol is the only thing effective. In addition, the anxiety which precedes withdrawal and/or delirium tremens may have exaggerated concerns in the patient with regard to his depersonalization symptoms.

Other Abused Substances

Although the stimulants cause depersonalization, it is the hallucinogens which produce the more pronounced and prolonged symptoms. Depersonalization may last long after the drug effect is over. Realization of this by users in past years has been a deterrent. LSD use in nonpsychotic individuals causes autonomic changes, kaleidoscopic visual hallucinations and illusions, hyperacusis, paresthesias, violent mood swings, body image distortions, and most particularly, feelings of estrangement and depersonalization.

Walker[29] reported two cases of depersonalization alteration with LSD use. The two cases emphasize the complexity of this issue. In one patient no depersonalization was present prior to the hallucinogen use, and the "trip" caused a severe depersonalization syndrome. In the second, the patient suffered from multineurotic symptoms including depersonalization, but these disappeared with LSD use and were replaced with an improved state of consciousness and greater affective accessibility. In the first, it increased alienation; in the second, it reduced it.

Marijuana use is more prevalent than that of the more potent hallucinogens. Annis and Smart[30] found that 14.8 percent of high school marijuana users reported one of the following symptoms when *not* using the drug: (a) visual perceptual distortions; (b) recurrent "highs"; (c) anxiety attacks. Thus, a history of marijuana use is critical to obtain, since it may be an etiologic factor even if not currently used. Urine and blood screens for cannabinols, phencyclidine hydrochloride (PCP), and other hallucinogens may be necessary in confirming a drug use pattern if the patient's reliability is in doubt. The rule is, if you think of ordering these tests, do so; if the patient does not improve, the clinician may regret the incompleteness of his initial examination and the truth will remain elusive.

Szynanski[31] reported four cases of severe depersonalization syndrome induced by marijuana. The prolonged symptoms in all four cases were identical to those experienced during the marijuana intoxication. One case finally evolved to schizophrenia; another developed more classical signs of a major depressive episode. The last received a personality disorder diagnosis. Only one of the four ended the treatment with an uncomplicated diagnosis of depersonalization disorder. All four were under considerable stress, and there was a suggestion that intrapsychic factors might be responsible for capturing and maintaining the symptom as a primary manifestation of the distress. Again, it is important to realize that none of the four patients showed evidence of mental disorder prior to the marijuana-induced depersonalization.

Medical Illnesses

Depersonalization can be induced by a number of stresses and pharmacologic treatments. Medical/surgical patients probably suffer depersonalization far more frequently than is reported. Depersonalization-derealization in postmyocardial infarction patients may be so severe that the person actually believes he is dead. Both pathophysiologic processes and the atmosphere of cardiac care units have been implicated as causes. In many hospital settings the high technology machinery around critically ill patients clearly contributes to an atmosphere which would support a derealized world view. Experiences of surgery and anesthesia profoundly affect patients' mutilation and death anxieties. Since the extremities of those circumstances invite examination, the literature on the subject is vast. How much depersonalization occurs in less threatening circumstances we can only speculate.

However, there are some medical conditions where depersonalization is a part of the clinical picture and is not a stress or drug-induced symptom. These are acute encephalopathic brain disorders like those caused by acute viruses (postinfectious encephalomyelitis, postvaccinal encephalomyelitis, acute perivascular myelinoclasis, or acute hemorrhagic leukoencephalitis). Here other stigmata of illness are always present.[32] Generalized systemic signs, particularly neurologic findings, or confusions of consciousness are typical. In the slow viral infections (scrapie, kuru, Creutzfeldt-Jakob disease), other findings are likely to precede or coexist with symptoms of consciousness change. An isolated case may occur with the compromise of the central nervous system beginning with depersonalization or depression. This is also the case with a demyelinating disorder like multiple sclerosis. However, rather than rush in with many expensive tests it would be wiser to watch the evolution of the illness. The possibility of encephalopathy as the cause of a new depersonalization syndrome is extremely unlikely.

With the epilepsies, however, the picture is different. For brevity we will focus on temporal lobe epilepsy where depersonalization-derealization is common. As syphilis was in past years, now TLE is the great imitator, if not in reality at least in the differential diagnostic imaginations of clinicians. Its manifestations are multiple and difficult to describe. Sherwin[33] reminds us that the diagnosis of TLE depends primarily on the nature of the clinical seizures which "tend to be characterized by complex sensory, motor, and autonomic disturbances, superimposed on a background of altered consciousness." Among the changes in consciousness are a number of ictal memory disturbances. Déjà vu and jamais vu are highly characteristic memory disturbances in TLE. With these come dreamy states characterized by depersonalization and detachment. A sense of being dead may accompany the depersonalization.[34]

Again, a patient who presents in the emergency room with depersonalization may not warrant the elusive pursuit of TLE unless some of the other phenomena are present. These might include amnesia, forced thinking, interictal memory disturbances, olfactory hallucinations, aggressiveness, and a cluster of features consistent with an "epileptic personality." This personality includes great variability, emotional lability, personality inconsistencies, etc. TLE is a more generalized phenomena than depersonalization alone.

Surgical Complications

As mentioned above, depersonalization-derealization may be found in patients who have been subjected to the stress of cardiac surgery. Clinicians trained in Eastern medicine with its focus on chakras or specific energy centers might explain the estranging symptoms as a predictable result of manipulation of the heart and the space it occupies, the spiritual center of the human body.[35] Regardless of clinical orientation, the deathlike depersonalization episodes do occur, but their frequency is greatly diminished by careful preparation of the patient and postsurgical sensitivity to the experience of patienthood.

Physical Trauma

Psychic trauma always accompanies physical trauma in the conscious patient. A good example of a condition of great physical-psychological stress is the combat experience which produces posttraumatic stress disorder. Here depersonalization-derealization is one of the complex of anxiety symptoms involving chronic anxiety, panic, labile depressive features, irritability, explosive outbursts, the fear of stimulation, repetitive nightmares, etc. Alcohol and other substance abuse may be a complicating factor. The alienation which contributes to this malaise experienced by many Vietnam war veterans often makes them reluctant to discuss their experiences or even help the examiner discover the connection between the current symptoms and military experience. Since the onset of the posttraumatic stress syndrome is delayed, it is important to ask about military service, wounds, combat stress, etc.

Psychiatric Differential Diagnosis

We have mentioned that depersonalization-derealization and the other nonpsychotic disturbances of reality may occur in the prodromal stage of schizophrenia or major depressive episodes. Here the clinical course will elucidate the diagnosis and the treatment. In some depressives, depersonalization may be the primary symptom. Here clinical wisdom and empirical trial of antidepressants may clarify both diagnosis and treatment. Freeman and Melges[36] have described depersonalization and temporal disintegration in acute mental illness. In schizophrenia, when florid symptoms are present, the diagnosis is not difficult but the evolution of the full syndrome may be gradual (as long as years) and systematic treatment prior to a final psychotic break may cover or retard the emergence of this manifestation. If the clinician suspects a schizophrenic diagnosis and the mental status fails to reveal hard signs, the rule is to examine the patient's total functioning over an extended time. Is there evidence of social withdrawal? Are school grades or work performance declining? Have friends and family noted personality changes? Is the patient underachieving?

These can provide rough indicators of the presence or absence of an ego-impairing illness.

The clarity of this line of inquiry is blurred in the character disorders, the last group of psychiatric patients in which nonpsychotic disorders of reality are often reported. Here a familiarity with the features of the histrionic, the passive-dependent, the antisocial, and the borderline personalities will help the clinician. This group presents in emergency rooms with many other complaints and deserves study so that they may be recognized. Personality disorders may be complexly symptomatic in a chronic, stable fashion. Although the patients often seem markedly unstable, they are in less danger than they appear to be. Their symptoms are woven into the social matrix of their lives and often serve transparently obvious manipulative purposes. Again, alcohol and substance abuse are common conditions.

All of the above are situations where depersonalization is a symptom, not a syndrome. One condition described in the literature deserves study as more than a symptom. It is the phobic anxiety depersonalization syndrome.[37] Although the DSM-III has tried to include only noncontroversial entities so that therapeutic specificity will be increased, a group of patients with similar characteristics present in emergency rooms, outpatient clinics, and clinicians' offices. The phobic anxiety (or anxiety phobic) depersonalization syndrome begins with anxiety or panic and the powerfully distressing autonomic symptoms which accompany panic. The patient may attribute these symptoms to a physical condition like a heart attack. Later a fear of loss of control or fear of insanity produces a marked vigilance. This leads to staying in safe places, close to home, a behavior which develops into phobic response. The patient severely limits his experience and creates a self-imposed sensory isolation. This situation leads to emotional estrangement, an "as if" sense of life, and eventually to frank depersonalization and derealization.

This syndrome is a challenge to a clinician. At first it may look as if the patient needs little more than reassurance. Perhaps the precipitating circumstance has been a minor influenza or an unimportant sensory change such as one's arm falling asleep across the back of a chair. Linton and Estock[38] feel that this syndrome must be examined in terms of the patient's cognitive perceptual style, stage of development, past learning history, situational variables, and state of the organism. In their studies, these patients are extroverted persons — the home base of their egos is relatively closer to, more dependent on, external reality for optimal functioning — withdrawal appears to be unfortunate; they seem to need strong stimulus nutrient from the environment and without their stimulus nutrient they experience feelings of estrangement and depersonalization.

SUMMARY

With nonpsychotic disorders of reality, we are looking at a range of adaptive and maladaptive changes in the experience of body/self/world without a major loss of reality testing. Clinicians are most often dealing with the pathologic dysphoric experiences, particularly depersonalization and derealization. The presence of these symptoms should encourage a vigorous and complete psychiatric examination, for they may be brief and unimportant or the harbinger of a serious debilitating mental or emotional disorder. Although clinicians may not be called to treat the altered states of consciousness associated with meditation, hypnosis, or sensory deprivation, they should have a curiosity about these conditions as they reveal mechanisms of the mind and elucidate the pathways to self-deception and sickness, as well as new vision.

REFERENCES

1. Levy JS, Wachfel PL: Depersonalization: an effort at clarification. *Am J Psychoanal* 1978;38:291-300.
2. Walsh RN: Depersonalization: definition and treatment. *Am J Psychiatry* 1975;132:8.
3. Freud S: A disturbance of memory on the Acropolis. *Int J Psychoanal* 1941;22:93-101.
4. Levitan HJ: The depersonalization process. *Psychoanal Q* 1970;39:449-470.
5. Jacobson E: *Depression* . New York, New York Institute Press, 1971.
6. Guntrip H: *Schizoid Phenomena, Object Relations and the Self.* New York, International Universities Press, 1969.
7. Feigenbaum D: Depersonalization as a defense mechanism. *Psychoanal Q* 1931;139(6):4-1.
8. Searl MN: A note on depersonalization. *Int J Psychology* 1932;13:329-347.
9. Stewart WA: Depersonalization. *J Am Psychoanal Assoc* 1964;12:171-186.
10. Bird B: Feeling of unreality. *Int J Psychoanal* 1957;38:256-265.
11. Bergler E: Further studies on depersonalization. *Psychiatr Q* 1950;24:269-277.
12. Nunberg H: *Practice and Theory of Psychoanalysis.* Nervous and Mental Monographs No. 74. New York, Coolidge Foundation, 1948.

13. Oberndorf CP: The genesis of the feeling of unreality. *Int J Psychoanal* 1934;15:271-295.

14. Oberndorf CP: The role of anxiety in depersonalization. *Int J Psychoanal* 1950;31:1-5.

15. Stamm JL: Altered ego states: an aid to depersonalization. *J Am Psychoanal Assoc* 1962;10:762-783.

16. West LJ: Disassociative reaction, in Kaplan H (ed): *Comprehensive Textbook of Psychiatry* . Baltimore, Williams & Wilkins Co, 1967.

17. Blank RH: Depression, hypomania and depersonalization. *Psychoanal* 1954;23:20-37.

18. Milner PM: *Physiological Psychology* . New York, Holt, Rinehart & Winston, 1970.

19. Jaynes J: *The Origin of Consciousness in the Breakdown of the Bicameral Mind* . Boston, Houghton Mifflin Co, 1975.

20. Pribram K, in Wilber K (ed): *The Holographic Paradigm and Other Paradoxes* . Shambala, 1982, p 2.

21. Noyes RJ, Kletti R: Depersonalization in response to life threatening danger. *Compr Psychiatry* 1977;18: 375-384.

22. McKellar A: Depersonalization in a 16-year-old boy. *South Med J* 1978;71:1580-1588.

23. Kennedy R: Self induced depersonalization syndrome. *Am J Psychiatry* 1976;133:1326-1328.

24. Wineburg E, Straker N: An episode of acute, self-limiting depersonalization following a first session of hypnosis. *Am J Psychiatry* 1973;130:98-100.

25. Simpson M: Another approach to self-induced depersonalization. *Am J Psychiatry* 1977;134:1445-1450.

26. Fewtrell WD: Relaxation and depersonalization. *Br J Psychiatry* 1984;145:217.

27. Gabbard GO, Twemlow SW, Jones FC: Differential diagnosis of altered mind/body perception. *Psychiatry* 1982;45:361-369.

28. Liebowitz MR, McGrath P, Bush SC: mania occurring during treatment for depersonalization: a report of two cases. *J Clin Psychiatry* 1980;41:23-34.

29. Waltzer H: Depersonalization and the use of LSD: a psychodynamic study. *Am J Psychoanal* 1972;32:45-52.

30. Annis HM, Smart RG: Adverse reactions and recurrences from marijuana use. *Br J Addict* 1973;68:315-319.

31. Szynanski HV: Prolonged depersonalization after marijuana use. *Am J Psychiatry* 1981;138:2.

32. Beeson P, McDermmott W, Wyngaarden J: *Cecil Textbook of Medicine* . Philadelphia, WB Saunders, 1979.

33. Sherwin I: *Psychiatric aspects of temporal lobe epilepsy.* Weekly Psychiatry Update Series, No. 23. Princeton, Bionedre, Inc.

34. Greenberg DB, Hochberg FH, Murray GB: The theme of death in complex partial seizures. *Am J Psychiatry* 1984;141:1587-1589.

35. Mishlove J: *The Roots of Consciousness* . New York, Random House, 1975.
36. Freeman AM, Melges FT: Depersonalization and temporal disintegration in acute mental illness. *Am J Psychiatry* 1977;134:6
37. Ambrosino S: Phobic anxiety: depersonalization syndrome. *NY State J Med* 1973;73:419-425.
38. Linton PH, Estock RE: The anxiety phobic depersonalization syndrome: role of the cognitive-perceptual style *Dis Nerv Syst* 1977;38:138-141.

10 Suicide

Stephen M. Soreff

SUICIDE (Sui, Self + *Caedo*, to kill)   The act or instance of taking one's own life voluntarily and intentionally.

Case report   A 22-year-old, brilliant, lonely college student begins to cut his wrist. His uncle had committed suicide; he has recently broken up with his girlfriend; and he is about to enter a graduate program. Living alone, he feels desperate, depressed, and hopeless. Self-destruction offers an escape, a signal, and a solution.

FEATURES

Mood

A number of feelings characterize the suicidal person.

Depression stands as the pivotal, most common, and major emotion in the suicidal person. It features not only a quality of sadness, melancholy, and unhappiness, but also a feeling of desperation and despair. The sense of prolonged, unrelenting, unending, pervasive, crushing, undiminished dysphoric pain, which is at once both immediate and protracted, propels the person into self-destruction.

Anger emerges as another critical affect. Patients may feel frustration, annoyance, and resentment toward their spouses, families, relatives, friends, and the world. They are angry at themselves. They struggle with rage; they have a sense of revenge; and they hate themselves and those about them. Their death becomes the ultimate defiance and repudiation.

Detachment represents another common feeling. Patients note an affect of distance, unreality, and depersonalization as they contemplate their deaths. They "watch" themselves cut themselves or take pills. They are detached emotionally from both themselves and their surroundings.

A *calmness* develops in certain suicidal patients. Once they have reached a death decision, plan, and scheme, they are relaxed, suddenly comfortable, and purposeful. A 40-year-old man, manic-depressive, depressed phase, inpatient, after weeks of anguish, withdrawal, and "no progress," became more open and at ease. He asked to return to work. While out on a pass he killed himself.

Thoughts

Suicidal behavior results from a variety of perceptual experiences. These elements of the thought content both mirror the patients' moods and cause the affect.

Hopelessness stands as the cardinal perception in suicidal patients.[1] These patients view themselves as beyond hope and see the future as totally bleak. Not only do they see no future but what they perceive is continued, increasing, intolerable despair and pain. There is no light at the end of the tunnel, only an endless, prolonged black void.

Meaninglessness emerges as another key sense.[2] The patients reflect upon their lives, their world, their existence, and their living as being without meaning. They lack direction; their struggles are without purpose. They think not only "Why live," but also, "Why not die?"

Helplessness ranks as another principal suicide self-perception. These individuals see themselves as beyond help and look upon any intervention as futile. They are so bad nothing or no one will make a difference.

Ambivalence also represents a major pivotal concept in suicidal patients. On the other hand, they see themselves as hopeless and worthless, yet they wonder, just maybe something will change. They enter into a suicidal activity, eg, taking pills, half hoping to die and half hoping to be saved and helped. The classic movie scene of the man on the ledge captures the dramatic ambivalence of the patient and the situation. In their suicidal struggle dwells a cry for help.[3]

Alteration remains an important orientation in suicidal behavior for some patients. They hope through their suicide attempt to change their environment, call attention to their plight, or get a lover back. Or they see their death as hurting certain people. One common fantasy is, "At my graveside my family will finally realize how they wronged me."

Preoccupation marks yet another mental mechanism for some suicidal patients. For them, an obsessive quality develops as they continually dwell upon suicide. They fantasize about death, funerals, and ways of dying. One 45-year-old woman spent an entire year mentally preparing, reviewing, and scheming her suicide.

Death as a *solution*, either suddenly concluded or emerging after long contemplation, represents a powerful mental construct in many suicidal patients. Whatever the stresses, suicide may become the only perceived alternative. These individuals may be locked into that method and ultimately may focus exclusively upon it. Further, for many of these patients the suicide solution will not only help them, but they believe it will also benefit their families. In essence, their death will remove a family burden. This orientation is particularly lethal.

Homicidal ideation may surface in the thinking of the suicidal patients. It has two causes, both linked to the patients' depression. First, patients perceive someone or some group as responsible for their misery. Hence, striking back becomes a solution. Second, patients believe that not only is their world terrible and unbearable, but also that the whole world is bleak. As a result they will kill themselves and others. They do not want to leave others behind to suffer. This deadly view may lead to a homicide followed by suicide.

Delusions may lead to suicidal behavior. The extremes of hopelessness, worthlessness, meaninglessness, and helplessness move into delusional thinking. Also, a number of other psychotic delusions may trigger a self-destructive response. One schizophrenic man perceived that only his death would save the world from nuclear war. A manic woman seeing herself as the Messiah "sacrificed" herself for a better world.

Hallucinations may also be responsible for suicidal behavior. The most deadly are the *command hallucinations,* usually the auditory type. Here the patients experience verbal orders to kill themselves. A woman heard God ordering her to kill herself. She cut her wrists and waited to be taken.

Disorientation as well as memory difficulty may lead to a variety of self-destructive activities. These include leaving the gas stove on, walking in traffic, and taking too many pills. Patients with organic mental deficits may, through lack of insight and poor judgment, create lethal situations and live in dangerous circumstances.

Behavior

The act of suicide galvanized the mood and thought processes into a dramatic, compelling, focused behavior. Such behavior has a number of components. First is the preparation; second is the act itself; third is the response to the act.

Prior to suicide, many patients engage themselves in a number of significant activities. Preparation for their death constitutes one major group of actions. These include writing notes, making their wills, arranging for care of their children or pet animals, giving away property, and leaving their jobs. Further, some may procure the implements of their death: stockpiling pills, purchasing a gun, obtaining a rope, or getting a hose. Also occurring at this time period, many patients will see a physician.[4]

The act of suicide can be viewed in two dimensions: active versus passive and lethality. Active suicidal behavior involves steps actually taken by patients to kill themselves, eg, taking pills, cutting themselves, or shooting themselves. Passive suicidal behavior means patients bring about their deaths by *not* doing something, eg, not taking insulin, not going to hemodialysis, or refusing their digitalis. Halfway between these extremes stands the act of deliberate starvation. Lethality represents the other dimension to suicidal behavior.[5] Certain methods are more lethal than others. Hanging, shooting, burning, and jumping often leave little opportunity to intervene. The gap between attempt and success in these methods is quite close. In contrast, other ways, especially an overdose, often permit treatment and reversal of the attempt.

Finally, the patients vary in their response to their suicidal actions. Some will immediately recognize the deadly consequence of the behavior and seek help. A young woman took an overdose; she realized the "silliness" of her conduct and she called a friend. Others will perceive their attempt as not fatal and will try to complete the act in another way. A man, realizing that lacerating his wrists would not bring about his death, tried to throw himself out of the window.

Physical Examination and Laboratory Findings

A number of general observations and considerations will be advanced before discussing specific situations and findings. First, immediate life-saving steps must be taken in any suicide attempt: attention to breathing, blood pressure, bleeding, and cardiac status (with some drugs). Second, patients may attempt to kill themselves several ways simultaneously. A 35-year-old man took an overdose of antidepressants, then drove his car into a tree. Third, the patients being treated for suicide attempt should be accompanied at all times to circumvent any further self-destructive behavior.

In the physical examination, the physician should focus on a number of facets. Pulse and blood pressure remain critical measurements and reveal both shock and hypertensive crisis. Attention to respirations will help to detect a respiratory arrest. Temperature is important: anticholinergic drugs produce hyperthermia, and opiates cause a lowered body temperature.[6] General inspection will show evidence of lacerations, hanging, and trauma. The county jail sent a prisoner to the ER after he cut his wrists in a suicide attempt. The intern discovered during the physical examination that the man had also lacerated his thighs. Specific suicide methods require particular considerations: attention, care, and studies. Different medications employed for an overdose dictate different studies: barbiturates, plasma barbital concentration; digitalis; a plasma digitalis level, an ECG; aspirin, a plasma salicylate concentration; tricyclic antidepressants, a serum level, serum electrolytes, and an ECG; and lithium carbonate, a serum lithium level. A hanging attempt dictates cervical roentgenograms.

Interviewer's Reaction

Interviewers struggle with a host of often conflicting reactions as they deal with and confront suicidal patients and their actions. First, there is response to help: to stop the behavior and to treat the immediate condition. They find themselves sympathetic and caring. Yet, many interviewers feel a sense of frustration and annoyance. They experience anger at people who deliberately harm themselves when there are so many naturally ill patients to treat! On another level, the suicidal patients challenge a basic tenet of Western civilization and keystone concept stressing the relevance and reverence of life.[7] Third, the interviewers may develop a sense of questioning: Why did it happen? Who would do such a thing? What was achieved? Fourth, they may experience a sense of fascination with suicide. Indeed, the extensive literature on self-destruction, the tenth leading cause of death in these United States, indicated a degree of intrigue and curiosity about the subject.

Pathogenesis

Psychodynamics A number of powerful psychodynamic determinants contribute to or cause the suicide ideation and behavior. These constitute the individual background to self-destructive activities. They constitute the human drama, the personal struggle, and the intimate conflicts which often have a lethal result.

Depression and loss remain the major determinants of suicide. The most important cause of all depression is loss. The loss may take a variety of forms: diminished self-esteem, unemployment, divorce, death, separation, leaving home, or illness. The loss may be real or perceived. In the former, the person experiences a genuine setback, such as breaking up with a lover. In the latter, the individual fails to achieve an ideal, a perfect grade, or an unobtainable mark. Of interest, that individual is considered by all about him a success. The sense of hopelessness particularly ultimately correlates with a lead to a suicide.[8]

In *reunion,* patients connote suicide as a way of joining a dead person. Their death will reunite them with a loved one. Such a notion is the motive behind some suicide pacts; they will go together in order to be together forever. Widows and widowers may voice the wish and hope to join their departed. Suicides of this type may often occur on the anniversary of the loved one's death.

Escape for many patients stands as the determinant of their suicide. They want to move beyond a host of problems: family conflicts, marital stresses, physical illness, pain, isolation, overwhelming pressures, employment demands, financial strains, or a "world gone mad." To them death means the end of something intolerable.

Suicide as a *positive* event and *solution* represents an affirmative concept one step beyond escape. In this construct advanced by Lifton, these patients view suicide both as leading to peace and representing an admirable conclusion to life.[9] In contrast to suicide meaning an escape, it becomes a value, a goal, and an achievement. Not infrequently, patients with this view have been exposed to suicide within their family.

Suicide becomes a method to express *anger* and *revenge*. It is used as a tool to hurt others, to inflict pain, and to gain vengeance. Frequently, suicide notes will spell out how much the patient had suffered and the hope that the death will produce anguish, torment, grief, and remorse. Suicide represents a vivid, undeniable hostile message.

Control is another key component of suicidal threats and behavior. This control operates on many levels. At one level some people use suicide as a method of obtaining what they want. "If you leave me, I will kill myself" represents a simple formula by which certain individuals remain banded together. On a deeper level, some employ suicide as the last full measure of their control of their lives. They will say they have lost all alternatives and options in their life except to choose when they will die. Death is the only element under their control. A 65-year-old man with chronic obstructive pulmonary disease contemplated the options of risky surgery for a lung mass or chemotherapy. He felt trapped, alone, and overwhelmed. He saw suicide as the only way to control his life.

Killing the object within designates a classic psychoanalytic explanation for suicide. Freud put forth the theory of suicide symbolizing the destruction of an internalized object, person.[10,11] In this equation, the patients incorporate a love object into their selves. Ultimately, as with all objects, it is ambivalently held. They then focus on the hated aspects. Death provides a way to rid themselves of this object. In another form, the suicidal patients may come to see themselves as truly bad, dirty, and unredeemable. They view their "inner selves," the one nobody "really knows," as vile, terrible, contaminating, and condemned. They must kill themselves to destroy the internal evil.

Suicide means *atonement* for some patients. They have sinned; they must die. Their offenses may be imagined or real. In the former, some patients evolving a psychotic depression come to view themselves as such sinners, liars, and cheats, that their salvation requires their death. In the latter, patients who kill believe they should also die. During a severe altercation a 55-year-old, depressed man shot and killed his wife. Recognizing what he had just done, he turned the gun on himself. Later in the emergency department he said, "I must die; an eye for an eye; a tooth for a tooth."

Patriotism represents another reason for suicide. This embodies the concept of not only dying for one's country, idea, faith, or belief, but also of actively, deliberately sacrificing themselves for the cause. The kamikaze pilots in World War II and car bomb drivers of the Middle East provide exceptionally destructive examples of this.

Increased *risk factors* to suicide include sex, age, developmental factors, psychiatric hospitalization, prior suicidal behavior, and physician visits. First, more women than men attempt suicide; however, more men than women actually kill themselves.[12] Also, certain groups have high suicide rates, eg, American Indians.[13] Second, in terms of age, the risk of suicide increases with advancing age. The rise commences in the 40-year-old group and rises progressively into the 60-year-old-and-beyond group.[14]

Also, there has been a recent dramatic increase in adolescent and young adult suicides.[15-17] Third, there are a number of important developmental factors. Patients with family histories of suicides are at high risk.[1] Fourth, psychiatric hospitalization and especially recent (within 1 month) discharge correlate with suicide.[20] Fifth, about 25% of those patients who attempt suicide will ultimately kill themselves.[21] Sixth, many patients prior to suicide will have had contact with a physician or an emergency department.

Biologic Explanation

The biologic contribution to suicide has both a global explanation as explored in earlier chapters and a number of specific relationships. In depression, the catecholamine hypothesis provides a biochemical genesis for melancholia, hopelessness, and despair and thus sets the affective context for self-destructive behavior. In psychosis, suicidal activities may develop within the constellation of major biochemical changes such as an increase of dopamine or norepinephrine. In paranoia, causative organic deficits may account for suicide reactions.

A number of specific relationships between biochemical alterations and self-destructive events have been reported. These represent a more focused approach and suggest a more concentrated fertile area of emerging research in suicidology. Targum et al have found a significant number of abnormal dexamethasone suppression tests among patients with unipolar depression who had made suicide attempts.[22] In contrast, other studied patients with unipolar depression without self-destructive behavior do not demonstrate cortisol escape during the dexamethasone suppression. They suggest such cortisol breakthrough designates and signals a high-risk group within the group of unipolar depressed patients.

The important relationship betwen suicidal behavior and serotonin has been advanced. Brown et al have found a correlation between a low CSF 5-hydroxyindoleacetic acid (5-HIAA), a metabolite of serotonin, and both aggression and self-destructive behavior.[23] They studied hospitalized patients with borderline personality disorders. They report not only was there a significant decrease in the CSF serotonin metabolic level, but also the CSF metabolite levels of norepinephrine and dopamine bore no relationship to suicidal behaviors. Finally, Ostroff et al, in looking at psychiatrically hospitalized group patients, reported those who made serious suicide attempts had both a significantly higher cortisol level determined by a 24-hour urine analysis and a lower norepinephrine/epinephrine ration than the nonsuicidal patients.[24] The high urinary cortisol levels suggest great psychic distress. They further discuss the concept that a high norepinephrine/epinephrine ratio correlates with aggression outwardly directed, whereas a low ratio reflects inward directed anger with suicidal consequences.

Genetics

A family history of suicide represents a major determinant of an individual's suicidal behavior.[25] Particularly relevant is when the suicide was a parent and occurred when the patient was young.[26] The suicide suggests an historical family solution. Often such suicides are maintained as secrets, further heightening their power. A 45-year-old engineer hung himself. His older brother had committed suicide when he was 45 years old. The younger brother had always closely identified with his brother, idealized him, and struggled to lead a similar life. The suicide within the family becomes a legend, a focus, a signal event, a scar, and a mark. All these elements converge into the surviving family members. The survivors not only carry the pain, the anguish, the guilt, the memory, and the uncertainty, but also, more significantly, they harbor the subtle prophecy and dread foreshadowing across their futures.[27]

The genetic feature in suicide represents one of the factors in schizophrenia, manic-depressive illness, and alcoholism. All three diseases carry with them significant risk of suicide. All three have been shown to have a genetic component and pattern.[28-31]

Seymour Kety has advanced the theory that suicide may have its own inheritance pattern not necessarily associated with those of schizophrenic and depressive illnesses.[32] He supports this position with demonstrated monozygotic concordance rates for suicide but no significant concordance in dizygotic twins and biochemical studies. He has provided an important area for research.

Environment

Living alone ranks as a critical risk factor in suicide. The causes of single life are legion: divorce, widowhood, separation, seclusion by individual preference, and assignment. Yet, regardless of the reason, living alone often promotes isolation, withdrawal, and disengagement. It further enhances a situation where detection and intervention are either not available or delayed. The sequence of suicide followed by a discovery of the person days later develops frequently in single living circumstances.

The response of significant others to the patient's plight, despair, threats of suicide, and actual self-destructive behavior stands as a crucial environmental determinant.[33] In two ways, family, friends, coworkers, and companions can actually advance suicide. First, they react with indifference to the patient. They ignore the pain, the talk, and the attempt. A girl tried to tell her parents of her boyfriend's rejection. They only continued to watch television. She took some aspirin and got their attention. Second, the significant others, for a variety of reasons, ranging from rage to devotion, actually promote suicide. A family brought an aging relative to dialysis three times a week, traveling 80 miles each way. They denied ever being annoyed by the trip or the inconvenience, yet they also frequently provided the patient with salty food, which caused fluid overload and congestive heart failure.

Lack of *community ties* also heightens the suicide risk. This correlates with the solitary life and a dangerous response by significant others. The alienated, the isolated, the disenfranchised, and the disconnected live on the peripheral society, dwell at the margin, and exist in the shadows.

Unemployment represents a pivotal element in suicide.[34,35] The position and economic potential and capacity stand as highly visible, tangible, and specific evidence of one's place in our society. Loss of a job means a rupture of all the social aspects and supports which come with work. Long-term unemployment means chronic depression, alienation, and disengagement. It leads to hopelessness and helplessness culminating, in some situations, in suicide. The acute insult, pain, loss and humiliation of employment termination can be catastrophic for some individuals. A 35-year-old woman was fired. She went home and took a fatal overdose.

A number of *occupations* have been associated with high rates of suicide. Often cited are the professions of medicine, dentistry, and law.[36] These groups share high levels of responsibility, perfectionistic strivings, moments of isolation, heavy time pressure, and work commitments. All those qualities may contribute to excessive death rates. Law enforcement officials also have a high incidence of suicide.[37] Factors there include divorce, alcohol, alienation, and availability of handguns.

Specific situations and circumstances have high rates of suicide. Jails and prisons have this phenomenon.[38] An extraordinary number of suicides occur during the first 24 hours of the confinement. Elements of despair, hopelessness, fear, and isolation contribute to the suicides.[39] The most important quality of these and other potentially lethal situations is that the patients feel trapped. Be it in the service, at camp, at school, or in a certain group, the persons perceive themselves as helplessly trapped.

Societal changes may also contribute to suicide. Durkheim observed that not only did suicide rates increase during periods of economic depression, but also during periods of an expanding economy.[40] He used the term *anomie* to describe the condition of society in a state of flux: rules changing, standards altering, and ideas evolving. For people becoming uncertain and unsure, suicides reflect shifting values.

Availability of *guns* ranks as a decisive factor which turns an attempt into death. The presence of firearms proves to be a particularly lethal component. Its effect is both immediate and irreversible. Other potentially fatal situations include high buildings, heights, and bridges.

DIFFERENTIAL DIAGNOSIS

Nonpsychotropic Drugs

Nonpsychotropic drugs, as described in Chapter 2, may cause depression, which subsequently leads to suicide. Patients experiencing hopelessness, helplessness, and despair induced by medications, do not recognize their state as drug-precipitated. To them suicide is the consequence of their profound, relentless misery. They see no end of the pain. Not only do they fail to realize the reversible nature of their sadness, but also all too frequently their physicians have failed to warn them or to notice the depression.

Psychotropic Drugs

Discontinuance of either antipsychotic drugs or antidepressants may cause the emergence of suicidal behavior. In the case of the antipsychotic medication, the patients may have experienced remissions of their psychotic processes while on the drugs.[41] However, once terminated, they may again develop auditory hallucinations, persecutory delusions, withdrawal, or other schizophrenic symptoms. One 30-year-old man, within 6 weeks had command hallucinations every time he stopped his chlorpromazine, calling him evil and telling him to kill himself. In the case of antidepressants, either premature discontinuance or abruptly halting their use may plunge the patients back into a depression with its attendant suicide risk.[42]

Overdoses of psychotropic drugs stand as a persistent danger. This is especially true for the antidepressants.[43] Tricyclic antidepressant overdoses account for up to 37% of all intensive care unit acute poison-related admissions.[44] Physicians confront the paradoxical situation that the very medications which will help reverse the depression are the ones which may result in a fatal overdose. The solution remains close monitoring of the patient, prescribing small amounts of drugs, and paying careful attention to the patient.

Alcohol

Alcohol *intoxication* stands as the great potentiator of depression. After a few drinks the "blue" person becomes melancholy, profoundly "down" and desperate. For alcohol, in and of itself, remains a pharmacological depressant. Further, under its influence, despair, morbid thoughts and wishes of death, and self-hatred may dramatically emerge. As a result, under the influence of alcohol, the depressed person becomes the suicidal patient. Not infrequently, one encounters the suicidal patient in the emergency department who has just taken an overdose, cut wrists, or attempted to jump, each while intoxicated, and who, upon obtaining sobriety, denies any suicidal ideation or pain. A 45-year-old, unemployed factory worker was brought to the emergency department after he shot himself in the abdomen while intoxicated, damaging his stomach and left kidney. Still under the influence of alcohol in the trauma, he stated, "I was aiming for my heart." The next day, after surgery and sober, he declared the entire episode to have been an accident and without any suicidal intent.

Chronic abuse of alcohol correlates highly with suicide. In one study 22% of suicides had a diagnosis of primary alcoholism.[45] Chronic alcoholism means losses: of job, family, spouse, friends, opportunities, and hopes. The Alcoholics Anonymous notion of "hitting bottom" reflects many setbacks, insults, and losses sustained during an alcoholic career. Particularly devastating and lethal is when an alcoholic encounters an acute significant loss, eg, divorce, widowhood, or death of a parent.[46]

Other Abused Substances

Suicides, suicidal behavior, and self-endangering and destructive activities occur at a high rate among the drug-abusing and addicted population. Miles calculates 10% of all suicide deaths as related to drug addiction and notes that this group has a suicide rate twenty times greater than those their age who do not abuse drugs.[47] The suicidal consequences represent both the results of the intoxication and the withdrawal. One may speculate on an underlying emptiness, depression, lack of pleasure, and anhedonia as part of the individual's reason for abusing substance use. Further, the losses of family, employment, and economic stability as a consequence of substance abuse promote suicidal behavior.

Amphetamine abuse results in suicide in two ways. First, used orally, and even more intravenously, amphetamines may precipitate a hypertensive crisis. Second, the withdrawal period from amphetamines is often marked by a profound, severe depression with avoidant behavior and excessive sleep with possibly suicidal consequences.

Barbiturate addiction carries with it a self-destructive potential. As the patients build up a tolerance for drugs and require an ever-increasing amount to satisfy their addictive needs, they move closer to dangerous and fatal risk. Certainly the combination of barbiturates and alcohol has proved particularly lethal. Barbiturates essentially move the patients into further depression and hopelessness.

Hallucinogens, eg, LSD may propel the intoxicated patient into suicide. Incidences of LSD-induced suicide have been noted.[48] Often the patient responds to terrifying, powerful, and forceful hallucinations with self-destructive reactions.

Opiates are commonly depicted as the major substance involved in suicide. The high suicide rate among users not only reflects the depression which follows the euphoria and the pain created by withdrawal symptoms, but also indicates accident factors. Often the death has been caused by the patients unknowingly injecting themselves with highly potent heroin. Alternately, the patients may be waning in opiate tolerance, making themselves fatally susceptible to their once normal habit. Of interest, there are two types of opiate overdose deaths.[49] In the first, the patients experience a sudden death syndrome, toxic, rather allergic in nature, and thought to be related to an arrhythmia. In the second, the patients die from hypoxia resulting from hypertension and respiratory difficulty. In the latter, the patients have constricted pupils.

Phencyclidine (PCP) propels the patients occasionally into destructive behavior. They may place themselves at risk by acting upon their hallucinations. They may wander into danger in their disorientation. Or they may kill themselves as they experience the depression associated with withdrawal.

Medical Illnesses

Medical illnesses correlate and contribute to suicidal behavior. Up to 70% of patients who kill themselves will have one or more active medical illnesses. Furthermore, in those with disease, there was a causative link between the illness and their suicides in 51% of the patients.[50] Suicide attempts in medically hospitalized patients dramatically underscore and highlight this major relationship.[52]

Two key factors forge the link between medical illness and suicidal behavior. The first stems from the fact that many diseases, eg, hypothyroidism, hepatic encephalopathy, and hypoadrenalism, cause depression by themselves.[53] From the disease-induced despair, suicidal activities emerge. The second revolves around the psychodynamic issues of loss and social stresses as a result of the illnesses. The individuals feel a sense of loss: of health, of options, and of well-being. They may also have a sense of rejection, conflict, and alienation from their family, friends, and coworkers. The result of both is depression.

Malignant diseases rank significantly in those patients who either attempt or complete suicide.[54] For many people, despite the advances, the terms "cancer" and "terminal" are synonymous. Cancerophobia remains extremely prevalent and contributory. For some cancer patients suicide seems the only way they may control their lives and destinies. Certainly, the pain, the isolation, the hopelessness, and the helplessness — all contribute to this relationship.

Psychosomatic diseases have been linked to suicide. In the work of Dorpat et al, 80 suicide deaths were examined.[55] Fifty-six of these patients (70%) had at least one active illness at the time of their death. Of the total 107 actual diseases in those patients, 47 (44%) were psychosomatic. The psychosomatic illnesses include peptic ulcer (17), rheumatoid arthritis (12), hypertension (11), asthma (2), hyperthyroidism (2), mucous colitis (1), cardiospasm (1), and ulcerative colitis (1). The psychosomatic diseases bridge the psychological and the physical gap. The underlying emotional pains coupled with the external problems of the disease may be a particular suicide-inducing combination.

Chronicity ranks as a very high suicide contributing factor. Patients' tolerance, optimism, and determination may often wane as the unrelenting, continual, unending reality of a number of illnesses begins to erode their hope. For many patients, their clinical course holds only promises of further complications, exacerbations, and lessening of function. One man, 47 years old with chronic organic pulmonary disease, became suicidal and depressed when he was admitted to the hospital for the third time in 4 months for respiratory infection. He bitterly complained that the first admission was a novelty, the second a setback, and the third meant the end. Abram et al reported the suicidal behavior of chronic dialysis patients as 400 times greater than the rate for the general population.[56] This finding emphasizes the self-destructive relationship to chronic disease.

Pain remains one of the most important contributors to suicide. Some patients prefer death to pain. A particularly lethal combination is a painful chronic disease. Chronic pain stands intimately related to depression and substance abuse.[57] Pain stands as an immediate, devastating, incapacitating sensation. It demands action; it compels attention; it precludes anything else; it eclipses the future. A 45-year-old man attempted to cut off his left arm. He had injured it in an industrial accident, had endured several only partially successful surgical procedures, had taken many "painkillers" without effect, could not sleep because of the pain, and felt his physician did not care. In his desperation he would have done "anything." Painful illness is clearly associated with suicidal activity.

Surgical Complications

Patients' *preoperative* reactions to their impending surgery may reflect suicidal considerations. For many individuals, surgery represents a source of great apprehension, fear, and dread. They liken it to being "put to sleep;" they see it as total loss of control; and they are terrified about being under the knife. They are afraid of postoperative pain, disfigurement, and dysfunction. As a result, some choose suicide to surgery. This particular choice is not infrequently made when the surgery is for cancer. For others who are already depressed, delay of surgery provides an avenue to acting out their self-destructive wishes.[58] They hope to cause their death by postponing an operation.

Certain *surgical procedures* seem particularly associated with depression and the attendant risk of suicide.[59] For some men, urologic surgery leading to impotence is a specific cause for profound depression. For some women, mastectomies and hysterectomies produce significant dysphoria with suicidal consequences. For many patients, surgery which results in demonstrable disfigurement, eg, operations to the head and neck, or an amputation, produces a major loss and suicidal behavior.

A number of *postoperative* complications may lead to suicidal behaviors. First is pain. Second delirium, administered opiates, alcohol withdrawal, or the intensive care unit, may yield to destructive threats and activities as the patient struggles to gain control in a rapidly changing world. Third, patients may choose suicide as they begin to appreciate the surgical results or the possibility of future procedures. Fourth, some patients may become suicidal as they sense and suffer the postoperative withdrawal of attention by their physicians and family. A 50-year-old man four days after successful cardiac surgery threatened to jump from his hospital window. He later explained all he wanted was his doctor, wife, and son to notice him. He felt abandoned as everything "healed" uneventfully.

Trauma

Suicidal behavior may lead directly to accidents with their resultant trauma.[60] Not only do stresses cause accidents, but also in certain cases these accidents represent a suicide attempt or completion. Some automobile accidents are, indeed, actually suicides.[61] Other traumatic situations and events also are a consequence of specific self-destructive behavior.[62] A depressed, 40-year-old man with manic-depressive illness, depressed phase, drove his car into an interstate bridge abutment. He perceived his "accidental" death would be more acceptable to his family and covered by his insurance.

Some patients *respond to their trauma* and the ensuing disfiguration, immobilization, pain, and loss by becoming suicidal. Trauma often involves major and significant changes and losses. Patients may lose function, their jobs, their attractiveness, their mobility, and control of their lives. The results of accidents — facial scars, body mutilation, traction, or protracted bouts of surgery — prove to be devastating, intolerable, and overwhelming. Depression follows in the wake of trauma. As patients struggle to confront the accident's results and implications, they may become suicidal. A young professional golfer approaching the peak of her career, was struck by a car as she crossed an intersection. As she began to comprehend the consequences of the trauma — she could not return to her tour — she contemplated suicide. An active young man who became paraplegic following a diving accident killed himself after his discharge from the rehabilitation unit.

Head trauma may lead to suicidal behavior in several ways. First, the resultant depression for some patients may produce self-destructive activities. Second, the patients' disorientation and memory deficits may cause them to enter dangerous situations: walking in traffic or leaving the gas stove on. Third, head trauma can produce drug automatism.[63] In this condition the patients may continue to ingest medications with a resultant overdose. Automation involves purposeful behavior without total consciousness or insight or recall.

Psychiatric Diagnosis

Patients with any psychiatric diagnosis may engage in suicidal behavior or kill themselves. Indeed, suicide cuts across all categories. Yet, statistics continually demonstrate high incidence in certain diagnoses. This section will focus on those groups and emphasize their self-destructive capacities. Further, the diagnostic criteria follow those articulated in the *Diagnostic and Statistical Manual of Mental Disorders* [DSM-III].[64]

Schizophrenic patients may kill themselves and are at increased risk for suicide.[65] The schizophrenic disorder involves delusions; grandiose, religious, or nihilistic; auditory hallucinations; loose associations; at least a 6-month duration of active illness; and deterioration in the sphere of living and activities. The symptoms and signs suggest suicidal consequences. Suicide occurs relatively early in the course of the disease, especially in contrast to alcoholism.[66]

Some schizophrenic patients responding to the acute phase of their illness and symptoms may become self-destructive. They may be following the dictates of command hallucinations demanding and ordering the act. They may involve a bizarre delusion suggesting their family's destiny and their community depend upon their death. They may attempt suicide to escape their thoughts quarreling within their heads; or they may seek suicide to avoid the disintegration of their ego boundaries.

Suicide in chronic schizophrenic patients represents often a response to their deterioration, the protracted symptoms, and the resultant depression of both. Chronic schizophrenic patients experience social, work, and recreation losses. They may have periods of hospitalizations, difficulty maintaining employment, and family disruptions. They may have endured symptoms for long periods. As a consequence, some of these patients will be depressed. Depression does occur within the schizophrenic patient's life and world.[67] A 40-year-old man with a chronic schizophrenic illness prepared to kill himself. He had been unemployed for years and "knew" he was too paranoid to work. He had been divorced, lived alone, and required neuroleptics to control his "wild" thoughts. He not only hated his past and his illness, but also could not contemplate a future.

In **bipolar disorders,** manic-depressive illness, suicide occurs at a high rate. Although self-destructive acts do happen during the *manic* phase, eg, as a result of a grandiose scheme to save the universe, suicidal behavior represents a consequence of the *depressed phase.* The depressed phase leading to suicide not only has the weight loss, sleep disturbances, feelings of worthlessness, no energy, and psychomotor changes, but also psychotic features. Psychotic features include hallucinations or delusions dominated by required punishment, guilt, nihilism, or individual inadequacy. It is often advanced that the most dangerous time in the depressed phase occurs as the patients begin to get better. As they emerge from the depth of despair, they also finally have the energy to act upon their self-destructive fantasies. Since manic-depressive illness is a genetic disease, many of these patients will not only have relatives with it, but also may have family histories of suicides. Certainly some patients with manic-depressive illness, especially before the advent of lithium treatment, may have considered suicide as they surveyed a future of major hills and valleys.

A **major depression** has all the attendant symptoms of the *depressed phase* without the recurrent history. Again, the patients experience a world which is black, a future which is bleak, and a self which is worthless. The initial precipitant may be real but the depression becomes profound, and pronounced. A 45-year-old woman responded to a move, the marriage of her last daughter, and loss of her employment with a major depression. She resented the move, felt anguish over her daughter, and guilt about the job. She could not sleep, be alone, eat, or enjoy herself. She hated herself for "not being stronger" and wondered if they all would be better off without her. She considered suicide. Patients during the period following a depression recovery remain at suicide risk.[68]

Dysthymic disorder also correlates with suicidal activity.[69] Here the patients have sustained periods of depression during the prior 1 to 2 years, and although they are dysphoric for up to several weeks to months, it is not of such severity or duration to warrant the diagnosis of major depression. In the depressed episodes they experience at least three of the following: sleep disturbance, fatigue, low self-esteem, diminished productivity, decreased attention, social wihdrawal, no interest in pleasurable activities, irritability, nonresponsiveness to compliments, diminished activity, pessimistic life view, tears, and suicidal or death recurrent thoughts.[64] The patients do not have psychotic features, eg, hallucinations or delusions. The sense of chronic depression permeates these persons.

Adjustment disorder with depressed mood represents an acute reaction to a defined, definite, and usually limited stress and loss. Although the initial response may be severe, the origin is readily identifiable and the patients usually reconstitute rapidly. One often encounters these in the emergency department as one sees patients reacting to specific losses by suicide attempts. Stresses include rejection by lovers, divorces, loss of employment, or fights with spouses.

Persons with certain personality disorders may be prone to suicidal behavior.

Persons with an antisocial personality disorder kill themselves at high rates.[70] This incidence reflects the dramatic clash of consequences of their lifestyle and their basic personality. The antisocial personality is characterized before 15 years of age by truancy, running away, lying, casual repeated sexual intercourse, thefts, substance abuse, and starting fights; and after 18 years of age by difficulty sustaining employment, irresponsible parenting, illegal activity, no enduring sexual relations, aggressiveness, impulsiveness, and recklessness. As a result of these features, the antisocial persons find themselves in trouble, in jail, unemployed, and divorced. They may become suicidal when confronted with the consequences.[71]

Patients with **borderline personality disorders** often engage in suicidal activity. Indeed, self-destructive behavior constitutes part of the DSM-III criteria for this diagnosis. These patients' characteristics include impulsiveness, unstable and intense interpersonal patterns, anger, disturbance of identity, affective lability, and protracted feelings of emptiness. The suicide, the self-mutilation, and the self-destructiveness not only represent a response to the social losses sustained, but also the reaction to their profound, intense, seemingly limitless internal sense of "nothingness," void, and emptiness.

Delirium involves an acute global disorientation which may result in a self-destructive act. The delirium features perceptual disturbances, altered sleep-wake cycles, often psychomotor heightened activity. In the rapidly changing, unstable, and frightening world, the patients may injure themselves.

Dementia involves self-destruction in two ways: accidental and as a depression consequence. Intellectual losses, memory deficits, concrete thinking, judgment impairment, higher cortical function disturbances, and personality changes characterize this diagnosis. The impaired judgment may lead patients into dangerous situations, eg, leaving their cigarettes lighted in bed, getting lost away from home in cold weather, or leaving on the burner on a stove. Many patients become depressed as they realize they are losing their "mind." They would prefer to kill themselves than suffer the gradual erosion of their intellectual capacity and ability.

The previous sections on *alcohol and other substance abuse* cover the substance dependence diagnoses and their effects. The dependence itself is characterized by three qualities. First, it is pathologic. The patients cannot control the use. They cannot stop. Second, the use has led to work or social impairment. Third, the patients have developed either tolerance to the substance, requiring higher doses for the drug's effect, or experience withdrawal signs and symptoms when they stop the drug.

Suicide stands as a compelling dramatic threat, attempt, and all too frequently completed action. Its genesis emerges from the convergence of the person, the personality, the biology, the family, and the predicament.

REFERENCES

1. Beck AT, Kovacs M, Weissman A: Hopelessness and suicidal behavior. *JAMA* 1975;234:1146-1149.
2. Frankl VE: *The Unheard Cry for Meaning.* New York, Simon & Schuster, 1979.
3. Faberow HL, Shneidman ES: *The Cry for Help.* New York: McGraw-Hill Book Co, 1965.
4. Murphy GE: Suicide and attempted suicide. *Hosp Pract* 1977;12:73-81.
5. Beck AT, Beck R, Kovacs M: Classification of suicidal behaviors: I. Quanitifying intent and method lethality. *Am J Psychiatry* 1975;132:285-287.
6. Slaby AE, Lieb J, Tancredi LR: *Handbook of Psychiatric Emergencies,* ed 2. Garden City, NY, Medical Examination Publishing Co, 1981.
7. Slater P: *Footholds.* New York, EP Dutton & Co, 1977.
8. Beck AT, Steer, RA, Koracs M, et al: Hopelessness and eventual suicide: a ten-year prospective study of patients hospitalized with suidical ideation. *Am J Psychiatry* 1985;142:559-563.
9. Lifton R: *The Broken Connection.* Beaverton, Ore, Touchstone, 1980.
10. Freud S: Mourning and melancholia, in *Standard Edition of the Complete Psychological Works,* Strachey J (trans). London, Hogarth Press, Ltd., 1935-1965, vol 14, pp 247-252.
11. Litman RE: Sigmund Freud on suicide, in Shneidman ES, *Essays in Self-Destruction.* New York, Science House, 1967, pp 324-344.
12. Weissman MW: The epidemiology of suicide attempts. *Arch Gen Psychiatry* 1974;30:737-746.
13. Hochkirchen B, Jilek W: Psychosocial dimensions of suicide and parasuicide in Amerindians of the Pacific Northwest. *J Operational Psychiatry* 1985;16:24-28.
14. Final mortality statistics, in National Center for Health Statistics: *Vital Statistics of the United States.* Hyattsville Md, National Center for Health Statistics, 1978, vol 29, No. 6 (suppl 2).
15. Hellon CP, Solomon MI: Suicide and age in Alberta, Canada, 1951 to 1977. *Arch Gen Psychiatry* 1980;37:505-510.
16. Sudak HS, Ford AB, Rushforth HB: Adolescent suicide: an overview. *Am J Psychother* 1984;38:350-363.
17. Rushforth NB, Ford AB, Sudak HS, et al: Increasing suicide rates in adolescents and young adults in an urban community: 1958 to 1982, in Sudak HS, Ford AB, Rushforth NB (eds): *Suicide in the Young.* Boston, John Wright-PSG Inc, 1984, pp 45-68.

18. Zung WWK: Suicide prevention by suicide detection. *Psychosomatics* 1979,20:149-159.
19. Green AH: Self-destructive behavior in battered children. *Am J Psychiatry* 1978;135:579-582.
20. Roy A: Risk factors for suicide in psychiatric patients. *Arch Gen Psychiatry* 1982;39:1089-1095.
21. Maris RW: *Pathways to Suicide: A Survey of Self-Destructive Behaviors*. Baltimore, Johns Hopkins University Press, 1981.
22. Targum SD, Rosen L, Capodanno AE: The dexamethasome suppression test in suicidal patients with unipolar depressions. *Am J Psychiatry* 1983;140:877-879.
23. Brown GL, Ebert MH, Goyer PT, et al: Aggression, suicide, and serotonin: relationships to CSF amine metabolites. *Am J Psychiatry* 1982;139:741-746.
24. Ostroff F, Giller E, Banese K, et al: Neuroendocrine risk factors of suicidal behavior. *Am J Psychiatry* 1982;139:1323-1325.
25. Dublin CI: *Suicide: A Sociological and Statistical Study*. New York, Ronald Press, 1963.
26. Cain AC, Fast I: Children's disturbed reactions to parent suicide. *Am J Orthopsychiatry* 1966;36:873-880.
27. Shneidman ES: Prevention, intervention, and postvention of suicide, in Ross JF: The management of the presuicidal, suicidal, and postsuicidal patient. *Ann Intern Med* 1971;75:453-458.
28. Kety SS: Genetic aspects of schizophrenia. *Psychiatr Ann* 1976;6:6-15.
29. Mendlewica J, Linkowski P, Guroff JF, et al: Color blindness linkage to bipolar manic-depressive illness. *Arch Gen Psychiatry* 1979;36:1442-1447.
30. Egeland JA, Sussex JH: Suicide and family loading for affective disorders. *JAMA* 1985;254:915-918.
31. Winokur G, Reich T, Rimmer J, et al: Alcoholism III: diagnosis and familiar psychiatric illness in 259 alcoholics. *Arch Gen Psychiatry* 1970;23:104-111.
32. Kety SS: Interactions between stress and genetic processes, in Zales MR (ed): *Stress in Health and Disease*. New York, Brunner/Mazel, 1985, pp 115-129.
33. Soreff S: *Management of the Psychiatric Emergency*. New York, John Wiley & Sons, 1981.
34. Roy A: Specificity of risk factors for depression. *Am J Psychiatry* 1981;138:959-961.
35. Platt S: Unemployment and suicidal behavior: a review of the literature. *Soc Sci Med* 1984;19:93-115.
36. Blachly PH, Disher W, Roduner G: Suicide by physicians. *Bull Suicidology 1-18* 1969.
37. Heiman MF: Suicide among police. *Am J Psychiatry* 1977;134:1286-1290.
38. Topp DO: Suicide in prison. *Br J Psychiatry* 1979;134:24-27.

402

39. Smialek JE, Spitz WV: Death behind bars. *JAMA* 1978;240:2563-2564.
40. Durkheim E: *Suicide.* Glencoe, Ill, Free Press, 1951.
41. Davis JM: Overview: maintenance therapy in psychiatry and schizophrenia. *Am J Psychiatry* 1975;132:1237-1245.
42. Davis JM: Overview: maintenance therapy in psychiatry: II. *Affective Disorders* 1976;133:1-13.
43. Boehnert MT, Lovejoy FH: Value of the QRS duration versus the serum drug level in predicting seizures and ventricular arrhythmias after an acute overdose of tricyclic antidepressants. *N Engl J Med* 1985;313:474-479.
44. Kathol RG, Henn FA: Tricyclics: the most common agent used in potentially lethal overdoses. *J Nerv Ment Dis* 1983;171:250-252.
45. Morrison JR: Suicide in a psychiatric practice population. *J Clin Psychiatry* 1982;43:348-352.
46. Murphy GE, Armstrong JW, Hermele SL, et al: Suicide and alcoholism. *Arch Gen Psychiatry* 1979;36:65-69.
47. Miles CP: Conditions predisposing to suicide: a review. *J Nerv Ment Dis* 1977;164:231-246.
48. Kolb LC: *Modern Clinical Psychiatry,* ed 8 Philadelphia, WB Saunders Co, 1973.
49. Shine D: Substance abuse, in Kravis TC, Warner LC (eds): *Emergency Medicine.* Rockville, Md, Aspen Pub, 1983, pp 493-516.
50. Fawcett J: Suicidal depression and physical illness. *JAMA* 1972;219:1303-1306.
51. Reich P, Kelly MI: Suicide attempts by hospitalized medical and surgical patients. *N Engl J Med* 1976;294:298-301.
52. Jefferson IW, Marshall JR: *Neuropsychiatric Features of Medical Disorders.* New York, Plenum Medical Book Co, 1981.
53. Valenstein E, Heilman FM: Emotional disorders resulting from lesions of the central nervous system, in Heilman KM, Valenstein E (eds): *Clinical Neuropsychology.* New York, Oxford University Press, 1979, pp 413-438.
54. Faberow NL, Shneidman ES, Leonard CV: Suicide among patients with malignant neoplasms, in Shneidman ES, Faberow NL, Litman RE (eds): *The Psychology of Suicide.* New York, Science House, 1970.
55. Dorpat TL, Anderson WF, Ripley HS: The relationship of physical illness to suicide, in Resnik HLP (ed): *Suicidal Behaviors, Diagnosis and Management.* Boston, Little, Brown, & Co, 1968, pp 209-219.
56. Abram HS, Moore GL, Westervelt FB: Suicidal behavior in chronic dialysis patients. *Am J Psychiatry* 1971;127:1199-1207.
57. Katon W, Egan K, Miller D: Chronic pain: lifetime psychiatric diagnosis and family history. *Am J Psychiatry* 1985;142:1156-1160.
58. Andrew JM: Delay in surgery: patients' motivations, in Howells JC (ed): *Modern Perspectives in the Psychiatric Aspects of Surgery.* New York, Brunner/Mazel, 1976, pp 77-108.

59. Bukberg JB, Straker N: Psychiatric consultation with the ambivalent cancer surgery candidate. *Psychosomatics* 1982;23:1043-1050.
60. Tsuang MT, Boor M, Fleming JA: Psychiatric aspects of traffic accidents. *Am J Psychiatry* 1985;142:538-546.
61. Schmidt CW, Shaffer JW, Zlotowitz HI, et al: Suicide by vehicular crash. *Am J Psychiatry* 1977;134:175-178.
62. Hutcherson RR, Kreuger DW: Accidents making suicide attempts. *J Trauma* 1980;20:800-801.
63. Good MI: The concept of drug automatism. *Am J Psychiatry* 1976;133:948-952.
64. American Psychiatric Association: *Diagnostic and Statistical Manual of Mental Disorders,* ed 3. Washington, American Psychiatric Association, 1980.
65. Drake RE, Gates C, Whitaker A, et al: Suicide among schizophrenics: a review. *Compr Psychiatry* 1985;26:90-100.
66. Winokur G, Tsuang M: The Iowa 500: Suicide in mania, depression, and schizophrenia. *Am J Psychiatry* 1975;132:650-651.
67. Roy A: Depression in the course of chronic undifferentiated schizophrenia. *Arch Gen Psychiatry* 1981;38:296-297.
68. Avery D, Winokur G: Suicide, attempted suicide, and relapse rates in depression. *Arch Gen Psychiatry* 1978;35:749-753.
69. Friedman RC, Corn R, Aronoff MS, et al: The seriously suicidal adolescent: affective and character pathology, in Sudak HS, Ford AB, Rushforth HB (eds): *Suicide in the Young.* Boston, John Wright-PSG Inc, 1984, pp 209-226.
70. Helgason J: Epidemiology of mental disorder in Iceland. *Acta Psychiatr Scand Suppl* 1964;174:1-258.
71. Hendin H: Growing up dead: student suicide. *Am J Psychother* 1975;19:327-338.

11 Violence

George McNeil
Stephen M. Soreff

Violence is an integral part of the human condition. It is usually recognizable but not so readily given to definition. It may be thought of as "that which causes harm." Though such harm is usually physical, no one would debate the violence inherent in acts such as rape and child molestation: acts that do not always inflict physical injury.

While there is a large differential diagnosis that may underlie the act of violence, it must be stressed that violence is not necessarily a symptom of illness. Yes, violence may be born, for example, out of the psychotic disorganization of schizophrenia; it may also be an act of someone simply bad or immoral.

The conclusion that someone is "bad" seems, however, to abrade psychiatric sensitivities; hence, our need to *explain* even the most heinous behavior. To the credit of our science, all behavior may ultimately be explained by concatenation of biological and psychodynamic data. However, such explanation does not in itself denote illness, because it does not take into account the element of free will that operates in all but those with severe psychiatric impairment. In the absence of free will, no one would be responsible for their acts; biological and psychic determinism would reign supreme. And as in Orwell's *1984*, there would be no crime only "sickness."

> **Case report**   An 18-year-old man was brought to the emergency room by his parents who had noted the recent onset of withdrawn behavior. In addition, the patient had become increasingly

suspicious and was particularly concerned about being approached by homosexuals. These changes began when he left home for the first time to attend college and necessitated his leaving college. While being interviewed in a small room by a male medical student, the patient became increasingly anxious, struck the student, and fled the room.

FEATURES

Mood

It is not surprising that *anger* provides the most common substrate for violence. This feeling may be conscious and directed toward the object of the violence, as when violence is an act of vengeance. Conversely, anger may arise out of the mists of the unconscious and may be displaced and directed at people undeserving of the patient's wrath (people such as medical personnel or total strangers).

Fear may also provide an impetus for violence. In the case described above, delusional fears of homosexual attack were precipitated by the student's physical proximity. In cases where the threat of physical harm is real (eg, assault by a would-be robber), fear may be seen as an entirely normal response; and preemptive violence (or flight) are similarly normal and adaptive.

Thought

The thought content of the violent patient may be marked by preoccupation with violence. To the extent that violent fantasies can be aired and violent plans determined, the interviewer may decrease the potential for new violence. At the very least such exploration helps to determine the need for restraining the patient (hospitalization, notification of intended victims, etc).

More specifically, the thought content and thought processes of the violent patient may suggest one of the number of psychiatric illnesses (see "Psychiatric Differential Diagnosis" below). Illogical, "nonsensical" thinking with thought blocking suggests schizophrenia. Effusive speech with tangential thinking and flight of ideas suggest mania. Paranoid delusions, in the absence of other pathologic findings, suggest a paranoid disorder.

Behavior

It is behavior that defines the violent patient. His behavior may take the form of impulsive lashing out with fists, feet, teeth, or other offensive instruments immediately at hand. Such is apt to be the case with the patient suffering from a psychotic organic brain syndrome or severe functional psychosis. On the other hand, violence may be premeditated and may involve various tools of destruction: knives, guns, etc. More subtle forms of violence include rape and sexual abuse of children. This sort of planned, organized violent behavior is most consistent with the more integrated mental state seen in the paranoid disorders and in the antisocial personality.

Most curious and by far most frightening is the group violence that has its ultimate expression in war. With cultural sanction it seems that the most hideous violence can occur in the absence of psychopathology and worse, in the absence of overriding moral restraint.

Physical Examination and Laboratory Findings

With the exception of the signs of sympathetic autonomic arousal that accompany the act of violence, there are no physical findings specific to the violent patient. However, in view of the common association between violence and organic brain syndrome (see "Differential Diagnosis"), a careful history and physical examination should be undertaken. Laboratory studies should be done as dictated by the clincial setting and by the enormous diversity of physical disorders that may produce violence in the setting of delirium and dementia. Even in the face of a normal physical examination, it might be argued that the patient with episodic violent outbursts should have an EEG. The association between temporal lobe epilepsy and violence will be discussed below.

Interviewer's Reaction

The sensible interviewer will react to the violent patient with some degree of fear. The clinician who does not heed this response increases his chances of being victimized by the patient.

Fear of the violent patient should lead to the question of whether or not the patient is carrying weapons. If the armed patient refuses the dispassionate but firm demand that these be surrendered, fear should dictate a retreat from the patient.

The clinician may find his own anger and hostility piqued by the violent patient. In this setting it may be tempting to wade in and "mix it up" with the patient. This is hardly ever indicated, and physical heroics ought to be left to police and others more suited for them. In the case of the violent patient who is not armed and poses no imminent threat, the clinician may find himself in the position of staying the hand of others inclined to use force with the violent patient. The use of such force is likely to escalate the patient's violent leanings and should, where possible, be avoided.

PATHOGENESIS

Psychodynamic Explanation

Freud[1] felt that aggression is an inevitable, instinctual part of human behavior. Although his early work stressed the primacy of *eros*, an instinct directed at sustaining and reproducing life, he later introduced a more pessimistic view of the human condition that counterposed *eros* and *thanatos*. In part a product of Freud's observation of the grim events of World War I, *thanatos* was described as a destructive instinct, one whose energies militated toward death. In Freud's view, violence or aggression simply represents an outward displacement of inexorable *thanatos*.

If all are heir to instinctual violence, why is it, then, that some are more successful than others in eschewing violent behavior? Theoretically, the healthy well-functioning ego keeps such "unacceptable" impulses at bay, just as it does with the press of sexual impulses. Instinctual aggression may simply be repressed (posing a risk for depression in Freud's view, see chapter 2), or it may be handled by other ego defenses at more or less psychic cost to the patient. Optimally, these instincts may be handled through sublimation, in which case aggression may take the form of hard work and competitive striving. On the other hand, if the functioning of the ego is critically impaired, as in psychotic illness, instinctual aggression may more readily gain expression.

Biochemistry The biochemical correlates of violence are poorly understood and are, no doubt, complex. Mann et al have done some intriguing work with postmortem brain specimens of suicide victims (suicide may be seen as the ultimate expression of violence turned against the self).[2] Their findings suggested a deficiency in presynaptic serotonin nerve terminals. Brown et al studied a group of patients with histories of suicidal and aggressive behavior and found that these behaviors were significantly associated with each other and with low spinal fluid 5-hydroxyindoleacetic acid (5-HIAA, a metabolite of serotonin).[3] Whether decreased serotonin turnover has broader relevance to violent behavior remains to be seen. The role of other neurotransmitters and neuromodulators remains speculative.

Genetic Contribution

It is almost axiomatic that violence runs in families.[4,5] The precise roles of "nature" (genetics) and "nurture" (environment, see below) are often difficult to dissect. It does seem clear that a cluster of disorders predisposing toward violence tends to exist in certain families and to cross generational boundaries.[4] Antisocial personality disorder, alcoholism, and hysteria are overrepresented in these families and (it comes as little surprise) in the criminal population.

Perhaps the best support for the role of genetics in violence comes from studies of offspring adopted away from antisocial parents.[4,5,7] Despite being reared by parents unaffected by antisocial personality disorder, such offspring have been demonstated to show a significant incidence of the disorder.

The significance of the XYY chromosome pattern remains unclear.[4] Studies of violent criminals have suggested an etiologic role for this abnormality. However, men with the XYY pattern also seem to be overrepresented in psychiatric institutions and institutions for the mentally retarded.[8]

Mental retardation, in general, may increase the likelihood of violent behavior.[6,9] The inability of the retarded individual to negotiate complicated or frustrating situations is probably related to this.

Environment

The family is both a common arena for violence and a culture medium for future violence.[10] A most potent predictor of violence in children seems to be the family's acceptance of violence as a normative means of settling conflict. By way of confirming this common-sense assumption, Lewis et al studied 21 homicidally aggressive children and found that violent fathers, and mothers who had attempted suicide (violence against the self), were overrepresented in the study group.[11] In reviewing his experience with young patients suffering from episodic dyscontrol, Harbin found a strong tendency toward inconsistent parental values *vis a vis* violence.[12] He also found that families of such parents tended to be erratic in setting limits to violent behavior.

Cultural norms may also affect the expression of violence. For example, the curious American fascination with guns is associated with an appalling prevalence of gun-related violence. Such violence is relatively rare in Great Britain and other societies with more rigorous gun control.

The extent to which television reflects cultural ideals may be argued, but the preeminent role of this medium in American culture is nearly beyond dispute. The role of televised violence in fostering real-life violence is debated, but such an association seems real.[13] Anecdotal reports of bizarre acts of violence, mimicking televised depictions of similar acts, argue for a causal link at least in some cases.

Rarely, the cultural prescription of individual violence may be more specific. *Amok* is a phenomenon largely limited to the Malay archipelago consisting of violent, indiscriminate assaults lasting up to a few hours and followed by amnesia for the episode.[14] These episodes, which often result in the deaths of victims and of the perpetrator, are usually seen in response to situational stress and are apt to be associated with feelings of anger, fear, shame, or grief. Though officially proscribed and seen as an act of madness, amok still appears to enjoy subtle cultural sanction.[14]

Group pressures for violent behavior may override individual morality. This phenomenon is seen in Golding's depiction of innocents abroad in *Lord of the Flies*.[15] On a larger and more horrid scale it was seen in the extermination of millions of Jews under the cloak of German nationalism.

Several more concrete environmental factors may lend to the occurrence of violence; namely *crowding,* excessive *noise,* and *heat*.[16] Ardrey's observations of aggression in animals imply an innate proprietary need for "territory" that is likely to take the form of violence toward intruders.[17] Can such observations be extrapolated to the human animal? Studies seeking to show a causative link between crowding and violence have yielded mixed results.[16] Freedman et al have attempted to reconcile these by suggesting that in the face of other stimuli likely to cause violence, crowding may exert an enabling or enhancing effect.[18] Similarly, while a causative link between "noise pollution" and violence is difficult to establish, an enabling or enhancing role seems likely.[16]

Along with noise, crowding, and social ferment, heat has often been an apparent factor in the occurrence of riots. Can the "long, hot summer" precipitate violence? Again, available evidence suggests that while heat, per se, cannot explain violent behavior, it may be one of a chain of variables that may join to produce violence.[16]

DIFFERENTIAL DIAGNOSIS

Drugs

A great many drugs may be associated with violence in the setting of intoxication or drug-induced delirium.[19] In the acute confusional state the ego's defenses against unfettered aggression may tumble. In addition, the patient with impaired sensorium is likely to be frightened and may misperceive the actions of neutral or even helping figures as threats. Violence in this setting may then serve as a misdirected self-preservative function. Drugs that are associated with such psychotic disturbances have previously been listed (see chapter 3).

The association between alcohol and violence is common enough to deserve special attention.[20] While the mechanism for this is not entirely clear, it is clear that alcohol has a disinhibiting effect. The moral constraints of the superego often seem to dissolve in this drug, allowing the emergence of aggressive and other base impulses.

The paradoxical violence associated with minor tranquilizer use (particularly in the elderly) may have a similar pathogenesis.[21]

Among the other drugs of abuse (see Chapter 3), phencyclidine hydrochloride stands out as an agent that seems to have a special proclivity for igniting violence.[22] In view of the fact that drug abuse is often a correlate of antisocial character disorder, it is not unreasonable to question the role of characterologic predisposition in drug-related violence. Fauman and Fauman asked just this question in a study of 16 chronic phencyclidine abusers.[23] They found that drug-related violence in this group occurred independent of a prior history of violence, suggesting a direct, causative role for phencyclidine.

On the other hand, Keckich has reported a case of homicidal violence associated with neuroleptic-induced akathisia in a man with antisocial character disorder.[24] Here it was felt that the character disorder and a history of overt hostility played a significant causative role.

Finally, the role of testosterone or other androgens in the genesis of violence bears mention.[6] One needs simply to consider the population of our jails and prisons to see that violence is a behavior more natural to the male of our species. Moreover, castration or other antiandrogen therapies

Table 11-1
Differential Diagnosis of Violence

I. Drugs
   Drug intoxication
   Drug-induced delirium (toxic psychosis)
   Disinhibiting drugs (alcohol, sedative-tranquilizers)
   Phencyclidine
   Testosterone
II. Medical illnesses
   Any illness causing delirium
   Disease of the limbic and temporal lobes,
      especially those associated with complex
      partial seizures
   Premenstrual syndrome
   Mininal brain dysfunction
III. Psychiatric illness
   Organic psychosis any etiology
   Brief reactive psychosis
   Schizophrenia
   Bipolar affective illness
   Paranoid disorders
   Antisocial personality disorder

---

have proved successful in selected cases of intractable violence (particularly sexual violence).

Medical Illnesses

Violence may be a nonspecific by-product of psychotic delirium associated with a host of medical illnesses (see chapter 3). It may also be seen as a product of the fear and desperation associated with certain acute disease states. For example, the patient with acute bronchospasm — terrified and "fighting to breathe" — may lash out at medical personnel.

More directly involved in the pathogenesis of violence are certain diseases of the CNS, specifically those involving the temporal and limbic lobes.[6,25,26] Violent episodes have been described in vascular, infectious, neoplastic, or other disease processes involving these areas.

The relationship between violence and *complex partial seizures* (temporal lobe epilepsy, psychomotor epilepsy) continues to be debated.[27,28] It is generally agreed that there is an interictal personality profile associated with this disorder and that this profile includes emotional lability and a proclivity toward open anger and aggression.[29] More obscure is the question of *ictal* violence, violence that is an immediate, direct result of cortical dysrhythmia. Such violence would be associated with amnesia for the act (unlike the interictal violence noted above) and would logically be associated with diminished responsibiltiy for the act (a crucial legal issue). after careful review of this question, Delgado-Escueta et al have concluded that ictal violence does occur, but that such violence almost always consists of poorly organized, often stereotypic aggression (eg, spitting, scratching, lashing out with a fist).[27] More integrated, complex acts of violence, such as those involved in murder, armed robbery and other crimes, are extremely unlikely to be seizure phenomena.

Another disorder that has gained the attention of forensic workers is *premenstrual syndrome.* It has long been part of anecdotal wisdom that many women are given to increased irritability around the time of menstruation. Dalton, on the other hand, has reported three women involved in crimes of violence (manslaughter, arson, assault) during this time.[30] All three had long histories of violence during the premenstruum and all three responded dramatically to treatment with progesterone.

Finally, *minimal brain dysfunction* has been linked with violence.[4,31] This disorder is often diagnosed in children with learning and interpersonal difficulties, difficulty concentrating (hence, "attention deficit disorder," synonymous with MBD), and hyperactivity. The natural history of the disorder is such that these children may become impaired adults with affective lability and a tendency to alcohol and drug abuse and to irritability, and, at times, violence. Such adults, who may be difficult to distinguish from the population with antisocial character disorder, respond to treatment with amphetamine (like children with MBD), without an addictive pattern.[32]

Surgery

Violence associated with surgical illness or with the postoperative period may be expected to occur in the setting of delirium. For a more through dicussion of organic psychosis associated with surgery, see chapter 3.

Trauma

With the exception of trauma that damages the limbic or temporal lobes of the brain, the link between physical violence and trauma is indirect. Organic psychosis may be a sequel to trauma (see chapter 3), and violence may be born out of this state.[33] Severe trauma may also be asssociated with *brief reactive psychosis* (see chapter 3) which in turn may have violent features. Depending upon the character makeup of the patient (see below), violence may be a response to the frustration of chronic disability as a sequela to trauma.

Psychiatric Illnesses

Notwithstanding the public ferment created by the more infamous of the criminally insane, it is by no means clear that mental illness begets violence. There has been noted an increasing arrest rate among mental patients. Sosowsky, following a group of California state hospital patients, documented an arrest rate for violent crime nearly ten times that of the general population.[34] Such data, however, need to be interpreted with caution. As deviant behavior becomes increasingly identified as "sick," are we simply hospitalizing more criminals?

In a different sort of epidemiologic study, Craig reviewed the records of 876 consecutive state hospital admissions and found that 11% of these patients had been assaultive before admission.[35] Breaking the patients into diagnostic categories, Craig suggested the *schizophrenic males* and patients with *organic brain disease* were more highly predisposed toward violence. A similar review of violence among geriatric psychiatric inpatients has suggested that the functional psychoses *(schizophrenia* and *mania*, particularly when marked by *paranoid* features) are associated with the highest risk of violence. [36]

On the other hand, Tardiff and Koenigsberg reported a large series of psychiatric outpatients, of whom 3% had been assaultive prior to their clinic evaluations.[37] Most of these patients were not psychotic, but they tended to be young and male and to have diagnoses of childhood or adolescent disorders or of personality disorder. The authors note the bias of their patient sample away from more severe psychiatric illness. (Psychotic patients tend to bypass the process of clinic intake and to be hospitalized.)

A review by London and Taylor of 187 men found not guilty by reason of insanity found a high percentage (34%) of bipolar affective illness.[38] *Violent* crime, however, was most heavily associated with *alcohol abuse, other drug abuse,* and *organic mental syndrome.* This is consonant with earlier findings by Guze that serious crime is associated with drug and alcohol abuse and with antisocial personality disorder but not with schizophrenia or affective illness.[39,40]

To the extent that people with *antisocial personality disorder* are identified as mentally ill, violence will be increasingly associated with mental illness. Like all character disorders, this is marked by chronic, maladaptive behavior that has its onset during or before the teenage years. This particular disorder is distinguished by antisocial behavior which, if not criminal, is on the fringe of criminality and brings the perpetrator into conflict with authority. The person with antisocial personality disorder (called the sociopath or the psychopath in past diagnostic schemata) is highly impulsive, tolerates frustration poorly, and has no sense of loyalty to anyone but himself. He is apt to be assaultive and may have a history of multiple arrests. He has little conscious sense of guilt. Often superficially engaging, he may be skilled at "conning" others (including medical personnel) for his own gain. Psychiatry, which has lent much to the understanding of this disorder, offers little in the way of treatment.

REFERENCES

1. Freud S: Introductory lectures on psychoanalysis, in Strachey J (ed): *Standard Edition of the Complete Psychological Works of Sigmund Freud,* Strachey J (trans), London, Hogarth Press, 1963.
2. Mann JJ, Stanley M, McBride PA: Suicide and a specific serotonin receptor lesion, abstract New Research. Annual Meeting of the American Psychiatric Association, 1983.
3. Brown GL, Ebert MH, Goyer FF, et al: Agression, suicide, and serotonin: relationships to CSF amine metabolites. *Am J Psychiatry* 1982;139:741-746.
4. Menuck ME, Voineskos G: The etiology of violent behavior. *Gen Hosp Psychiatry* 1981;3:37-47.
5. Cloninger CR, Reich T. Guze SB: The mulifactorial model of disease transmission: II. Sex differences in the familial transmission of sociopathy (antisocial personality). *Br J Psychiatry* 1975;127:11-22.
6. Goldstein M: brain research and violent behavior. *Arch Neurol* 1974;30:1-35.
7. Cadoret RJ: Psychopathology in adopted-away offspring of biologic parents with antisocial personality. *Arch Gen Psychiatry* 1978;35:176-184.
8. Hook EB: Behavioral implications of the human XYY genotype. *Science* 1973;179:139-150.
9. Kolb LC: *Modern Clinical Psychiatry,* ed 8. Philadelphia, WB Saunders Co, 1973.
10. Barnhill LR: Clinical assessement of intrafamilial violence. *Hosp Community Psychiatry* 1980;31:543-547.

11. Lewis DO, Shanok SS, Grant M, et al: Homicidally aggressive young children: neuropsychiatric and experiential correlates. *Am J Psychiatry* 1983;140:148-153.

12. Harbin HT: Episodic dyscontrol and family dynamics. *Am J Psychiatry* 1977;134:1113-1116.

13. Editorial: Teenagers and television violence. *Lancet* 1979;1:591-592.

14. Carr JE, Eng KT: In search of the true amok: amok as viewed within the Malay culture. *Am J Psychiatry* 1976;133(11):1295-1299.

15. Golding W: *Lord of the Flies.* New York, Coward McCann & Geoghegan, 1978.

16. Baron RA: Aggression, in Kaplan HI, Freedman AM, Sadock BJ (eds): *Comprehensive Textbook of Psychiatry,* ed 3. Baltimore, Williams & Wilkins Co, 1980.

17. Ardrey R: *The Territorial Imperative.* New York, Atheneum, 1966.

18. Freedman JL, Levy AS, Buchanan RW, et al: Crowding and human aggressiveness. *J Exp Soc Psychology* 1972;8:528.

19. Rabin PL, Koomen J: The violent patient—differential diagnosis and management. *J Tenn Med Assoc* 1982;75:313-317.

20. Gerson LW, Preston DA: Alcohol consumption and the incidence of violent crime. *J Stud Alcohol* 1979;40:307-312.

21. Slaby AE, Lieb J, Trancredi LR: *Handbook of Psychiatric Emergencies,* ed 2. New York, Medical Examination Publishing Co, 1981.

22. Rada RT: The violent patient: rapid assessment and management. *Psychosomatics* 1981;22:101-109.

23. Fauman MA, Fauman BJ: Violence associated with phencyclidine abuse. *Am J Psychiatry* 1979;136:1584-1586.

24. Keckich WA: Neuroleptics, violence as a manifestation of akathisia. *JAMA* 1978;240:2185.

25. Lion JR, Bach-y-rita G, Ervin FR: Violent patients in the emergency room. *Am J Psychiatry* 1969;125;1706-1711.

26. Simon RH, Desilva M: Intracranial tuberculoma coexistent with uncinate seizures and violent behavior. *JAMA* 1981;245:1247-1248.

27. Delgado-Escueta AV, Mattson RH, King L, et al: The nature of aggression during epileptic seizures. *N Engl J Med* 1981;305:711-716.

28. Lewis DO, Pincus JH, Shanok SS, et al: Psychomotor epilepsy and violence in a group of incarcerated adolescent boys. *Am J Psychiatry* 1982;139:882-887.

29. Bear D, Arana G: Nonfunctional disorders of emotion. *Neurol Neurosurg Weekly Update* 1978;1:1-7.

30. Dalton K: Cyclical criminal acts in premenstrual syndrome. *Lancet* 1980;1:1070-1071.

31. Anstett RE, Wood L: The patient exhibiting episodic violent behavior. *J Fam Pract* 1983;16:605-609.

32. Stringer AY, Josef NC: Methylphenidate in the treatment of aggression in two patients with antisocial personality disorder. *Am J Psychiatry* 1983;140:1365-1366.

33. Goldstein K: *After-effects of Brain Injuries in War.* New York, Grune & Stratton, Inc, 1942.
34. Sosowsky L: Explaining the increased arrest rate among mental patients: a cautionary note. *Am J Psychiatry* 1980;137:1602-1605.
35. Craig TJ: An epidemiologic study of problems associated with violence among psychiatric inpatients. *Am J Psychiatry* 1982;139:1262-1266.
36. Petrie WM, Lawson E, Hollender MH: violence in geriatric patients. *JAMA* 1982;248:443-444.
37. Tardiff K, Koenigsberg HW: Assaultive behavior among psychiatric outpatients. *Am J Psychiatry* 1985;142:960-963.
38. London WP, Taylor BM: Bipolar disorders in forensic setting. *Compr Psychiatry* 1982;23:33-37.
39. Guze SB, Goodwin DW, Crane JB: Criminality and psychiatric disorders. *Arch Gen Psychiatry* 1969;20:583-591.
40. Guze SB, Woodruff RA, Clayton PJ: Psychiatric disorders and criminality. *JAMA* 1974;227:641-642.

INDEX